Imaging of the Pediatric Abdomen and Pelvis

Editors

JONATHAN R. DILLMAN
ETHAN A. SMITH

MAGNETIC RESONANCE IMAGING CLINICS OF NORTH AMERICA

www.mri.theclinics.com

Consulting Editors
SURESH K. MUKHERJI
LYNNE S. STEINBACH

November 2013 • Volume 21 • Number 4

ELSEVIER

1600 John F. Kennedy Boulevard • Suite 1800 • Philadelphia, Pennsylvania, 19103-2899

http://www.mri.theclinics.com

MRI CLINICS OF NORTH AMERICA Volume 21, Number 4
November 2013 ISSN 1064-9689, ISBN 13: 978-0-323-24227-1

Editor: John Vassallo (j.vassallo@elsevier.com)
Developmental Editor: Yonah Korngold

Magnetic Resonance Imaging Clinics of North America (ISSN 1064-9689) is published quarterly by Elsevier Inc., 360 Park Avenue South, New York, NY 10010-1710. Months of issue are February, May, August, and November. Business and Editorial Offices: 1600 John F. Kennedy Blvd., Ste. 1800, Philadelphia, PA 19103-2899. Customer Service Office: 3251 Riverport Lane, Maryland Heights, MO 63043. Periodicals postage paid at New York, NY and additional mailing offices. Subscription prices are $375.00 per year (domestic individuals), $581.00 per year (domestic institutions), $190.00 per year (domestic students/residents), $420.00 per year (Canadian individuals), $755.00 per year (Canadian institutions), $545.00 per year (international individuals), $755.00 per year (international institutions), and $275.00 per year (international and Canadian students/residents). International air speed delivery is included in all *Clinics* subscription prices. All prices are subject to change without notice. **POSTMASTER:** Send address changes to *Magnetic Resonance Imaging Clinics*, Elsevier Health Sciences Division, Subscription Customer Service, 3251 Riverport Lane, Maryland Heights, MO 63043. Customer Service (orders, claims, online, change of address): Elsevier Health Sciences Division, Subscription Customer Service, 3251 Riverport Lane, Maryland Heights, MO 63043. Tel:1-800-654-2452 (U.S. and Canada); 314-447-8871 (outside U.S. and Canada). Fax: 314-447-8029. E-mail: journalscustomerservice-usa@elsevier.com (for print support); journalsonlinesupport-usa@elsevier.com (for online support).

Reprints. For copies of 100 or more of articles in this publication, please contact the Commercial Reprints Department, Elsevier Inc., 360 Park Avenue South, New York, NY 10010-1710. Tel.: 212-633-3874; Fax: 212-633-3820; E-mail: reprints@elsevier.com.

Magnetic Resonance Imaging Clinics of North America is covered in the *RSNA Index of Imaging Literature, MEDLINE/PubMed (Index Medicus),* and *EMBASE/Excerpta Medica.*

Printed in the United States of America.

Contributors

CONSULTING EDITORS

SURESH K. MUKHERJI, MD, FACR
Professor and Chairman; W.F. Patenge
Endowed Chair, Department of Radiology,
Michigan State University, East Lansing,
Michigan

LYNNE S. STEINBACH, MD, FACR
Professor of Radiology and Orthopaedic
Surgery, University of California-San
Francisco, San Francisco, California

EDITORS

JONATHAN R. DILLMAN, MD
Assistant Professor of Radiology, Section of
Pediatric Radiology, Department of Radiology,
C.S. Mott Children's Hospital, University of
Michigan Health System, Ann Arbor, Michigan

ETHAN A. SMITH, MD
Clinical Assistant Professor, Section of
Pediatric Radiology, Department of Radiology,
C.S. Mott Children's Hospital, University of
Michigan Health System, Ann Arbor, Michigan

AUTHORS

MELKAMU ADEB, MD
Division of Body Imaging, Department of
Radiology, The Children's Hospital of
Philadelphia, Philadelphia, Pennsylvania

MAHMOUD M. AL-HAWARY, MD
Section of Abdominal Radiology, Division of
Abdominal Imaging, Department of Radiology,
University of Michigan Health System, Ann
Arbor, Michigan

SUDHA A. ANUPINDI, MD
Assistant Professor of Radiology, Department
of Radiology, The Children's Hospital of
Philadelphia, Perelman School of Medicine,
University of Pennsylvania, Philadelphia,
Pennsylvania

MARK BITTMAN, MD
Department of Radiology, Cohen Children's
Medical Center of New York, North Shore-
Long Island Jewish Medical Center, New Hyde
Park, New York

DAVID A. BLOOM, MD, FACR
Associate Professor of Radiology and
Pediatrics, Department of Radiology, Oakland
University William Beaumont School of

Medicine, Beaumont Children's Hospital,
Royal Oak, Michigan

MICHAEL CARR, MD, PhD
Division of Urology, Department of Surgery,
The Children's Hospital of Philadelphia,
Perelman School of Medicine, University of
Pennsylvania, Philadelphia, Pennsylvania

POOJA R. CHOPRA, BA
School of Medicine, University of Missouri—
Kansas City, Kansas City, Missouri

JESSE COURTIER, MD
Assistant Clinical Professor of Radiology,
Department of Radiology, UCSF Benioff
Children's Hospital & San Francisco General
Hospital, UCSF School of Medicine,
San Francisco, California

KASSA DARGE, MD, PhD
Chief, Division of Body Imaging; John Hope
Chair for Radiology Faculty Development,
Department of Radiology, The Children's
Hospital of Philadelphia, Perelman School of
Medicine, University of Pennsylvania,
Philadelphia, Pennsylvania

JONATHAN R. DILLMAN, MD
Assistant Professor of Radiology, Section of
Pediatric Radiology, Department of Radiology,
C.S. Mott Children's Hospital, University of
Michigan Health System, Ann Arbor, Michigan

DAVID DINAN, MD
Department of Medical Imaging, Nemours
Children's Hospital, Orlando, Florida

NATHAN D. EGBERT, MD
Radiology Resident, Department of Radiology,
University of Michigan Health System, Ann
Arbor, Michigan

MOHAMED A. ELTOMEY, MD
Lecturer of Radiology and Faculty of Medicine,
Radiology and Medical Imaging Department,
Tanta University, Tanta, Egypt

MONICA EPELMAN, MD
Vice-Chair, Department of Medical Imaging,
Nemours Children's Hospital, Orlando, Florida

MICHAEL S. GEE, MD, PhD
Sections of Pediatric Imaging and Abdominal
Imaging and Intervention, Department of
Radiology, Massachusetts General Hospital,
Harvard Medical School, Boston,
Massachusetts

MATTHEW R. HAMMER, MD
Section of Pediatric Radiology, Department of
Radiology, C.S. Mott Children's Hospital,
University of Michigan Health System, Ann
Arbor, Michigan

CHRISTOPHER P. KEUP, MD
Departments of Radiology, Children's Mercy
Hospitals and Clinics, and The University of
Missouri—Kansas City, Kansas City, Missouri

MARIA F. LADINO-TORRES, MD
Clinical Assistant Professor, Section of
Pediatric Radiology, Department of Radiology,
C.S. Mott Children's Hospital, University of
Michigan Health System, Ann Arbor, Michigan

CHARLES A. LAWRENCE, MD
Assistant Professor, Departments of
Radiology, Children's Mercy Hospitals and
Clinics, and The University of Missouri—
Kansas City, Kansas City, Missouri

EDWARD Y. LEE, MD, MPH
Chief, Division of Thoracic Imaging; Director,
Magnetic Resonance Imaging, Department of
Radiology, Boston Children's Hospital and
Harvard Medical School, Boston,
Massachusetts

MARC A. LEVITT, MD
Professor and Director, Department of Surgery,
Colorectal Center, Cincinnati Children's
Hospital Medical Center, University of
Cincinnati College of Medicine, Cincinnati, Ohio

PETER S. LIU, MD
Assistant Professor of Radiology and Vascular
Surgery, Department of Radiology, University of
Michigan Medical Center, Ann Arbor, Michigan

LISA H. LOWE, MD
Professor, Departments of Radiology,
Children's Mercy Hospitals and Clinics, and
The University of Missouri—Kansas City,
Kansas City, Missouri

DEEPA R. PAI, MD
Clinical Assistant Professor, Section of
Pediatric Radiology, Department of Radiology,
C.S. Mott Children's Hospital, University of
Michigan Health System, Ann Arbor, Michigan

DANIEL J. PODBERESKY, MD
Associate Professor, Department of Radiology,
Cincinnati Children's Hospital Medical Center,
University of Cincinnati College of Medicine,
Cincinnati, Ohio

FELICIA RATNARAJ, BA
School of Medicine, The University of
Missouri—Kansas City, Kansas City, Missouri

DAVID M. SADA, MD
Michael E. DeBakey VA Medical Center,
Houston, Texas

SURAJ D. SERAI, PhD
Department of Radiology, Cincinnati Children's
Hospital Medical Center, University of
Cincinnati College of Medicine, Cincinnati, Ohio

SABAH SERVAES, MD
Residency and Fellowship Director; Director,
Computed Tomography, Department of
Radiology, The Children's Hospital of
Philadelphia, Perelman School of Medicine,
University of Pennsylvania, Philadelphia,
Pennsylvania

ETHAN A. SMITH, MD
Clinical Assistant Professor, Section of
Pediatric Radiology, Department of Radiology,
C.S. Mott Children's Hospital, University of
Michigan Health System, Ann Arbor,
Michigan

OWENS TERREBLANCHE, MD (FC Rad)
Visiting Research Fellow, Department of
Radiology, UCSF Benioff Children's Hospital &
San Francisco General Hospital, UCSF
School of Medicine, San Francisco,
California

ALEXANDER J. TOWBIN, MD
Assistant Professor, Department of Radiology,
Cincinnati Children's Hospital Medical Center,
University of Cincinnati College of Medicine,
Cincinnati, Ohio

SARA O. VARGAS, MD
Department of Pathology, Boston Children's
Hospital, Boston, Massachusetts

RANJITH VELLODY, MD
Assistant Professor of Radiology, Department
of Radiology, University of Michigan Medical
Center, Ann Arbor, Michigan

Contents

Although the spectrum of renal masses in children has some overlap with that of adults, it is important to understand the renal pathologic processes specific to the pediatric population, as well as their characteristic imaging appearances and clinical presentations. This article reviews benign and malignant renal masses in children, with an emphasis on magnetic resonance imaging and clinical features that are specific to each lesion type.

Duplex renal collecting systems are common congenital anomalies of the upper urinary tract. In most cases they are incidental findings and not associated with additional pathologies. They demonstrate, however, higher incidences of hydroureteronephrosis, ureteroceles, and ectopic ureters. The most comprehensive morphologic and functional evaluation of duplex systems can be achieved using magnetic resonance urography. Functional magnetic resonance urography allows better separation of the renal poles, thus more accurate calculation of the differential renal functions compared with renal scintigraphy. Magnetic resonance urography is the study of choice when upper urinary tract anatomy is complex or when functional evaluation is needed.

This article addresses the current technique and protocols for magnetic resonance (MR) enterography, with a primary focus on inflammatory bowel disease (IBD) and a secondary detailed discussion of other diseases of the small bowel beyond IBD. A brief discussion of MR imaging for appendicitis is included, but the evaluation of appendicitis does not require an enterographic protocol. The focused key points and approach presented in this article are intended to enhance the reader's understanding to help improve patient compliance with the MR enterographic studies, overcome challenges, and improve interpretation.

Both benign and malignant pelvic masses are encountered in the pediatric population. Although ultrasonography remains the modality of choice for initial evaluation of a pediatric pelvic mass, in selected cases magnetic resonance (MR) imaging can add important diagnostic information. MR imaging has several advantages over ultrasonography and computed tomography, including superior contrast resolution and an ability to characterize abnormalities based on unique tissue characteristics. MR evaluation assists in lesion characterization, presurgical planning, and staging when a malignancy is suspected. MR imaging also offers a nonionizing imaging modality for long-term follow-up of patients undergoing therapy for malignant pelvic masses.

Although many Müllerian duct anomalies do not require treatment, surgical intervention is sometimes necessary to enable sexual activity or to preserve fertility. The identification of these anomalies is important for optimal clinical management or surgical treatment. Magnetic resonance (MR) imaging is a robust method for adequately evaluating and characterizing uterine and vaginal anomalies. The information provided by MR imaging allows for a more complete understanding of the malformation, facilitating management decisions and potentially changing the outcome. In this article, the embryology, classification, and MR imaging findings of Müllerian duct and related anomalies in children and adolescents are reviewed.

Magnetic Resonance Imaging of Anorectal Malformations 791

Daniel J. Podberesky, Alexander J. Towbin, Mohamed A. Eltomey, and Marc A. Levitt

Anorectal malformation (ARM) occurs in approximately 1 in 5000 newborns and is frequently accompanied by anomalies of the genitalia, gynecologic system, urinary tract, spine, and skeletal system. Diagnostic imaging plays a central role in ARM evaluation. Because of the lack of ionizing radiation, excellent intrinsic contrast resolution, multiplanar imaging capabilities, technical advances in hardware, and innovative imaging protocols, magnetic resonance (MR) imaging is increasingly important in assessment of ARM patients in utero, postnatally before definitive surgical correction, and in the postoperative period. This article discusses the role of MR imaging in evaluating ARM patients.

Magnetic Resonance Imaging of Perianal and Perineal Crohn Disease in Children and Adolescents 813

Matthew R. Hammer, Jonathan R. Dillman, Ethan A. Smith, and Mahmoud M. Al-Hawary

Noninvasive, nonionizing, multiparametric magnetic resonance (MR) imaging of the pelvis using a field strength of 3-T now provides a comprehensive assessment of perineal involvement in pediatric Crohn disease. MR imaging accurately evaluates inflammatory disease activity, and allows determination of the number and course of fistula tracts as well as their relationships to vital perianal structures, including the external anal sphincter, helping to guide surgical management and improve outcomes. This article provides an up-to-date review of perineal MR imaging findings of Crohn disease in the pediatric population, including fistulous disease, abscesses, and skin manifestations. Imaging technique is also discussed.

Advanced Techniques in Pediatric Abdominopelvic Oncologic Magnetic Resonance Imaging 829

Ethan A. Smith

Advances in the treatment of pediatric abdominopelvic malignancies have increased survival drastically. Imaging is critical in initial tumor characterization/staging, assessment of treatment response, and surveillance following therapy. Magnetic resonance imaging (MRI) is playing an increasing role in the care of these patients due to its lack of ionizing radiation, superior contrast resolution and the ability to characterize tumors based on tissue characteristics (e.g., T1 and T2 relaxation times). Modern MR techniques also allow for assessment of tumors based on functional characteristics. This article is focused on emerging MRI technologies and potential applications in the imaging of pediatric abdominopelvic malignancies.

Magnetic Resonance Angiography of the Pediatric Abdomen and Pelvis: Techniques and Imaging Findings 843

Ranjith Vellody, Peter S. Liu, and David M. Sada

Although traditional catheter-based angiography has been the gold standard for pediatric abdominal and pelvic vascular imaging for the past several decades,

advances in magnetic resonance angiography (MRA) have made it a viable alternative. MRA offers several advantages in that it is noninvasive, can be performed without ionizing radiation, and does not necessarily rely on contrast administration. The
ability of modern MRA techniques to define variant vascular anatomy and detect
vascular disease may obviate traditional angiography in some patients.

MAGNETIC RESONANCE IMAGING CLINICS OF NORTH AMERICA

DOWNLOAD Free App!

Review Articles
THE CLINICS

NOW AVAILABLE FOR YOUR iPhone and iPad

PROGRAM OBJECTIVE
The goal of Magnetic Resonance Imaging Clinics of North America is to keep practicing physicians up to date with current clinical practice by providing timely articles reviewing the state of the art in patient care.

TARGET AUDIENCE
All practicing physicians and healthcare professionals who provide patient care utilizing findings from Magnetic Resonance Imaging.

LEARNING OBJECTIVES
Upon completion of this activity, participants will be able to:
1. Discuss MRI of pediatric abdomen, pelvis, liver, and kidney.
2. Discuss MRI of anorectal malformations.
3. Describe magnetic resonance urography in evaluation of duplicated renal collecting systems.

ACCREDITATION
The Elsevier Office of Continuing Medical Education (EOCME) is accredited by the Accreditation Council for Continuing Medical Education (ACCME) to provide continuing medical education for physicians.

The EOCME designates this enduring material for a maximum of 15 *AMA PRA Category 1 Credit*(s)™. Physicians should claim only the credit commensurate with the extent of their participation in the activity.

All other health care professionals requesting continuing education credit for this enduring material will be issued a certificate of participation.

DISCLOSURE OF CONFLICTS OF INTEREST
The EOCME assesses conflict of interest with its instructors, faculty, planners, and other individuals who are in a position to control the content of CME activities. All relevant conflicts of interest that are identified are thoroughly vetted by EOCME for fair balance, scientific objectivity, and patient care recommendations. EOCME is committed to providing its learners with CME activities that promote improvements or quality in healthcare and not a specific proprietary business or a commercial interest.

The planning committee, staff, authors and editors listed below have identified no financial relationships or relationships to products or devices they or their spouse/life partner have with commercial interest related to the content of this CME activity:
Melkamu Adeb, MD; Mahmoud M. Al-Hawary, MD; Sudha A. Anupindi, MD; Mark Bittman, MD; David A. Bloom, MD; Michael Carr, MD, PhD; Pooja R. Chopra; Jesse Courtier, MD; Kassa Darge, MD, PhD; Jonathan R. Dillman, MD; David Dinan, MD; Nathan D. Egbert, MD; Mohamed A. Eltomey, MD; Monica Epelman, MD; Michael S. Gee, MD, PhD; Matthew R. Hammer, MD; Brynne Hunter; Christopher P. Keup, MD; Maria F. Ladino-Torres, MD; Sandy Lavery; Charles A. Lawrence, MD; Edward Y. Lee, MD, MPH; Marc A. Levitt, MD; Peter S. Liu, MD; Lisa H. Lowe, MD; Jill McNair; Suresh K. Mukherji, MD; Deepa R. Pai, MD; Lindsay Parnell; Daniel J. Podberesky, MD; Felicia Ratnaraj; David M. Sada, MD; Suraj D. Serai, PhD; Sabah Servaes, MD; Ethan A. Smith, MD; Lynne S. Steinbach, MD, FACR; Karthik Subramaniam; Owens Terreblanche, MD; Alexander J. Towbin, MD; John Vassallo; Sara O. Vargas, MD; Ranjith Vellody, MD.

The planning committee, staff, authors and editors listed below have identified financial relationships or relationships to products or devices they or their spouse/life partner have with commercial interest related to the content of this CME activity:
Daniel J. Podberesky, MD is a consultant/advisor for GE; is on speaker's bureau for Toshiba; receives royalties/patents for Amirsys. Alexander J. Towbin, MD receives royalties/patents from Amirsys, and has stock ownership in Merge Healthcare.

UNAPPROVED/OFF-LABEL USE DISCLOSURE
The EOCME requires CME faculty to disclose to the participants:
1. When products or procedures being discussed are off-label, unlabelled, experimental, and/or investigational (not US Food and Drug Administration (FDA) approved); and
2. Any limitations on the information presented, such as data that are preliminary or that represent ongoing research, interim analyses, and/or unsupported opinions. Faculty may discuss information about pharmaceutical agents that is outside of FDA-approved labelling. This information is intended solely for CME and is not intended to promote off-label use of these medications. If you have any questions, contact the medical affairs department of the manufacturer for the most recent prescribing information.

TO ENROLL
To enroll in the *Magnetic Resonance Imaging Clinics of North* Continuing Medical Education program, call customer service at 1-800-654-2452 or sign up online at http://www.theclinics.com/home/cme. The CME program is available to subscribers for an additional annual fee of $223 USD.

METHOD OF PARTICIPATION
In order to claim credit, participants must complete the following:
1. Complete enrolment as indicated above.
2. Read the activity.
3. Complete the CME Test and Evaluation. Participants must achieve a score of 70% on the test. All CME Tests and Evaluations must be completed online.

CME INQUIRIES/SPECIAL NEEDS
For all CME inquiries or special needs, please contact elsevierCME@elsevier.com.

Foreword

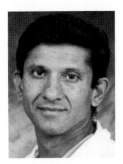

Suresh K. Mukherji, MD, FACR
Consulting Editor

One of the most rapid growth areas is in pediatric magnetic resonance (MR) imaging. This is likely due to a combination of factors that include avoidance of ionizing radiation, technical advances that permit enhanced imaged quality with faster acquisitions, which reduce the need for sedation. An indicator of the growing acceptance of MR occurred at our home institution. The recently constructed University of Michigan C.S. Mott Children's Hospital actually has more MRI than CT scanners (!), indicating our feeling that the future growth in MR will exceed CT.

I would like to thank Drs Jonathan Dillman and Ethan Smith for guest editing this edition of *Magnetic Resonance Imaging Clinics of North America*. They have done a wonderful job assembling twelve comprehensive articles covering a wide range of pediatric abdominopelvic MRI topics.

These articles are authored by well-respected, national and international leaders in the field of pediatric radiology. The articles are written in a manner such that all radiologists can understand their important content. I would like to thank all of the authors for their outstanding contributions. I am very confident that the readers will find this issue to be informative and relevant to daily clinical practice.

Suresh K. Mukherji, MD, FACR
Department of Radiology
Michigan State University
824 Service Road
East Lansing, MI 48824, USA

E-mail address:
mukherji@rad.msu.edu

Magn Reson Imaging Clin N Am 21 (2013) xiii
http://dx.doi.org/10.1016/j.mric.2013.07.010
1064-9689/13/$ – see front matter © 2013 Published by Elsevier Inc.

mri.theclinics.com

Preface

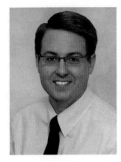
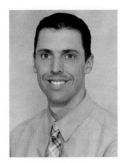

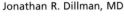

Jonathan R. Dillman, MD   Ethan A. Smith, MD

Editors

It has been our pleasure to serve as guest editors for the current issue of *Magnetic Resonance Imaging Clinics of North America* entitled, "Imaging of the Pediatric Abdomen and Pelvis." We are thrilled to present numerous contemporary review articles presenting the use of state-of-the-art abdominopelvic MRI techniques in children and adolescents. In our pediatric radiology practice, the use of magnetic resonance imaging (MRI) for the evaluation of abnormalities of the abdomen and pelvis continues to steadily increase. In recent years, many new MRI applications have entered routine pediatric clinical practice. In fact, in several instances at many institutions, MRI has supplanted the previous imaging standard (eg, MR enterography replacing either computed tomography enterography or fluoroscopic studies for evaluation of inflammatory bowel disease).

Increasing utilization of abdominopelvic MRI in the pediatric population is likely due to several factors. Of course, a major driver of increasing use is the fact that MRI does not require ionizing radiation, thus avoiding any potential harmful adverse effects. However, there are other reasons to explain this increased utilization. Relatively recent hardware and software advances have led to much improved image quality due to increased signal-to-noise ratio, contrast-to-noise ratio, and spatial resolution. Taken together, these advances have allowed for substantial improvements in image quality when imaging the pediatric abdomen and pelvis. Parallel imaging techniques and newly developed pulse sequences have allowed for decreased imaging times with a resultant reduced need for sedation and general anesthesia.

We are also particularly excited about the increasing availability and use of 3-Tesla MRI scanners for imaging of the pediatric abdomen and pelvis. In our practice, we now commonly prefer higher field strength imaging in younger children (including neonates and infants) as abdominopelvic image quality seems overall superior to imaging performed at lower field strengths. Numerous examples of MRI of the abdomen and pelvis at 3-Tesla are presented in this issue. One such instance where 3-Tesla high-spatial-resolution MRI is critical is in the assessment of perianal and perineal Crohn disease, as shown in the article, "Magnetic resonance imaging of Perianal and Perineal Crohn Disease in Children and Adolescents."

The present issue is a collection of twelve unique review articles covering a wide range of pediatric abdominopelvic MRI topics. These articles are authored by well-respected, national and international leaders in the field of Pediatric Radiology. It is our hope that readers will find the image-rich material provided in these articles to be informative and relevant to daily clinical practice.

Briefly, articles in the present issue include the following:

1. In the article entitled, "Magnetic Resonance Imaging of the Pediatric Liver: Benign and Malignant Masses," key imaging findings of

Magn Reson Imaging Clin N Am 21 (2013) xv–xvii
http://dx.doi.org/10.1016/j.mric.2013.07.009
1064-9689/13/$ – see front matter © 2013 Published by Elsevier Inc.

mri.theclinics.com

common benign and malignant liver masses are presented. The authors also devote substantial attention to the use of hepatocyte-specific contrast material for focal liver lesion characterization (an "off-label" practice in the pediatric population).

2. In the article entitled, "Magnetic Resonance Imaging of the Pediatric Liver: Imaging of Steatosis, Iron Deposition, and Fibrosis," established and cutting-edge techniques for imaging diffuse liver diseases using both qualitative and quantitative approaches are described. The authors detail available noninvasive MRI-based methods for evaluation of hepatic fat, iron deposition, and fibrosis and discuss advantages and disadvantages of these different techniques.

3. In the article entitled, "Magnetic Resonance Imaging of the Pediatric Pancreaticobiliary System," the use of magnetic resonance cholangiopancreatography (MRCP) is extensively reviewed. The authors present MRCP techniques, including advantages and disadvantages, and indications for imaging, as well as present the imaging appearances of numerous common and uncommon conditions affecting the pancreaticobiliary system.

4. In the article entitled, "Magnetic Resonance Imaging of the Pediatric Kidney: Benign and Malignant Masses," both the clinical and imaging features of benign and malignant renal masses that occur in children and adolescents are presented. Imaging technique is also reviewed.

5. In the article entitled, "Magnetic Resonance Urography in Evaluation of Duplicated Renal Collecting Systems," the authors discuss appropriate terminology for duplicated upper urinary tracts as well as pertinent embryology. The various clinical presentations and imaging appearances of duplicated renal collecting systems are also presented in detail.

6. In the article entitled, "Magnetic Resonance Enterography: IBD and Beyond," a comprehensive review of MRI of the bowel in children is presented. Variations on the basic MR enterography protocol are discussed, and the advantages and disadvantages of each are described. The article also includes a review of inflammatory bowel disease classification and image interpretation and concludes with a discussion of potential applications of MR enterography beyond imaging of inflammatory bowel disease.

7. In the article entitled, "Magnetic Resonance Imaging of Pediatric Pelvic Masses," the authors provide a broad review of both benign and malignant pediatric pelvic masses and stress the advantages of MRI for initial diagnosis, staging, and imaging surveillance. MR imaging characteristics of specific masses are reviewed and imaging technique is discussed.

8. In the article entitled, "Müllerian Duct and Related Anomalies in Children and Adolescents," common and uncommon developmental anomalies of the uterus and vagina are described. Relevant embryology, classification, and imaging findings are presented in a systematic manner.

9. In the article entitled, "Magnetic Resonance Imaging of Anorectal Malformations," the increasing roles of MRI in the evaluation of anorectal and other complex pelvic malformations prenatally and postnatally prior to definitive surgical repair are presented in detail. Expected and unexpected postoperative MRI findings are also described.

10. In the article entitled, "Magnetic Resonance Imaging of Perianal and Perineal Crohn Disease in Children and Adolescents," perineal and perianal imaging findings of Crohn disease in the pediatric population are presented, including fistulous disease, abscesses, and skin manifestations. Perianal anatomy, classification of perianal Crohn disease lesions, and MRI technique are also reviewed.

11. In the article entitled, "Advanced Techniques in Pediatric Abdominopelvic Oncologic Magnetic Resonance Imaging," the author reviews the role of MRI in the management of pediatric cancer patients, including a review oncologic MR imaging protocol issues. The article also presents cutting-edge MR imaging techniques, including diffusion-weighted imaging, whole-body MRI, dynamic contrast-enhanced MRI, and positron emission tomography-MRI.

12. In the article entitled, "Magnetic Resonance Angiography of the Pediatric Abdomen and Pelvis: Techniques and Imaging Findings," the authors provide a comprehensive review of the various noncontrast and contrast-enhanced techniques for vascular MR imaging. The second half of the article focuses on common and uncommon vascular anatomic variants and pathologic conditions that occur in the pediatric population.

We would like to sincerely thank all of the authors, who spent countless hours contributing to this effort. We would also like to acknowledge Pamela Hetherington, who shepherded both the authors and the editors through the preparation of this issue. It is our hope that readers of these works learn as much about state-of-the-art pediatric abdominopelvic MRI as we have while assembling this issue!

Jonathan R. Dillman, MD
Section of Pediatric Radiology
Department of Radiology
University of Michigan Health System
C.S. Mott Children's Hospital
Ann Arbor, MI 48109, USA

Ethan A. Smith, MD
Section of Pediatric Radiology
Department of Radiology
University of Michigan Health System
C.S. Mott Children's Hospital
Ann Arbor, MI 48109, USA

E-mail addresses:
jonadill@med.umich.edu (J.R. Dillman)
ethans@med.umich.edu (E.A. Smith)

Magnetic Resonance Imaging of the Pediatric Liver
Benign and Malignant Masses

Christopher P. Keup, MD[a], Felicia Ratnaraj, BA[b],
Pooja R. Chopra, BA[b], Charles A. Lawrence, MD[a],
Lisa H. Lowe, MD[a],*

KEYWORDS

- MR imaging - Children - Liver - Masses - Malignancy - Gadoxetate disodium

KEY POINTS

- Magnetic resonance imaging is a useful tool for characterizing both benign and malignant pediatric liver lesions.
- Characteristic patterns of signal intensity and postcontrast enhancement can narrow the differential diagnosis and help determine whether a liver lesion is likely benign or malignant.
- Use of hepatocyte-specific contrast agents, such as gadoxetate disodium, can provide additional information to help refine the differential diagnosis for focal liver lesions.

INTRODUCTION

Primary hepatic neoplasms constitute approximately 5% to 6% of all pediatric intra-abdominal masses, most of which (approximately two-thirds) are malignant.[1] Overall, malignant primary hepatic tumors account for 1% to 2% of all childhood cancers.[2] It is important, therefore, to systematically approach and accurately characterize hepatic masses to ensure the best possible clinical management strategy (**Table 1**).

In children, magnetic resonance (MR) imaging is particularly desirable for evaluating liver lesions because of the lack of ionizing radiation and superb soft tissue contrast resolution compared with traditional multiphase computed tomography (CT) protocols. The potential disadvantages of sedation and scan time may be offset by the ability of MR imaging to provide more clinically relevant information when compared with CT. The recent development and implementation of hepatocyte-specific contrast agents (HSA), such as gadoxetate disodium, further strengthens the role of MR imaging in hepatic lesion characterization.

Thus, understanding how pathologic features of hepatic neoplasms are represented in imaging helps the radiologist to better characterize the lesions, which ideally leads to proper work-up and treatment of liver lesions. This article discusses key MR imaging findings of common benign and malignant pediatric lesions (**Tables 2 and 3**) and focuses on the utility of new HSA to help achieve optimal diagnostic accuracy.

IMAGING TECHNIQUE/PROTOCOL

MR imaging has some distinct advantages compared with CT and ultrasound (US), which include lack of ionizing radiation (compared with CT), more specific soft tissue characterization, dynamic postcontrast imaging, and more complete evaluation of the biliary system. The lack of

Disclosures: The authors have nothing to disclose.
[a] Departments of Radiology, Children's Mercy Hospitals and Clinics, and The University of Missouri—Kansas City, Kansas City, MO, USA; [b] School of Medicine, University of Missouri—Kansas City, Kansas City, MO, USA
* Corresponding author. Department of Radiology, 2401 Gillham Road, Kansas City, MO 64108.
E-mail address: lhlowe@cmh.edu

Magn Reson Imaging Clin N Am 21 (2013) 645–667
http://dx.doi.org/10.1016/j.mric.2013.06.003
1064-9689/13/$ – see front matter © 2013 Elsevier Inc. All rights reserved.

Table 1
Approach to evaluation of pediatric hepatic masses[a]

| **Usually Solitary** | *versus* | **Usually Multifocal** |

Hepatoblastoma[b]

Hepatocellular carcinoma[b]

Fibrolamellar hepatocellular carcinoma

Undifferentiated embryonal sarcoma

Focal nodular hyperplasia[b]

Hepatic adenoma[b]

Inflammatory pseudotumor

Mesenchymal hamartoma

Embryonal rhabdomyosarcoma

Malignant rhabdoid tumor

Metastasis (neuroblastoma, Wilms,

lymphoma, and so forth.)

Nodular regenerative hyperplasia

Infantile hemangiomas

History of chronic liver disease

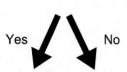

Yes   No

HCC   All others

Elevated alpha-fetoprotein

Yes

HCC or Hepatoblastoma

[a]Age and clinical setting can be used to further narrow differential diagnosis
[b]Although these lesions are most often solitary, multifocal presentation is common

ionizing radiation becomes increasingly important when multiphase (including delayed phase) imaging is needed to assess the enhancement characteristics of focal lesions. MR imaging is particularly useful for the characterization of cystic and solid lesions, which are commonly indeterminate in nature at both CT and US, facilitating the formulation of a focused differential diagnosis. Another

Table 2
Benign pediatric hepatic masses: summary of age, associated laboratory data, and common imaging findings

Neoplasm	Ultrasound	CT	MR Imaging
Infantile hemangioma • <1 y old • AFP normal (caveat: normally elevated first few months of life)	Hypoechoic or mixed echogenicity Doppler shows increased diastolic flow	Peripheral early phase postcontrast enhancement with homogenous or centripetal fill in (note, larger lesions may not entirely fill in because of fibrosis or hemorrhage)	T2W hyperintense T1W hypointense Early phase postcontrast enhancement with homogenous or delayed fill in Hypointense on delayed postcontrast imaging using HSA (20 min)
Mesenchymal hamartoma • <2 y old • AFP normal (caveat: normally elevated first few months of life)	Mixed echogenicity depending on mixture of cystic and solid portions	Multicystic ± solid components that enhance with IV contrast material	Cystic areas are T2W hyperintense and T1W hypointense Solid portions enhance Hypointense on delayed postcontrast imaging using HSA (20 min)
Focal nodular hyperplasia • >2–5 y old • AFP normal • History of prior abdominal malignancy	Hyperechoic, isoechoic, or hypoechoic Central scar is hyperechoic	Homogenous with arterial postcontrast enhancement Isoattenuating or nearly isoattenuating on noncontrast and delayed postcontrast imaging Central scar shows delayed enhancement	T1W hypointense/ isointense T2W hyperintense/ isointense T2W hyperintense central scar that shows delayed enhancement Arterial-phase postcontrast hyperenhancement Isointense on delayed venous imaging Hyperintense/ isointense to normal liver on delayed imaging using HSA (20 min)
Hepatic adenoma • >10 y old • Associated with anabolic steroids or oral contraceptive pills	Hyperechoic, isoechoic, or hypoechoic depending on amount of lesional hemorrhage and lipid and underlying liver disease	Heterogeneous because of lipid and/ or hemorrhage Variable heterogeneous postcontrast enhancement	Heterogeneously hyperintense on T1W and T2W because of hemorrhage and/or lipid Heterogeneous arterial-phase postcontrast enhancement Hypointense on delayed postcontrast imaging using HSA (20 min)

(continued on next page)

Table 2
(continued)

Neoplasm	Ultrasound	CT	MR Imaging
Nodular regenerative hyperplasia • Older patients • Underlying condition, such as Budd Chiari, chronic portal venous occlusion, connective tissue disease, or myeloproliferative disorder	Hyperechoic, isoechoic, or hypoechoic	Hyperenhancing or hypoenhancing (depending on postcontrast imaging phase)	Variable T2W signal intensity Isointense to hyperintense on T1W May show arterial postcontrast enhancement Hyperintense/isointense on delayed postcontrast imaging using HSA (20 min)
Inflammatory pseudotumor • Any age • Diagnosis requires strong clinical suspicion	Heterogeneous (mixed echogenicity) Patchy or sparse Doppler blood flow	Heterogeneous postcontrast enhancement (enhancement may increase on delayed imaging)	Heterogeneous T1W and T2W signal intensity Heterogeneous postcontrast enhancement (enhancement may increase on delayed imaging) Hypointense on delayed postcontrast imaging using HSA (20 min)

Abbreviations: AFP, alpha-fetoprotein; IV, intravenous; T1W, T1-weighted; T2W, T2-weighted.

specific advantage of MR imaging compared with CT is with the evaluation of the biliary tree because bile duct masses, wall thickening, and filling defects are all better visualized with this modality.

Disadvantages of MR imaging include the length of scan time compared with CT or US and its sensitivity to patient motion, possibly necessitating sedation or general anesthesia in pediatric patients. Other disadvantages may include incompatibility with indwelling ferromagnetic devices; susceptibility artifacts and distortion from metallic implants, such as spinal hardware; and limited characterization of calcification/bone. In most clinical imaging situations, the benefits of MR imaging outweigh these disadvantages. The authors' protocol for imaging of the pediatric liver is presented in **Table 4**.

BENIGN PEDIATRIC LIVER LESIONS
Infantile Hemangiomas

Infantile hemangiomas are the most common tumor of infancy, occurring in up to 10% of infants.[3–6] Recent data suggest that they are comprised of primitive blood vessels derived from angioblasts or placental stem cells that may implant on the fetus in utero.[7,8] Infantile hemangiomas are most common in premature female Caucasian infants, those with a low birth weight, and those whose gestation was complicated by placental disruption or chorionic villous sampling.[5,9] Although they can occur throughout the body, infantile hemangiomas are most frequently cutaneous, with the liver being the most common extracutaneous site.[9] Hepatic lesions are seen in up to 13% of children with skin lesions.[10]

Recent histopathological discoveries have caused vascular anomalies in children, including infantile hemangiomas, to be reclassified according to a biologic classification system first proposed in 1982.[11] In this system, lesions are divided into 2 basic categories: neoplasms (masses that proliferate and grow by undergoing mitosis) and vascular malformations (congenitally deformed vessels that do NOT undergo mitosis). Infantile hemangiomas are true neoplasms that undergo mitosis during their proliferative phase, followed by gradual involution. They have been found to contain a unique pathologic marker, glucose transporter protein isoform 1 (GLUT1), which is not found in any other tissue, except for the human placenta.[12] This system was accepted

Table 3
Malignant pediatric hepatic masses: summary of age, associated laboratory data, and common imaging findings

Neoplasm	Ultrasound	CT	MR Imaging
Hepatoblastoma • <2 y old • Elevated AFP	Heterogeneous Predominantly solid ± Calcification/ ossification	Predominantly solid ± necrotic or cystic areas ± Calcification/ ossification Heterogeneous postcontrast enhancement ± Vascular invasion	Heterogeneous T1W and T2W Heterogeneous postcontrast enhancement ± Vascular invasion Hypointense on delayed postcontrast imaging using HSA (20 min)
Hepatocellular CA • >5 y old • Often history of chronic liver disease • AFP usually elevated	Heterogeneous Predominantly solid	Predominantly solid May contain necrotic or cystic areas Postcontrast arterial- phase hyperenhancement with delayed wash out	Heterogeneous T1W and T2W Postcontrast arterial- phase hyperenhancement with delayed wash out ± Vascular invasion Hypointense on delayed postcontrast imaging using HSA (20 min)
Metastasis • Neuroblastoma, Wilms tumor, Lymphoma, and so forth • Can be hypovascular or hypervascular • Normal AFP	Solid, cystic, or mixed solid/cystic Generally multiple lesions	Solid, cystic, or mixed solid/cystic Generally multiple lesions Hypoenhancing or hyperenhancing on postcontrast imaging depending on tumor of origin and imaging phase	Solid, cystic, or mixed solid/cystic Generally T1W hypointense to isointense and T2W hyperintense Hypoenhancing or hyperenhancing on postcontrast imaging depending on tumor of origin and imaging phase Hypointense on delayed postcontrast imaging using HSA (20 min)
Fibrolamellar CA • Adolescents and young adults • No underlying liver disease • Normal AFP	Solid Central scar ± echogenic calcification/ ossification	Solid Postcontrast arterial- phase hyperenhancement ± wash out Hypoenhancing central scar ± calcification	Solid Variable T1W and T2W T2W hypointense, hypoenhancing central scar Postcontrast arterial- phase hyperenhancement ± wash out Hypointense on delayed postcontrast imaging using HSA (20 min)

(continued on next page)

Table 3
(continued)

Neoplasm	Ultrasound	CT	MR Imaging
UES • 6–10 y of age • Normal AFP	Heterogeneous Predominantly solid	Commonly appears cystic and solid Heterogeneous postcontrast enhancement with septations and mural nodularity ± Hemorrhage	Commonly appears cystic and solid Variable T1W and T2W Heterogeneous postcontrast enhancement with septations and mural nodularity Hypointense on delayed postcontrast imaging using HSA (20 min)
ERMS • <6 y of age • Elevated bilirubin • Normal AFP	Solid, cystic or mixed solid/cystic Tumor may be observed in dilated bile ducts	Heterogeneous postcontrast enhancement Enhancing tumor may be observed in dilated bile ducts	T1W hypointense and T2W hyperintense Heterogeneous postcontrast enhancement Enhancing tumor may be observed in dilated bile ducts Hypointense on delayed postcontrast imaging using HSA (20 min)
Rhabdoid tumor • <2 y of age • Similar to ATRT of brain • Normal AFP	Heterogeneous Mixed solid and cystic	Mixed solid and cystic Heterogeneous postcontrast enhancement	Variable T1W and T2W Hypointense on all postcontrast phases, including delayed HAS imaging (20 min)

Abbreviations: AFP, alpha fetoprotein; ATRT, atypical teratoid/rhabdoid tumor; CA, carcinoma; ERS, embryonal rhabdomyosarcoma; T1W, T1-weighted; T2W, T2-weighted; UES, undifferentiated embryonal sarcoma.

Table 4
Sample pediatric liver MR imaging protocol (using gadoxetate disodium[a])

Precontrast Imaging	Postcontrast Imaging
Coronal, single-shot fast spin echo (breath held or respiratory triggered)	Multiphase, axial, T1-weighted, 3D spoiled gradient-recalled echo with fat-saturation (breath held)
Axial, T2-weighted, fast spin echo with fat saturation (respiratory-triggered or navigator-gated or PROPELLER/BLADE technique)	Axial and coronal T1-weighted, 3D spoiled gradient-recalled echo with fat-saturation – 10- and 20-min delay (breath held)
Axial, T1-weighted, gradient-recalled echo (in and out of phase) (breath held)	—
Axial, T1-weighted, 3D spoiled gradient-recalled echo with fat saturation (breath held)	—
Axial, diffusion-weighted echo planar imaging (respiratory triggered or free breathing)	—

Abbreviation: 3D, 3 dimensional.
[a] Can be power injected at 1 to 2 mL/s at 0.025 mmol/kg through 22-g peripheral intravenous cannula (or larger).

by the International Society for the Study of Vascular Anomalies (ISSVA) in 1996 and is now widely used among pediatric subspecialists.[13] The utility of the ISSVA system lies in its ability to provide a systematic approach to vascular lesions that predictably correlates with history, lesion clinical course, imaging findings, accurate diagnosis, and treatment options.[14] Hassanein and colleagues[15] showed that 69% of children seen in a large vascular malformations clinic were initially given a wrong diagnosis leading to initial improper treatment in 20.6% of children. Hepatic hemangiomas are often further descriptively classified into 3 subtypes: focal, multifocal, and diffuse.[10,16] Other terms used include *hemangiomatosis* (indicating multiple hemangiomas) and *disseminated hemangiomatosis* (applied when hemangiomas occur in 3 or more organ systems).

Infantile hemangiomas generally present between 2 weeks and 2 months of age with one or more skin or hepatic lesions.[5] Lesions follow a predictable clinical course of initial proliferation over the first year of life followed by gradual involution that may extend into puberty. Although many children with infantile hemangiomas of the liver likely go undetected, these lesions may rarely come to attention because of a variety of associated complications, including high-output congestive heart failure, hypothyroidism, thrombocytopenia, hepatic failure, and respiratory distress caused by massive hepatomegaly.[9,17,18] The primary differential diagnosis of hepatic hemangioma is metastatic neuroblastoma, which can be easily excluded in most cases with urine catecholamine screening and abdominal US to assess for a primary adrenal or paraspinous mass.[19]

Although imaging of hepatic hemangiomas typically begins with sonography (**Fig. 1**), these lesions generally require additional cross-sectional imaging (preferably MR imaging), and rarely biopsy, for definitive diagnosis.[5,9] Infantile hemangiomas can demonstrate variable imaging features depending on their stage of development. Proliferative hemangiomas are generally well-defined, hypervascular, vigorously enhancing masses with internal flow voids. Multifocal lesions are usually small and uniform, whereas larger single lesions may contain central hemorrhage, necrosis, fibrosis, and, very rarely, calcifications.[5] Classically, these lesions are T1-weighted hypointense, T2-weighted hyperintense, and demonstrate postcontrast hyperenhancement (see **Fig. 1**). Postcontrast T1-weighted images usually show early peripheral enhancement (either continuous or discontinuous), with variable subsequent centripetal filling in more delayed venous phases.[20] This same pattern of enhancement has been described in adult hepatic lesions also known as hemangiomas (non-neoplastic GLUT1 negative vascular malformations). In infants, who often have numerous small hepatic hemangiomas, the pattern of centripetal enhancement is much less common and is not a reliable sign for diagnosis.[9] These lesions often flash fill, that is, they appear homogeneously hyperintense during the arterial-phase postcontrast imaging (**Fig. 2**). If a hepatocyte-specific contrast agent (HSA) is used, infantile hemangiomas vary in signal compared with the surrounding liver on the hepatocyte phase.[21,22] As lesions involute, which occurs after the first year of life, hepatic hemangiomas show progressively less enhancement.[10,17,23]

Because infantile hemangiomas undergo spontaneous involution, the prognosis is excellent and no treatment is needed in many cases. However, if life-threatening complications develop, a variety of treatment options are available that range from medical management with antiangiogenic drugs to surgery, percutaneous catheter embolization, and, very rarely, liver transplantation.[24,25] Although commonly used by many pediatric dermatologists, propranolol (a nonselective beta-blocker) is not yet approved by the Food and Drug Administration for this indication. Other antiangiogenic drugs used to treat hemangiomas include corticosteroids and more aggressive agents, such as vincristine.[9,26]

Mesenchymal Hamartoma

Mesenchymal hamartoma is the most common benign liver mass in children after infantile hemangioma. It usually occurs in children less than 2 years of age, and it is twice as common in boys as girls.[1] Patients may present with asymptomatic abdominal distention or complications related to mass effect, such as gastrointestinal obstruction.[27] The lesion is often a large, well-defined, solitary, predominantly cystic mass, measuring as large as 15 to 30 cm.[28] Multiple satellite lesions can also occur.[29]

Mesenchymal hamartoma results from uncoordinated proliferation of primitive mesenchyme in the periportal tracts. Often the mass proliferates by extending along the portal triads, which results in the compression of adjacent parenchyma. Fluid accumulation and cyst formation then develop in the resulting areas of atrophy and degeneration.[18,28] Lesions do not contain calcifications or hemorrhage.[18,28]

On imaging, mesenchymal hamartoma ranges from a cystic mass with thin or thick septations to a predominantly solid mass with a few small cysts. Cystic portions are avascular, and stromal portions are hypovascular.[30] MR imaging features

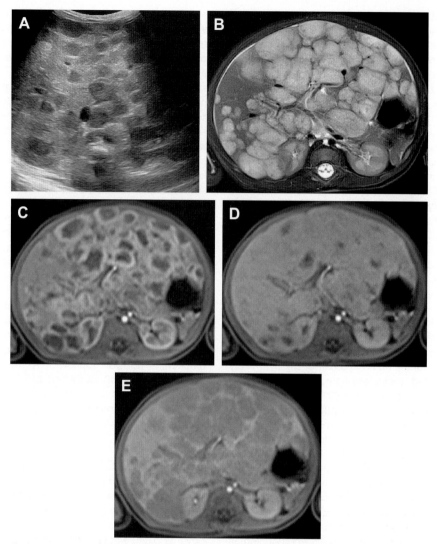

Fig. 1. Infantile hemangiomas in a 3-month-old boy with hepatomegaly and difficulty breathing. (*A*) Transverse gray-scale sonogram demonstrates many hypoechoic, well-defined, round and ovoid lesions throughout the liver. (*B*) Axial, T2-weighted, fat-saturated MR image confirms the presence of numerous homogeneous hyperintense liver masses. Axial gadoxetate disodium–enhanced, fat-suppressed, T1-weighted (*C*) arterial, (*D*) venous, and (*E*) 5-minute delayed-phase images reveal peripheral enhancement of lesions with centripetal filling in with contrast material over time. The lesions appear hypointense compared with normal liver parenchyma on delayed imaging because they do not retain contrast material.

depend on the amount of stroma within the mass and the protein content of the fluid in the cysts.[31] Solid portions of the lesion are hypointense to adjacent liver on T1- and T2-weighted sequences because of fibrosis.[30] Cystic portions demonstrate variable signal intensity on T1-weighted imaging depending on the protein content of the cyst fluid and are generally hyperintense on T2-weighted imaging. Postcontrast enhancement is limited to septations and stromal components (**Fig. 3**).[32,33]

The definitive treatment of mesenchymal hamartoma is surgical excision. If the mass is unresectable, partial resection or drainage with marsupialization may be used.[18,34] Overall, the long-term survival rate for mesenchymal hamartoma is 90%, even with incomplete resection.[35]

Focal Nodular Hyperplasia

Focal nodular hyperplasia (FNH) is a benign hamartomatous lesion that arises from polyclonal proliferation of hepatocytes, Kupffer cells, vascular structures, and biliary ductules. They may occur simultaneously with other benign lesions, such as

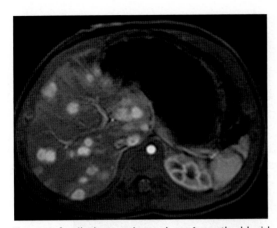

Fig. 2. Infantile hemangiomas in a 4-month-old girl with multiple liver lesions incidentally detected on US. Axial, T1-weighted, fat-suppressed, postcontrast image demonstrates homogeneous arterial-phase enhancement of multiple hepatic lesions, compatible with flash filling phenomenon. Lesions were homogeneously hyperintense on T2-weighted imaging (not shown). (*Courtesy of* Jonathan R. Dillman, MD, Section of Pediatric Radiology, Department of Radiology, C. S. Mott Children's Hospital, University of Michigan, Ann Arbor, MI.)

hepatic adenoma, and may result from vascular insults caused by trauma or chemotherapy.[36,37] FNH accounts for approximately 4% of all primary hepatic tumors in the pediatric population.[27] Histologically, FNH contains functioning hepatocytes, although the biliary ductules are malformed and nonfunctional.[20] FNH may present as a solitary, well-circumscribed, lobulated, and unencapsulated mass or as multiple masses in the setting of prior treated abdominal malignancy, such as Wilms tumor or neuroblastoma.[37]

On MR imaging, typical FNH is homogenous and isointense to slightly hypointense relative to normal liver on T1-weighted images and isointense to slightly hyperintense on T2-weighted sequences. Because the mass is comprised predominantly of hepatocytes, it appears similar to normal liver on unenhanced images and may not be visible in the absence of mass effect. In the setting of hepatic steatosis, the lesion is hyperintense on opposed-phase (out-of-phase), T1-weighted, gradient-recalled echo images caused by the lack of intracellular lipid (**Fig. 4**). Restricted diffusion may also occur.[38]

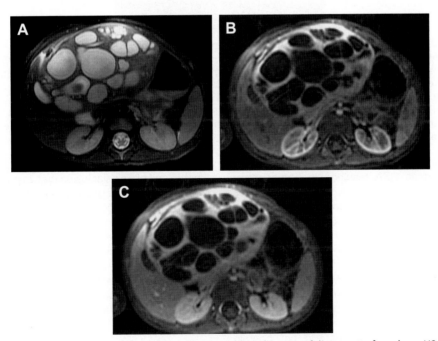

Fig. 3. Mesenchymal hamartoma in a 2-year-old boy with a history of liver cysts found on US. (*A*) Axial, T2-weighted, fat-saturated MR image demonstrates multiple hyperintense, well-defined cystic areas of varying size in the left hepatic lobe. Fat-suppressed, axial, T1-weighted images after administration of a traditional blood pool contrast agent in the (*B*) arterial and (*C*) delayed phases show septal hyperenhancement compared with normal adjacent liver. (*Courtesy of* Jonathan R. Dillman, MD, Department of Radiology, C. S. Mott Children's Hospital, University of Michigan, Ann Arbor, MI.)

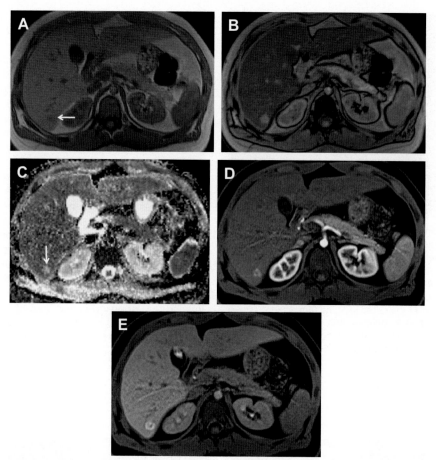

Fig. 4. Focal nodular hyperplasia in a 19-year-old young man with elevated liver transaminases discovered during follow-up of hypothalamic glioma. (*A*) Axial, T1-weighted, gradient-recalled echo in-phase MR image reveals a subtle hypointense right lobe lesion (*arrow*). (*B*) On out-of-phase imaging, the lesion has increased signal caused by the lack of lipid in the lesion compared with surrounding hepatic parenchyma. (*C*) Apparent diffusion coefficient image shows the lesion is hyperintense (*arrow*). (*D*) Axial, gadoxetate disodium–enhanced, fat-suppressed, T1-weighted arterial and (*E*) 20-minute delayed-phase MR images demonstrate retention of contrast material by the lesion that increases over 20 minutes. The hypointense central scar is most conspicuous on the 20-minute delayed image.

Characterization of suspected FNH is best performed with an HSA resulting in homogenous arterial-phase hyperenhancement that becomes isointense to adjacent liver on venous-phase images and remains isointense to hyperintense throughout the delayed (10–20 minute) hepatocyte phase (**Fig. 5**).[21,22] A central nonenhancing stellate scar comprised of malformed vascular structures in a myxoid and fibrous stroma can be seen with the use of an HSA.[22,35] By comparison, traditional blood pool MR imaging contrast agents may produce enhancement of the central scar on delayed images.[21,29] Liver lesions that do not contain functioning hepatocytes wash out long before the hepatocyte phase and are hypointense to the surrounding parenchyma. Besides FNH, the major differential consideration of a homogenously enhancing lesion on the hepatocyte phase is nodular regenerative hyperplasia (discussed later), a pathologically similar lesion that, in part, is distinguished by the lack of a central scar.

FNH does not produce derangements of laboratory values, and the lesion has no malignant potential or significant risk of hemorrhage. It grows slowly, remains asymptomatic, and is only discovered when imaging is performed for an unrelated purpose. In rare cases, surgical resection, ablation, or embolization is required to treat patients with symptoms related to mass effect or rapid growth.[35]

Nodular Regenerative Hyperplasia and Large Regenerative Nodules

Foci of nodular regenerative hyperplasia (NRH) are benign areas of hepatocellular proliferation in the

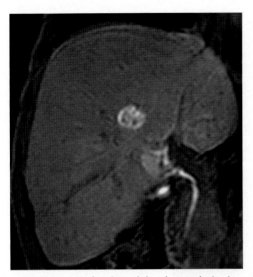

Fig. 5. Presumed focal nodular hyperplasia in an 11-year-old girl with history of Wilms tumor and renal cell carcinoma. Coronal, 20-minute delayed post-contrast (gadoxetate disodium), fat-suppressed, T1-weighted image shows that the lesion is hyperintense compared with normal liver, consistent with FNH. (*Courtesy of* Jonathan R. Dillman, MD, Section of Pediatric Radiology, Department of Radiology, C. S. Mott Children's Hospital, University of Michigan, Ann Arbor, MI.)

setting of generalized hepatocellular disease, cirrhosis, or insult from a variety of causes, such as hepatotoxic medications, collagen vascular disease, lymphoproliferative, or myeloproliferative disorders.[21,29] In children, NRH is often caused by vascular disturbances, such as the absence of the portal vein (Abernathy syndrome), chronic portal venous occlusion, and cardiac abnormalities.[39,40] NRH can occur at any age and is characterized by nodules of varying size from a few millimeters to several centimeters (so-called large or macroregenerative nodules). The pathogenesis of NRH is not fully understood but, as the name implies, involves a focal response to parenchymal or vascular insult with proliferation of functional hepatocytes. The insult can result in decreased blood flow to some acini, which subsequently atrophy. Adjacent acini with preserved flow may then undergo compensatory hyperplasia.[18] Some cases of NRH can be difficult to diagnose. Small nodules (<0.5 cm) may not be detected because they are compromised of functional hepatocytes and blend in with the surrounding normal liver.[27] Large regenerative nodules are commonly associated with postsinusoidal obstructive conditions, such as congestive cardiomyopathy and Budd-Chiari syndrome.[41]

On MR imaging, regenerative nodules are homogenous and isointense to normal liver or slightly hyperintense to abnormal liver on T1-weighted sequences. They are similarly isointense or slightly hypointense on T2-weighted sequences.[21,27,29] A rim of T1-weighted hypointensity or T2-weighted hyperintensity in addition to restricted diffusion can also be seen in NRH. Postcontrast T1-weighted imaging with an HSA results in early enhancement, which persists through the hepatocyte phase, similar to that seen with FNH (**Fig. 6**). The enhancement pattern can be hypointense, isointense, or hyperintense relative to the surrounding liver depending on the degree of underlying hepatocellular disease.[20,21,29]

There is no specific treatment of regenerative nodules other than to avoid hepatotoxic medications or exposures.[18,35] Large or coalescent nodules may hemorrhage or rupture, necessitating treatment.[35] Malignant transformation to hepatocellular carcinoma is a very rare complication.[35,39]

Hepatocellular Adenoma

Hepatocellular adenoma is a benign hepatic neoplasm, rare in children, that often presents as a well-circumscribed spherical or ovoid mass. It can occur as a result of the use of anabolic steroids in boys and oral contraceptives in girls, as sequela of chronic focal hepatic vascular disturbances, or in patients with diabetes mellitus or glycogen storage disease.[21,29,35] Multiple pathologic subtypes exist, most commonly the inflammatory hepatocellular subtype (40%–50% of all adenomas).[42] Hepatocellular adenomas often occur in women in their reproductive years; however, in the pediatric populations, they can be present in girls older than 10 years who use oral contraceptives.[43] Lesions can be single or multiple, with the term *adenomatosis* applied in the setting of 10 or more lesions.[21,29]

Patients with hepatocellular adenomas are often asymptomatic but can present with symptoms related to mass effect or hemorrhage, especially if larger than 5 cm.[42] There is a 5% to 10% risk of developing hepatocellular carcinoma.[42,44] Blood hepatic transaminase levels and alpha-fetoprotein (AFP) levels are usually normal.[45] Hepatocellular adenomas widely range in size, from less than 1 cm to greater than 15 cm.[46]

Imaging findings of hepatocellular adenoma are variable, depending on the amount of fat or hemorrhage within the mass.[47] They may be encapsulated or have a pseudocapsule with compression of adjacent hepatic parenchyma. Most hepatocellular adenomas are predominantly hyperintense to normal liver on T1-weighted and isointense to hyperintense on T2-weighted sequences.[42] T1-weighted signal hyperintensity is thought to be

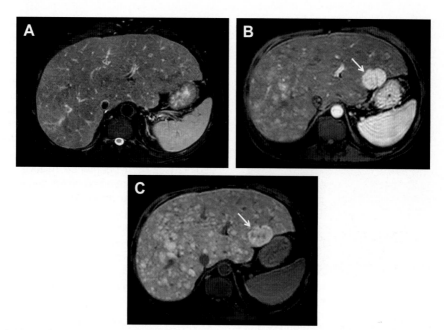

Fig. 6. Nodular regenerative hyperplasia in a 21-year-old young man with congenital heart disease status post Fontan palliation. MR imaging of the liver was performed as part of heart transplant evaluation. (*A*) Axial, T2-weighted, fat-saturated image shows no focal lesions. The liver is enlarged because of hepatic venous congestion, and it has a nodular contour. (*B*) Axial, gadoxetate disodium–enhanced, arterial-phase, fat-suppressed, T1-weighted image shows many arterially hyperenhancing liver nodules throughout both lobes that (*C*) remain hyperintense on 20-minute delayed-phase image. Random biopsy confirmed extensive nodular regenerative hyperplasia, whereas targeted biopsy of the dominant left lobe mass demonstrated FNH (*arrows*).

caused by hemorrhage, lipid, or glycogen deposition. T2-weighted signal hyperintensity may represent hemorrhage, fat, or areas of peliosislike changes at pathologic analysis.[48] Lipid-laden adenomas can be diffusely hyperintense on T1- and T2-weighted images, lose signal on T1-weighted, gradient-recalled echo, out-of-phase imaging, and may even demonstrate signal loss on fat-suppressed T2-weighted images (**Fig. 7**). Typically, hepatic adenomas demonstrate arterial enhancement on MR imaging with variable enhancement on delayed phase and may wash out by the portal venous phase (or more delayed phase).[42] If an HSA is used, these lesions typically fail to retain contrast material on the delayed hepatocyte phase, becoming hypointense to surrounding liver.

The treatment of hepatocellular adenomas depends on the size and symptoms. Discontinuation of oral contraceptives or dietary therapy in the setting of glycogen storage disease may cause adenomas to regress.[35] Adenomas greater than 5 cm in diameter or with hemorrhage and hemodynamic instability are frequently surgically resected or embolized. The risk of hemorrhage/rupture and malignant transformation increase when the adenoma reaches 5 cm or greater size.[42] The

inflammatory subtype has the highest risk of hemorrhage, approximately 30%, whereas the β-catenin-mutated subtype carries the highest risk of malignancy and is considered to be a borderline lesion between adenoma and hepatocellular carcinoma.[42] Adenomas of any size in male patients or patients with glycogen storage disease may also be resected because of the increased risk of malignant transformation in these patients.[42] Radiofrequency ablation is an additional treatment option if smaller than 4 cm.[42] Smaller adenomas may warrant follow-up imaging to ensure stability or biopsy if heterogeneous in signal intensity to exclude malignancy.[42]

Inflammatory Pseudotumor

Inflammatory pseudotumor, also known as inflammatory myofibroblastic tumor, is a rare and usually benign lesion that can occur throughout the body at any age but most commonly in young to middle-aged adults (mean age of 45 years in one study), with a male predominance.[49,50] The endoscopic retrograde cholangiopancreatography finding of periportal infiltration or biliary ductal strictures coupled with the clinical presentations of painless obstructive jaundice, fever, weight

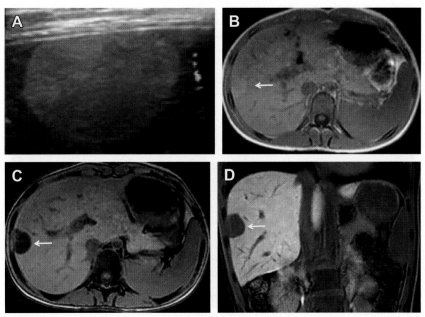

Fig. 7. Hepatocellular adenoma in a 12-year-old girl with chronic right heart failure caused by congenital heart disease. (*A*) Transverse US image demonstrates a large echogenic right lobe liver lesion. (*B*) Axial, T1-weighted, in-phase and out-of-phase (*C*) images reveal signal dropout on opposed phase, compatible with lipid-rich adenoma (*arrows*), which was biopsy confirmed. (*D*) The lesion is hypointense on axial, T1-weighted, fat-saturated, 20-minute delayed image after gadoxetate disodium administration (*arrows*). (*Courtesy of* Jonathan R. Dillman, MD, Section of Pediatric Radiology, Department of Radiology, C. S. Mott Children's Hospital, University of Michigan, Ann Arbor, MI.)

loss, and/or abdominal pain can mimic malignancy.[51] Inflammatory pseudotumor may arise from the hepatic parenchyma or bile ducts and has variable imaging characteristics. Strong clinical suspicion of this lesion is required.

Inflammatory pseudotumor is an encapsulated mass consisting of inflammatory cells, vascular elements, fibrous stroma, and spindle cells sometimes associated with a granulomatous reaction.[49] The pathogenesis of hepatic pseudotumor is unknown, but it is thought to be possibly related to infection, immune reaction, necrosis, phlebitis, and/or reaction to bile.[2] MR imaging findings vary and depend on the cellular composition. Lesions in which fibrosis predominates are hypointense on T1-weighted imaging and slightly hyperintense on T2-weighted imaging.[50] T2-weighted signal intensity can be affected by the degree of necrosis, inflammatory cellular infiltrate, and fibrosis within the lesion.[50] Intratumoral necrosis and desmoplastic reaction may cause capsular retraction, again mimicking malignancy.[52] Postcontrast images demonstrate delayed enhancement (**Fig. 8**).[51,53] Jeong and colleagues[52] describe a case in which enhancement persisted in the center of the lesion during the hepatocyte phase after HSA administration, possibly related to obstruction of biliary canaliculi.

Because there are no specific imaging characteristics to successfully exclude malignancy, the diagnosis is often made after resection with negative surgical margins.[50,51] Although some of these lesions are resectable, others may not be. Small, uncomplicated lesions may be managed more conservatively by treating with nonsteroidal antiinflammatory drugs or chemotherapy and monitoring for complications, such as biliary obstruction.[2,50,51]

MALIGNANT PEDIATRIC LIVER LESIONS
Hepatoblastoma

Hepatoblastoma, the most common primary hepatic tumor in children, is a malignant neoplasm of embryonic liver cells.[54] It is most common in children less than 5 years of age and is slightly more common in boys.[18,54–56] Hepatoblastoma is associated with many conditions, including prematurity/very low birth weight (<1500 g), Beckwith-Wiedemann syndrome, Gardner syndrome/familial adenomatous polyposis, glycogen storage disease type 1A, and trisomy 18.[54] Most children present with abdominal enlargement, anorexia, and weight loss.[18,54–56] Pulmonary metastases and vascular invasion of the hepatic vessels or inferior vena cava are common.[18,54–56]

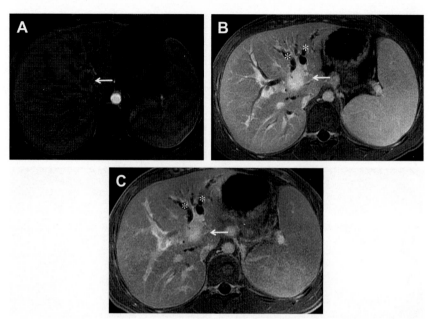

Fig. 8. Inflammatory pseudotumor in a 17-year-old girl with hyperbilirubinemia and jaundice. Axial, fat-suppressed, T1-weighted, postcontrast images after administration of a traditional blood pool agent reveal absent (*A*) arterial-phase enhancement with (*B*) subsequent hyperenhancement of the infiltrative periportal lesion (*arrows*) on portal and (*C*) late venous-phase images. Biliary dilatation (*asterisks*) is present because of central obstruction. (*Courtesy of* J. Knowlton, MD, Children's Mercy Hospital and Clinics, Kansas City, MO.)

Hepatoblastoma is almost always associated with elevated serum alpha-fetoprotein levels, which can be used to monitor the efficacy of therapy and tumor recurrence.[54–56]

Grossly, hepatoblastoma is a well-circumscribed single or commonly multifocal mass with lobulated borders and internal septa.[18,31,54,57–59] Hemorrhage and necrosis are common.[18,54,55] Histologically, hepatoblastomas are divided into 2 types: epithelial and mixed epithelial/mesenchymal.[54] The epithelial subtype is more common and can contain poorly or well-differentiated cells.[54]

Imaging of hepatoblastoma generally reflects its gross and microscopic histopathology. Lesions are well circumscribed, lobular, and often septated.[54] Enhancement and signal characteristics differ based on the amount of epithelial and mesenchymal components as well as the presence of necrosis and hemorrhage. The epithelial subtype tends to be homogenous, whereas the mixed subtype is more heterogeneous.[54] On MR imaging, the epithelial subtype is usually homogeneous, slightly hypointense on T1-weighted, and hyperintense on T2-weighted sequences.[54] The mixed subtype is heterogeneous, predominantly hypointense on T1-weighted sequences, and hyperintense on T2-weighted sequences (**Figs. 9** and **10**).[31,54,57,58] Fibrotic septa are typically

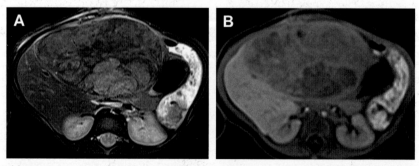

Fig. 9. Hepatoblastoma in a 9-month-old girl with liver mass discovered by pediatrician on physical examination. (*A*) Axial, fat-suppressed, T2-weighted, MR image demonstrates a heterogeneous, well-defined mass occupying the left hepatic lobe. (*B*) Axial, gadoxetate disodium–enhanced, fat-suppressed, T1-weighted, delayed-phase image shows heterogeneous enhancement within the mass that is less than the enhancement of the adjacent liver.

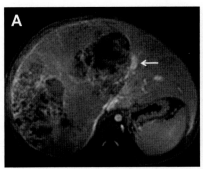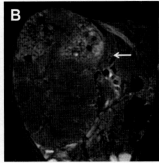

Fig. 10. Hepatoblastoma in a 1-year-old boy with increasing abdominal distention. (*A*) Axial, postcontrast (traditional blood pool agent), T1-weighted, fat-suppressed and (*B*) coronal, T2-weighted, fat-suppressed images demonstrate areas of heterogeneity, found to be mixed type at histology. Mass abuts middle hepatic vein (*arrows*). (*Courtesy of* Jonathan R. Dillman, MD, Section of Pediatric Radiology, Department of Radiology, C. S. Mott Children's Hospital, University of Michigan, Ann Arbor, MI.)

hypointense with both T1-weighted and T2-weighted sequences.[18,31,54,58,60] Calcifications (or ossifications) are more common in the mixed subtype and can represent mesenchymal differentiation into osteoid material or frank bone but are poorly visualized on MR imaging.[31,54] Tumor hemorrhage is most often hyperintense on T1-weighted imaging,[31,54,58] and vascular invasion may be identified as filling defects on postcontrast sequences or dedicated MR venography.[18,31,54,60] With standard blood pool contrast agents and HSA, the mass is usually hypointense to liver on all phases, but septa or the tumor periphery can show arterial-phase hyperenhancement.[21,61] Imaging during the hepatocyte phase is useful to evaluate for vascular involvement or tumor extension into the biliary tree.[21]

Staging of hepatoblastomas is required for treatment and the determination of prognosis. Quantification of involved liver segments, assessment of vascular invasion, and determination of distant disease are required according to PRETEXT (PRETreatment EXTent of disease

criteria defined by the International Childhood Liver Tumor Strategy Group).[62] Once staged using the PRETEXT system, hepatoblastomas are treated with surgical resection.[54] If the lesion is unresectable at diagnosis, neoadjuvant chemotherapy is initiated, which allows for a greater chance of future resection.[54,60] Transplantations are also performed in unresectable tumors.[54,55,60] The overall survival is 65% to 70% with specific prognosis depending on staging (**Table 5**).[18,54,58]

Hepatocellular Carcinoma

Despite its rarity in children, hepatocellular carcinoma (HCC) is the second most common primary hepatic malignancy after hepatoblastoma and the most common primary hepatic malignancy in adolescents.[16,21,54] Risk factors for the development of HCC include biliary atresia, familial cholestatic jaundice or progressive familial intrahepatic cholestasis, glycogen storage disease type 1, alpha-1 antitrypsin deficiency, Alagille syndrome, and liver cirrhosis secondary to chronic hepatitis B or C

Table 5
Hepatoblastoma survival by stage

	5-y Overall Survival Rate for Hepatoblastoma	
PRETEXT Stage	**Definition**	**Survival Rate (%)**
I	Three adjoining sectors free; tumor only in one sector	100
II	Two adjoining sectors free; tumor involves 2 adjoining sectors	91
III	One sector or 2 nonadjoining sectors free; tumor involves 3 adjoining or 2 nonadjoining sectors	68
IV	No free sector; tumor in all 4 sectors	57

Data from Pritchard J, Brown J, Shafford E, et al. Cisplatin, doxorubicin, and delayed surgery for childhood hepatoblastoma: a successful approach–results of the first prospective study of the International Society of Pediatric Oncology. J Clin Oncol 2000;18(22):3819–28.

infection.[54] Patients usually present with an abdominal mass that may be associated with pain, anorexia, and fever.[54,59] AFP levels are elevated in 70% of cases.[27] In adults, HCC is most commonly associated with cirrhosis.[16,21] In order from most common to least common, the 3 patterns of HCC at imaging include solitary, multifocal, and diffusely infiltrative.[54]

On MR imaging, HCC is usually slightly hyperintense on T2-weighted and variable in signal on T1-weighted images (**Fig. 11**).[47,54] In larger masses, heterogeneous signal intensity can be seen because of the areas of hemorrhage, calcification, fat, necrosis, or copper accumulation (copper retention occurs in abnormal hepatocytes of HCC compared with the surrounding liver).[47,54,55,63,64] After intravenous contrast material administration, early arterial enhancement is commonly seen followed by wash out on subsequent delayed phases.[27] If a capsule is present, it is hypointense on T1-weighted and T2-weighted sequences with subtle portal venous or delayed enhancement caused by the fibrous content.[54,65] Extracapsular extension and satellite nodules can also be visualized on MR imaging.[54] The use of an HSA may help facilitate the identification of satellite lesions, which are hypointense to liver in the hepatocyte phase.[21] An important caveat is that moderate or well-differentiated HCC may demonstrate uptake in the hepatocyte phase if the lesion contains functioning hepatocytes.[20] The presence of a hypointense capsule in the hepatocyte phase or a faint peripheral ring of venous or delayed enhancement may help distinguish HCC from a benign lesion.[66]

The definitive treatment of HCC is complete tumor resection, which provides the best chance for long-term survival.[54,59] Unfortunately, HCC in children is generally insensitive to chemotherapy.[54,67] Orthotopic liver transplant can be performed for some unresectable tumors.[54,59] Additionally, hepatic arterial chemoembolization has been successful in reducing tumors to resectable size.[68] The overall prognosis is poor, with a 5-year survival of 10% to 30%.[27,54,59]

Fibrolamellar Hepatocellular Carcinoma

Fibrolamellar hepatocellular carcinoma (FLC), a very rare malignant tumor, is a distinct histopathologic primary hepatocellular neoplasm. It is prevalent in adolescents without underlying hepatic disease and has no specific gender preference.[54] FLCs commonly present with a painful abdominal mass, nonspecific abdominal symptoms, and metastatic lymphadenopathy.[54,69]

Grossly, FLC is large, well circumscribed, and nonencapsulated.[54,65] Collagen deposition and fibrosis separate the tumor into lobules and form a macroscopic fibrous scar.[54,65] Calcifications can occur within the central scar.[54,65]

MR imaging shows slight T1-weighted signal hypointensity and T2-weighted signal hyperintensity; intense heterogeneous early enhancement with variable wash out can be seen on postcontrast imaging (**Fig. 12**).[54,70] The central scar is classically hypointense on T1-weighted and T2-weighted sequences and does not enhance.[27,54] Focal nodular hyperplasia occurs in the same age group as FLC, and it also contains a central scar. However, the scar in FNH can consist of myxoid, fibrous, or vascular stroma; enhances late with traditional agents; and is hyperintense on T2-weighted imaging.[54]

Surgical resection is the mainstay treatment of FLC. In some cases, liver transplant, chemotherapy, or even hepatic arterial chemoembolization are used.[54,71] The prognosis of FLC has been reported by some to be better than in conventional HCC, with a 5-year survival rate of 67% compared with 10% to 30% with HCC.[27,54,59]

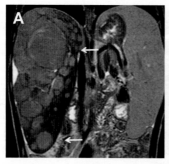
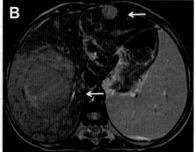

Fig. 11. Hepatocellular carcinoma in an 8-year-old boy with progressive familial intrahepatic cholestasis and portal hypertension based on presence of splenomegaly and small amount of ascites. (*A*) Coronal and (*B*) axial T2-weighted images reveal a large dominant mass in the right lobe with satellite lesions (*arrows*) in both lobes (multifocal hepatocellular carcinoma). (*Courtesy of* Jonathan R. Dillman, MD, Section of Pediatric Radiology, Department of Radiology, C. S. Mott Children's Hospital, University of Michigan, Ann Arbor, MI.)

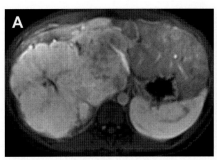 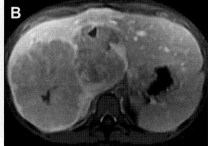

Fig. 12. Fibrolamellar hepatocellular carcinoma in a 19-year-old young woman with increasing abdominal distention. Axial, fat-suppressed, T1-weighted, postcontrast, MR images in the (*A*) arterial and (*B*) delayed phases using a traditional blood pool contrast agent demonstrate early avid enhancement and subsequent washout of a large mass arising from the right lobe. Note the lack of central scar enhancement. (*Courtesy of* Jonathan R. Dillman, MD, Section of Pediatric Radiology, Department of Radiology, C. S. Mott Children's Hospital, University of Michigan, Ann Arbor, MI.)

Undifferentiated Embryonal Sarcoma

Undifferentiated embryonal sarcoma (UES), a rare malignant neoplasm of mesenchymal origin, occurs most often in children between 6 and 10 years of age.[54,72–74] It is the third most common primary hepatic malignancy in the pediatric population after hepatoblastoma and HCC.[21] UES has a slight male predominance and metastasizes to lung, bone, brain, and skin.[1,54,73] Children present with abdominal mass or pain, fever, and weight loss.[54,74] Serum AFP levels are normal, although transaminases can be elevated.[54] UES more often involves the right lobe of the liver, and grossly is a well-circumscribed mass with a fibrous pseudocapsule.[54]

Paradoxically, UES is seen as a solid mass on US but commonly appears mostly cystic on other forms of cross-sectional imaging.[29] MR imaging reveals a mixed solid and cystic mass with possible foci of hemorrhage and necrosis.[30,54] Cystic foci and necrosis are hyperintense on T2-weighted images.[27] The fibrous pseudocapsule forms a hypointense rim on T1-weighted and T2-weighted sequences.[21,54,75] Hemorrhage is usually seen as focal areas of T1-weighted signal hyperintensity.[54,55] Fluid levels, internal debris, and septations, if present, are well visualized on MR imaging. After contrast administration, heterogeneous delayed enhancement, predominantly within the septations, is seen (**Fig. 13**).[76] The mass is hypointense to normal liver parenchyma on the hepatocyte phase.[21] MR imaging is preferred for planning tumor resection and detecting vascular invasion, biliary tree involvement, and local lymph node spread.[54]

Biopsy is needed for a definitive diagnosis.[54] Treatment includes complete surgical resection, with neoadjuvant chemotherapy making this possibility more likely.[54,74] However, 25% to 50% of

tumors are resistant to chemotherapy; in these cases, treatment with total liver resection and transplantation is indicated.[54,77] UES previously had an extremely poor prognosis (mean survival 12 months), but multimodality therapy with surgery and chemotherapy has led to improved survival (10 of 17 patients surviving 2.4–20.0 years after diagnosis in one study).[54,78]

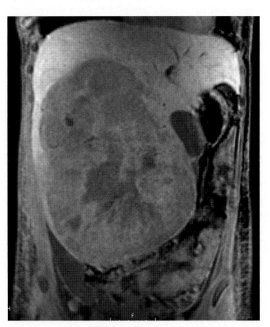

Fig. 13. Undifferentiated embryonal sarcoma in a 12-year-old girl with abdominal pain and mass palpated by pediatrician. Coronal, fat-suppressed, T1-weighted, postcontrast, MR image using a traditional blood pool contrast agent shows heterogeneous relative hypoenhancement of a very large, partly exophytic right lobe mass. (*Courtesy of* Ethan A. Smith, MD, Section of Pediatric Radiology, Department of Radiology, C. S. Mott Children's Hospital, University of Michigan, Ann Arbor, MI.)

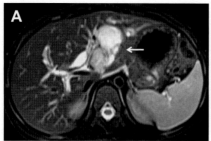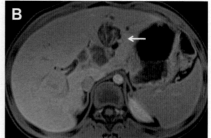

Fig. 14. Embryonal rhabdomyosarcoma in a 5-year-old boy with jaundice, abdominal pain, and itching. (*A*) Axial, fat-suppressed, T2-weighted, MR image demonstrates a hyperintense periportal and left lobe mass (*arrow*), likely within the biliary system. (*B*) Axial, fat-suppressed, postcontrast (gadoxetate disodium), T1-weighted image in the hepatocyte phase reveals hypoenhancement of the mass (*arrows*) with scattered internal septa that feature enhancement equal to adjacent liver. Mildly dilated, obstructed bile ducts are noted in both hepatic lobes.

Embryonal Rhabdomyosarcoma

Rhabdomyosarcoma is the most common soft tissue malignancy in pediatric patients.[54] A highly aggressive malignant neoplasm, it arises in the soft tissues of the body, including muscles, tendons, and connective tissues. It accounts for 3% of pediatric malignancies.[16] Embryonal rhabdomyosarcoma (ERMS), the most common subtype of rhabdomyosarcoma, accounts for 80% of cases and very rarely arises in the smooth muscle of the biliary tree.[54] Hepatic ERS comprises 1% of pediatric liver tumors.[54] Patients present with jaundice, abdominal distention, fever, hepatomegaly, nausea, and vomiting.[54] Laboratory analysis demonstrates elevated conjugated bilirubin, elevated alkaline phosphatase, and normal serum AFP.[54]

Typically diagnosed in children less than 5 years of age, ERS is a large tumor[54,79,80] with grapelike projections into the biliary duct lumen.[74] On MR imaging, this tumor is typically is T1-weighted hypointense and T2-weighted hyperintense often with associated obstructive biliary dilatation (**Fig. 14**).[54,80,81] A partially cystic obstructing lesion in the common bile duct and a mass adjacent to the duct causing mural irregularity can be seen on MR cholangiopancreatography (**Fig. 15**).[54,80,82]

Treatment includes a combination of surgical resection, radiation therapy, and chemotherapy, which result in a 5-year survival rate of 78% in cases with localized disease.[54,78,83] However, prognosis in the setting of metastatic disease remains extremely guarded (0% in one study).[83]

Malignant Rhabdoid Tumor

Malignant rhabdoid tumor (MRT) is an extremely rare but highly aggressive tumor that can arise in the central nervous system, kidneys, and soft tissues of children.[84] The lesion is related to the

atypical teratoid rhabdoid tumor of the central nervous system, most commonly found in the posterior fossa of the same age group.[85] MRTs present in children less than 2 years of age, with no gender preference.[84]

These lesions demonstrate impeded diffusion on diffusion-weighted MR imaging, a finding typical of highly cellular neoplasms. Although data are limited because of the rarity of the lesion, trends have shown MRT is heterogeneous, predominantly T2-weighted hyperintense, T1-weighted isointense to hypointense, and enhances following intravenous contrast material administration (**Fig. 16**). The presence of diffusion restriction may be helpful for distinguishing MRT from other hepatic masses, especially in the appropriate pediatric age group.[86,87]

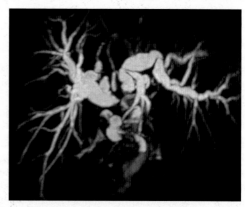

Fig. 15. Embryonal rhabdomyosarcoma in a 23-month-old boy with hyperbilirubinemia. Coronal, 3-dimensional, maximum-intensity-projection MRCP image shows high-grade biliary obstruction with filling defects in the extrahepatic biliary tree caused by tumor. (*Courtesy of* Jonathan R. Dillman, MD, Section of Pediatric Radiology, Department of Radiology, C. S. Mott Children's Hospital, University of Michigan, Ann Arbor, MI.)

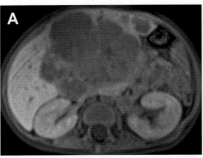
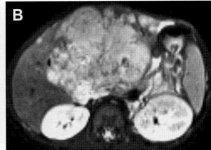

Fig. 16. Malignant rhabdoid tumor in an 11-month-old boy with a palpable abdominal mass. (*A*) Axial, fat-suppressed, delayed postcontrast (gadoxetate disodium), T1-weighted image in the 20-minute hepatocyte phase reveals a lobular left liver mass with hypoenhancement relative to adjacent liver. Mass was also hypoenhancing on all other postcontrast phases (not shown). (*B*) Diffusion-weighted MR image (b0) shows heterogeneous high signal intensity within the mass, which persisted on b500 and b1000 sequences (not shown) because of high cellularity within the mass.

No effective treatment regimen has been documented. So far, MRT has been shown to be very resistant to chemotherapy and radiation.[55,84,88] However, multimodal therapy consisting of ifosfamide, vincristine, and actinomycin may be of some benefit.[55] MRTs have an abysmal prognosis even with aggressive treatment because the reported mortality rate is 89%, with a mean survival of 15.3 weeks after diagnosis.[84] Younger age at diagnosis correlates with more advanced disease at the time of diagnosis and portends worse outcomes.[85]

Metastases

Metastatic lesions in the liver can occur in pediatric patients with hepatic and nonhepatic primary malignancies, most commonly Wilms tumor, neuroblastoma, and lymphoma.[21] Additionally, primary hepatic and biliary neoplasms can spread throughout the liver. The signal and enhancement characteristics of metastases depend on the primary tumor and whether it is hypovascular or hypervascular. In general, hypovascular metastases are mildly T2-weighted hyperintense and hypointense after intravenous contrast material injection on all phases (**Fig. 17**), whereas hypervascular metastases show arterial enhancement with rapid wash out and may appear hypointense on subsequent postcontrast phases (**Fig. 18**).[21,29] Lesional restricted diffusion on diffusion-weighted imaging and decreased apparent diffusion coefficient values correspond with high cellular density in the lesion.[89] Diffusion-weighted imaging may also be useful for detecting small hepatic metastases not seen on other pulse sequences. The treatment and prognosis of hepatic metastases depend on the histopathology and extent of neoplastic spread.

SUMMARY

MR imaging offers several advantages to CT and US when imaging benign and malignant pediatric hepatic tumors. Soft tissue characterization and

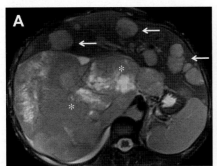
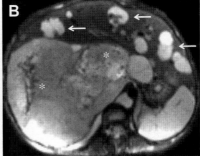

Fig. 17. Liver metastases in a 14-year-old girl with Wilms tumor. (*A*) Axial, fat-suppressed, T2-weighted, MR image shows multiple mildly hyperintense masses in the liver (*arrows*), which has been displaced anteromedially by a large heterogeneous right renal mass (*asterisks*). (*B*) Diffusion-weighted MR image reveals high signal intensity in the metastatic masses caused by dense cellularity (*arrows*). *Asterisks* denote primary right renal mass.

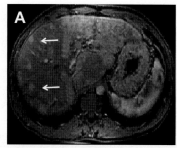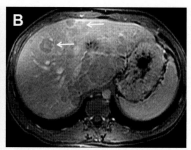

Fig. 18. Metastases in a 16-year-old boy with gastrinoma and Zollinger-Ellison syndrome. Axial, fat-suppressed, T1-weighted images demonstrate (*A*) arterial hyperenhancement with (*B*) wash out on venous-phase imaging after administration of traditional blood pool contrast agent within multiple hepatic lesions (*arrows*). Lesions were hyperintense on T2-weighted imaging (not shown). Also present is marked gastric fold thickening on all images from hypergastrinemia. (*Courtesy of* Jonathan R. Dillman, MD, Section of Pediatric Radiology, Department of Radiology, C. S. Mott Children's Hospital, University of Michigan, Ann Arbor, MI.)

the lack of ionizing radiation are two of its strongest characteristics. Although an exact diagnosis may not be achievable with every patient, MR imaging is a powerful tool that can offer a focused differential and help facilitate the choice of which lesions to biopsy or resect. The recent addition of HSAs further strengthens radiologists' capability to provide referring clinicians with focused and specific information.

What the referring physician needs to know
- MR imaging is a highly useful imaging modality for characterizing benign and malignant pediatric hepatic lesions
- MR imaging does not produce ionizing radiation (unlike CT), likely facilitating patient safety.
- MR imaging may not provide an exact radiologic diagnosis in every circumstance; but a focused differential diagnosis should be achievable, thereby guiding appropriate patient medical and surgical management.
- HSAs can help further characterize pediatric liver lesions, which were previously indeterminate.

REFERENCES

1. Jha P, Chawla SC, Tavri S, et al. Pediatric liver tumors–a pictorial review. Eur Radiol 2009;19(1): 209–19.
2. Soudack M, Shechter A, Malkin L, et al. Inflammatory pseudotumor of the liver: sonographic and computed tomographic features with complete regression. J Ultrasound Med 2000;19(7):501–4.
3. Bruckner AL, Frieden IJ. Hemangiomas of infancy. J Am Acad Dermatol 2003;48(4):477–93 [quiz: 494–6].
4. Koplewitz BZ, Springer C, Slasky BS, et al. CT of hemangiomas of the upper airways in children. AJR Am J Roentgenol 2005;184(2):663–70.
5. Restrepo R, Palani R, Cervantes LF, et al. Hemangiomas revisited: the useful, the unusual and the new. Part 1: overview and clinical and imaging characteristics. Pediatr Radiol 2011;41(7): 895–904.
6. Margileth AM, Museles M. Current concepts in diagnosis and management of congenital cutaneous hemangiomas. Pediatrics 1965;36(3):410–6.
7. Lo K, Mihm M, Fay A. Current theories on the pathogenesis of infantile hemangioma. Semin Ophthalmol 2009;24(3):172–7.
8. Khan ZA, Boscolo E, Picard A, et al. Multipotential stem cells recapitulate human infantile hemangioma in immunodeficient mice. J Clin Invest 2008; 118(7):2592–9.
9. Lowe LH, Marchant TC, Rivard DC, et al. Vascular malformations: classification and terminology the radiologist needs to know. Semin Roentgenol 2012;47(2):106–17.
10. Kassarjian A, Zurakowski D, Dubois J, et al. Infantile hepatic hemangiomas: clinical and imaging findings and their correlation with therapy. AJR Am J Roentgenol 2004;182(3):785–95.
11. Mulliken JB, Glowacki J. Hemangiomas and vascular malformations in infants and children: a classification based on endothelial characteristics. Plast Reconstr Surg 1982;69(3):412–22.
12. North PE, Waner M, Mizeracki A, et al. GLUT1: a newly discovered immunohistochemical marker for juvenile hemangiomas. Hum Pathol 2000; 31(1):11–22.
13. Nozaki T, Nosaka S, Miyazaki O, et al. Syndromes associated with vascular tumors and malformations: a pictorial review. Radiographics 2013; 33(1):175–95.
14. Van Aalst JA, Bhuller A, Sadove AM. Pediatric vascular lesions. J Craniofac Surg 2003;14(4): 566–83.
15. Hassanein AH, Mulliken JB, Fishman SJ, et al. Evaluation of terminology for vascular anomalies

in current literature. Plast Reconstr Surg 2011; 127(1):347–51.

16. Moore CW, Lowe LH. Hepatic tumors and tumor-like conditions. In: Slovis TL, editor. Caffey's pediatric radiology. 11th edition. Philadelphia: Mosby; 2008. p. 1929–43.

17. Christison-Lagay ER, Burrows PE, Alomari A, et al. Hepatic hemangiomas: subtype classification and development of a clinical practice algorithm and registry. J Pediatr Surg 2007;42(1):62–7 [discussion: 67–8].

18. Ishak KG, Goodman ZD, Stocker JT. Benign mesenchymal tumors and pseudotumors. In: Rosai J, Sobin L, editors. Atlas of tumor pathology: tumors of the liver and intrahepatic ducts. Washington, DC: Armed Forces Institute of Pathology; 2001. p. 71–157.

19. Rivard DC, Lowe LH. Radiological reasoning: multiple hepatic masses in an infant. AJR Am J Roentgenol 2008;190(Suppl 6):S46–52.

20. Courtier JL, Perito ER, Rhee S, et al. Targeted MRI contrast agents for pediatric hepatobiliary disease. J Pediatr Gastroenterol Nutr 2012;54(4):454–62.

21. Meyers AB, Towbin AJ, Serai S, et al. Characterization of pediatric liver lesions with gadoxetate disodium. Pediatr Radiol 2011;41(9):1183–97.

22. Ringe KI, Husarik DB, Sirlin CB, et al. Gadoxetate disodium-enhanced MRI of the liver: part 1, protocol optimization and lesion appearance in the noncirrhotic liver. AJR Am J Roentgenol 2010;195(1): 13–28.

23. Keslar PJ, Buck JL, Selby DM. From the archives of the AFIP. Infantile hemangioendothelioma of the liver revisited. Radiographics 1993;13(3):657–70.

24. Legiehn GM, Heran MK. Venous malformations: classification, development, diagnosis, and interventional radiologic management. Radiol Clin North Am 2008;46(3):545–97, vi.

25. Konez O, Burrows PE, Mulliken JB, et al. Angiographic features of rapidly involuting congenital hemangioma (RICH). Pediatr Radiol 2003;33(1): 15–9.

26. Denoyelle F, Leboulanger N, Enjolras O, et al. Role of propranolol in the therapeutic strategy of infantile laryngotracheal hemangioma. Int J Pediatr Otorhinolaryngol 2009;73(8):1168–72.

27. Adeyiga AO, Lee EY, Eisenberg RL. Focal hepatic masses in pediatric patients. AJR Am J Roentgenol 2012;199(4):W422–40.

28. Stocker JT, Ishak KG. Mesenchymal hamartoma of the liver: report of 30 cases and review of the literature. Pediatr Pathol 1983;1(3):245–67.

29. Duigenan S, Anupindi SA, Nimkin K. Imaging of multifocal hepatic lesions in pediatric patients. Pediatr Radiol 2012;42(10):1155–68 [quiz: 1285].

30. Ros PR, Goodman ZD, Ishak KG, et al. Mesenchymal hamartoma of the liver: radiologic-pathologic correlation. Radiology 1986;158(3): 619–24.

31. Powers C, Ros PR, Stoupis C, et al. Primary liver neoplasms: MR imaging with pathologic correlation. Radiographics 1994;14(3):459–82.

32. Mortele KJ, Ros PR. Benign liver neoplasms. Clin Liver Dis 2002;6(1):119–45.

33. Mortele KJ, Vanzieleghem B, Mortele B, et al. Solitary hepatic infantile hemangioendothelioma: dynamic gadolinium-enhanced MR imaging findings. Eur Radiol 2002;12(4):862–5.

34. Gow KW, Lee L, Pruthi S, et al. Mesenchymal hamartoma of the liver. J Pediatr Surg 2009;44(2): 468–70.

35. Chung EM, Cube R, Lewis RB, et al. From the archives of the AFIP: pediatric liver masses: radiologic-pathologic correlation part 1. Benign tumors. Radiographics 2010;30(3):801–26.

36. Hsee LC, McCall JL, Koea JB. Focal nodular hyperplasia: what are the indications for resection? HPB (Oxford) 2005;7(4):298–302.

37. Towbin AJ, Luo GG, Yin H, et al. Focal nodular hyperplasia in children, adolescents, and young adults. Pediatr Radiol 2011;41(3):341–9.

38. Battal B, Kocaoglu M, Akgun V, et al. Diffusion-weighted imaging in the characterization of focal liver lesions: efficacy of visual assessment. J Comput Assist Tomogr 2011;35(3):326–31.

39. Reshamwala PA, Kleiner DE, Heller T. Nodular regenerative hyperplasia: not all nodules are created equal. Hepatology 2006;44(1):7–14.

40. Al-Mukhaizeem KA, Rosenberg A, Sherker AH. Nodular regenerative hyperplasia of the liver: an under-recognized cause of portal hypertension in hematological disorders. Am J Hematol 2004; 75(4):225–30.

41. Hartleb M, Gutkowski K, Milkiewicz P. Nodular regenerative hyperplasia: evolving concepts on underdiagnosed cause of portal hypertension. World J Gastroenterol 2011;17(11):1400–9.

42. Katabathina VS, Menias CO, Shanbhogue AK, et al. Genetics and imaging of hepatocellular adenomas: 2011 update. Radiographics 2011;31(6): 1529–43.

43. Siegel MJ, Chung EM, Conran RM. Pediatric liver: focal masses. Magn Reson Imaging Clin N Am 2008;16(3):437–52, v.

44. Farges O, Dokmak S. Malignant transformation of liver adenoma: an analysis of the literature. Dig Surg 2010;27(1):32–8.

45. Brancatelli G, Federle MP, Vullierme MP, et al. CT and MR imaging evaluation of hepatic adenoma. J Comput Assist Tomogr 2006;30(5):745–50.

46. Grazioli L, Federle MP, Brancatelli G, et al. Hepatic adenomas: imaging and pathologic findings. Radiographics 2001;21(4):877–92 [discussion: 892–4].

47. Hussain SM, van den Bos IC, Dwarkasing RS, et al. Hepatocellular adenoma: findings at state-of-the-art magnetic resonance imaging, ultrasound, computed tomography and pathologic analysis. Eur Radiol 2006;16(9):1873–86.

48. Arrive L, Flejou JF, Vilgrain V, et al. Hepatic adenoma: MR findings in 51 pathologically proved lesions. Radiology 1994;193(2):507–12.

49. Fukuya T, Honda H, Matsumata T, et al. Diagnosis of inflammatory pseudotumor of the liver: value of CT. AJR Am J Roentgenol 1994;163(5):1087–91.

50. Venkataraman S, Semelka RC, Braga L, et al. Inflammatory myofibroblastic tumor of the hepatobiliary system: report of MR imaging appearance in four patients. Radiology 2003;227(3):758–63.

51. Tublin ME, Moser AJ, Marsh JW, et al. Biliary inflammatory pseudotumor: imaging features in seven patients. AJR Am J Roentgenol 2007; 188(1):W44–8.

52. Jeong JY, Sohn JH, Kim TY, et al. Hepatic inflammatory pseudotumor misinterpreted as hepatocellular carcinoma. Clin Mol Hepatol 2012;18(2): 239–44.

53. Kamaya A, Maturen KE, Tye GA, et al. Hypervascular liver lesions. Semin Ultrasound CT MR 2009; 30(5):387–407.

54. Chung EM, Lattin GE Jr, Cube R, et al. From the archives of the AFIP: pediatric liver masses: radiologic-pathologic correlation. Part 2. Malignant tumors. Radiographics 2011;31(2):483–507.

55. Meyers RL. Tumors of the liver in children. Surg Oncol 2007;16(3):195–203.

56. Woodward PJ, Sohaey R, Kennedy A, et al. From the archives of the AFIP: a comprehensive review of fetal tumors with pathologic correlation. Radiographics 2005;25(1):215–42.

57. Dachman AH, Pakter RL, Ros PR, et al. Hepatoblastoma: radiologic-pathologic correlation in 50 cases. Radiology 1987;164(1):15–9.

58. Helmberger TK, Ros PR, Mergo PJ, et al. Pediatric liver neoplasms: a radiologic-pathologic correlation. Eur Radiol 1999;9(7):1339–47.

59. Yu SB, Kim HY, Eo H, et al. Clinical characteristics and prognosis of pediatric hepatocellular carcinoma. World J Surg 2006;30(1):43–50.

60. Stocker JT. Hepatic tumors in children. Clin Liver Dis 2001;5(1):259–81, viii–ix.

61. Meyers AB, Towbin AJ, Geller JI, et al. Hepatoblastoma imaging with gadoxetate disodium-enhanced MRI–typical, atypical, pre- and post-treatment evaluation. Pediatr Radiol 2012;42(7):859–66.

62. Roebuck DJ, Aronson D, Clapuyt P, et al. 2005 PRETEXT: a revised staging system for primary malignant liver tumours of childhood developed by the SIOPEL group. Pediatr Radiol 2007;37(2): 123–32 [quiz: 249–50].

63. Ebara M, Fukuda H, Hatano R, et al. Relationship between copper, zinc and metallothionein in hepatocellular carcinoma and its surrounding liver parenchyma. J Hepatol 2000;33(3):415–22.

64. Matsuzaki K, Sano N, Hashiguchi N, et al. Influence of copper on MRI of hepatocellular carcinoma. J Magn Reson Imaging 1997;7(3):478–81.

65. Levy AD. Malignant liver tumors. Clin Liver Dis 2002;6(1):147–64.

66. Goodwin MD, Dobson JE, Sirlin CB, et al. Diagnostic challenges and pitfalls in MR imaging with hepatocyte-specific contrast agents. Radiographics 2011;31(6):1547–68.

67. Czauderna P, Mackinlay G, Perilongo G, et al. Hepatocellular carcinoma in children: results of the first prospective study of the International Society of Pediatric Oncology group. J Clin Oncol 2002; 20(12):2798–804.

68. Malogolowkin MH, Stanley P, Steele DA, et al. Feasibility and toxicity of chemoembolization for children with liver tumors. J Clin Oncol 2000; 18(6):1279–84.

69. Saab S, Yao F. Fibrolamellar hepatocellular carcinoma. Case reports and a review of the literature. Dig Dis Sci 1996;41(10):1981–5.

70. McLarney JK, Rucker PT, Bender GN, et al. Fibrolamellar carcinoma of the liver: radiologic-pathologic correlation. Radiographics 1999;19(2):453–71.

71. Liu S, Chan KW, Wang B, et al. Fibrolamellar hepatocellular carcinoma. Am J Gastroenterol 2009; 104(10):2617–24 [quiz: 2625].

72. Gourgiotis S, Moustafellos P, Germanos S. Undifferentiated embryonal sarcoma of the liver in adult. Surgery 2008;143(4):568–9.

73. Lack EE, Schloo BL, Azumi N, et al. Undifferentiated (embryonal) sarcoma of the liver. Clinical and pathologic study of 16 cases with emphasis on immunohistochemical features. Am J Surg Pathol 1991;15(1):1–16.

74. Stocker JT, Ishak KG. Undifferentiated (embryonal) sarcoma of the liver: report of 31 cases. Cancer 1978;42(1):336–48.

75. Yoon W, Kim JK, Kang HK. Hepatic undifferentiated embryonal sarcoma: MR findings. J Comput Assist Tomogr 1997;21(1):100–2.

76. Psatha EA, Semelka RC, Fordham L, et al. Undifferentiated (embryonal) sarcoma of the liver (USL): MRI findings including dynamic gadolinium enhancement. Magn Reson Imaging 2004;22(6): 897–900.

77. Okajima H, Ohya Y, Lee KJ, et al. Management of undifferentiated sarcoma of the liver including living donor liver transplantation as a backup procedure. J Pediatr Surg 2009;44(2):e33–8.

78. Bisogno G, Pilz T, Perilongo G, et al. Undifferentiated sarcoma of the liver in childhood: a curable disease. Cancer 2002;94(1):252–7.

79. Donnelly LF, Bisset GS 3rd, Frush DP. Diagnosis please. Case 2: embryonal rhabdomyosarcoma of the biliary tree. Radiology 1998;208(3):621–3.

80. Roebuck DJ, Yang WT, Lam WW, et al. Hepatobiliary rhabdomyosarcoma in children: diagnostic radiology. Pediatr Radiol 1998;28(2):101–8.

81. Nemade B, Talapatra K, Shet T, et al. Embryonal rhabdomyosarcoma of the biliary tree mimicking a choledochal cyst. J Cancer Res Ther 2007;3(1): 40–2.

82. Kitagawa N, Aida N. Biliary rhabdomyosarcoma. Pediatr Radiol 2007;37(10):1059.

83. Spunt SL, Lobe TE, Pappo AS, et al. Aggressive surgery is unwarranted for biliary tract rhabdomyosarcoma. J Pediatr Surg 2000;35(2):309–16.

84. Marzano E, Lermite E, Nobili C, et al. Malignant rhabdoid tumour of the liver in the young adult: report of first two cases. HPB Surg 2009;2009: 628206.

85. Morgenstern DA, Gibson S, Brown T, et al. Clinical and pathological features of paediatric malignant rhabdoid tumours. Pediatr Blood Cancer 2010; 54(1):29–34.

86. Abdullah A, Patel Y, Lewis TJ, et al. Extrarenal malignant rhabdoid tumors: radiologic findings with histopathologic correlation. Cancer Imaging 2010; 10:97–101.

87. Garces-Inigo EF, Leung R, Sebire NJ, et al. Extrarenal rhabdoid tumours outside the central nervous system in infancy. Pediatr Radiol 2009; 39(8):817–22.

88. Howman-Giles R, McCowage G, Kellie S, et al. Extrarenal malignant rhabdoid tumor in childhood application of 18F-FDG PET/CT. J Pediatr Hematol Oncol 2012;34(1):17–21.

89. Koh DM, Collins DJ. Diffusion-weighted MRI in the body: applications and challenges in oncology. AJR Am J Roentgenol 2007;188(6):1622–35.

Magnetic Resonance Imaging of the Pediatric Liver
Imaging of Steatosis, Iron Deposition, and Fibrosis

Alexander J. Towbin, MD*, Suraj D. Serai, PhD,
Daniel J. Podberesky, MD

KEYWORDS

- Liver • Fat fractionation • Hepatic fat quantification • Liver iron quantification • MR elastography

KEY POINTS

- Liver biopsy is considered the gold standard for quantifying hepatic fat content, hepatic iron content, and degree of hepatic fibrosis; however, it is limited by small sample size, risk of complication, subjectivity in interpretation, and poor patient acceptance.
- Hepatic fat quantification can be determined by multiple MR imaging methods. MR spectroscopy is considered the most accurate but other methods are used more commonly because of their ease of use.
- There are two general strategies for determining liver iron content by MR imaging: signal intensity ratio and relaxometry.
- MR elastography is an emerging technique that uses a shear wave to determine the stiffness of the liver parenchyma and quantify fibrosis.

Over the past decade, there have been numerous advances in MR imaging techniques used to image the liver. In the past, MR imaging assessment of the liver relied primarily on noncontrast T1- and T2-weighted images along with dynamic postcontrast sequences to characterize the liver parenchyma and underlying lesions. Although these sequences can offer the radiologist a morphologic assessment of the liver, they are not able to provide the functional data required to diagnose and manage diffuse hepatic disease as they present in their earliest, and potentially reversible, stages. This article provides an overview of modern pediatric liver imaging techniques, including methods used for hepatic fat quantification, hepatic iron quantification, and detection of hepatic fibrosis.

PATIENT PREPARATION AND IMAGING

There are several unique considerations when preparing to image pediatric patients. The first step of any pediatric imaging procedure is describing what will happen in an age-appropriate manner to the patient and his or her family. Child life specialists can be instrumental in this task, explaining

Funding Sources: None.
Conflict of Interest: Amirsys royalties, Merge Healthcare, shareholder (A.J. Towbin); None (S.D. Serai); Toshiba America Medical System, Professional Speaker Bureau member; General Electric Healthcare, Travel reimbursement; Philips Healthcare, Travel Reimbursement; Amirsys, royalties (D.J. Podberesky).
Department of Radiology, Cincinnati Children's Hospital Medical Center, 3333 Burnet Avenue, Cincinnati, OH 45229, USA
* Corresponding author.
E-mail address: Alexander.towbin@cchmc.org

Magn Reson Imaging Clin N Am 21 (2013) 669–680
http://dx.doi.org/10.1016/j.mric.2013.05.001

the procedure through play or demonstration. MR imaging is an ideal procedure for demonstration because the long scan times, relatively small scanner bore, and loud noises make it a difficult study for children to undergo without preparation. Mock scanners (scale or full-size models of the clinical scanners) have been used to prepare children for the experience of undergoing MR imaging.[1–6]

Simulation is another method used to prepare older children for an examination and is a key component of preparing patients for MR elastography (MRE). Before the examination, child life specialists show and allow the child to touch the passive driver, explain what the child will feel during scanning, and then place the vibrating passive driver on the child. The prescan simulation helps prepare patients for the sensation they will feel during scanning and helps to reduce patient anxiety and sudden movements at the start of the actual MRE sequence.[7]

Immobilization is important to obtain high-quality imaging. There are several techniques used to help children remain still. At the authors' institution, general anesthesia is used for most children younger than 3 years of age, whereas conscious sedation is used for most children between the ages of 3 and 6. In these young patients, conscious sedation or anesthesia helps to ensure cooperation and allows for controlled breathing while at the same time minimizing fear and anxiety. Distraction is the primary technique used to help older children and adolescents remain still during imaging. Video goggles allow patients to watch a television show or movie of their choice while they are being imaged.[8] Music can be listened to in lieu of video if the patient prefers.

Obtaining intravenous access can be difficult in children. Fortunately, the standard protocol for many of the functional imaging techniques of the liver does not require intravenous access. Typically, adult hepatobiliary imaging is performed after an overnight fast. In children who are not sedated, the authors ask that they take nothing by mouth for at least 4 hours before imaging.[7] This helps to minimize artifacts from bowel peristalsis and ensures a full gallbladder.[9]

During MR imaging, there are several factors that are modified for pediatric patients. The specific absorption rate is automatically maintained within acceptable limits by the scanner based on the patient's weight.[7] In addition, the scan field of view is set to a value depending on the size of the patient. Coils are also selected based on the size of the patient and the scanner. For most children, a cardiac coil is used for abdominal imaging. For larger patients, a torso coil can be used.[10]

HEPATIC FAT QUANTIFICATION

Hepatic fat quantification is most commonly used in the setting of nonalcoholic fatty liver disease (NAFLD). NAFLD is the most common cause of chronic liver disease in children, occurring with a prevalence of 8% to 9.6% of the general pediatric population.[11] It is more common in older children; obese children; males; and children of Hispanic, Asian, or caucasian descent.[11] Children typically present with protean symptoms including vague abdominal pain, irritability, fatigue, headache, and difficulty concentrating.[11] On physical examination, many patients are obese and may also have hypertension, hepatomegaly, and acanthosis nigricans.[11] Laboratory-based biomarkers of NAFLD include insulin sensitivity and elevated serum leptin.[11] In addition to these biomarkers liver enzymes may be elevated.

Pathologically, NAFLD is a general term encompassing a broad spectrum of disease ranging from steatosis, to steatohepatitis, fibrosis, and cirrhosis. Traditionally, NAFLD has been diagnosed by liver biopsy. Although biopsy is able to distinguish NAFLD from nonalcoholic steatohepatitis and other causes of fatty liver infiltration, it is an invasive procedure with inherent risks and potential complications. The rate of complications can vary depending on the operator and the type of biopsy procedure. Prior studies have shown that 1% to 3% of patients undergoing liver biopsy require subsequent hospitalization.[12,13] Other limitations of liver biopsy include its potential for sampling error, subjective interpretation/grading systems, and high amount of interobserver variation.[14,15] Ultimately, the limitations of liver biopsy along with its poor patient acceptance make it suboptimal for serial assessment of liver disease.

MR imaging–based hepatic fat quantification offers several advantages over biopsy and pathologic assessment. These advantages include its reproducibility, low degree of variability in interpretation, the ability to perform quantitative and qualitative assessment of hepatic fat, and its ability to assess the entire liver.[14] Perhaps the greatest advantage of imaging-based hepatic fat quantification is its noninvasive nature (**Box 1**).

Technique

MR imaging fat quantification can be performed using either MR spectroscopy or chemical shift imaging. MR spectroscopy is generally considered the gold standard for in vivo fat quantification because it is the most direct MR imaging method to separate liver signal into its water and fat components.[16,17] MR spectroscopy has several advantages when compared with chemical shift

> **Box 1**
> **Advantages of functional MR imaging compared with liver biopsy**
>
> - Noninvasive
> - Reproducible
> - Objective measure
> - Low degree of variability
> - Ability to assess entire liver
> - Ability to evaluate extrahepatic complications

imaging. First, it has a wide dynamic range allowing for quantification of any range of fat (0%–100%).[14,17] Because MR spectroscopy is very sensitive, it is able to detect subtle changes in hepatic triglyceride content during treatment.[14] The high sensitivity does not come at the cost of specificity. MR spectroscopy, unlike chemical shift imaging, is not susceptible to confounding effects from fibrosis, iron overload, or glycogen. Finally, MR spectroscopy is the only noninvasive method that is able to detect a necroinflammatory response.[14]

Even though there are many advantages of MR spectroscopy, it is not widely used in clinical practice. Spectral analysis methods are complex and require commercial postprocessing software to analyze the raw data.[14] This complexity can lead to variability in the results. In addition, the results can also vary depending on the MR imaging scanner, acquisition parameters, and method of analysis.[14] This potential lack of reproducibility makes it difficult for hospitals with multiple MR imaging scanners, possibly from different manufacturers, to reliably track hepatic fat content over time.

Because of its ease of performance and rapid acquisition, chemical shift imaging has become the preferred method of performing hepatic fat quantification. There are several methods that can be used to perform chemical shift imaging, although each method relies on the difference between the precession frequencies of fat and water protons to quantify hepatic fat content.[14] The frequency difference causes tissue voxels containing fat and water to lose signal in out-of-phase imaging. This signal loss can be compared with in-phase imaging, and the difference in signal is used to quantify the fat content.

The use of spin echo sequences for chemical shift imaging was first described in 1984.[18] In this technique, termed the Dixon method, a modified dual echo spin echo sequence was designed such that the first echo image is acquired when water and fat are in-phase with each other and the next echo image is acquired with water and fat in opposed-phase. For a voxel containing only water or fat, its net signal is the same on in-phase and opposed-phase acquisitions, because one component's signal is zero. In contrast, a voxel containing water and fat has different signals from the two acquisitions. Using this information, the in-phase and opposed-phase images are then added or subtracted to generate a water-only image and a fat-only image.[14] A quantitative fat-fraction value can be calculated from the generated water-only and fat-only images by taking a ratio of fat versus water and fat.[13]

This approach, termed the two-point Dixon method, is limited by its long acquisition times and sensitivity to magnetic field inhomogeneity.[14] To overcome the sensitivity to magnetic field inhomogeneity, a three-point Dixon method was developed, adding a third echo series of images to correct for the phase shifts that occurred between

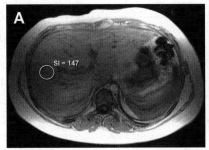
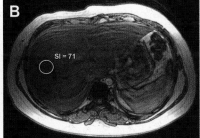

Fig. 1. A 14-year-old boy with obesity, type 2 diabetes mellitus, and elevated liver enzymes. (*A*) Axial in-phase image of the liver shows a normal contour of the liver. The liver has a signal intensity measurement (SI) of 147 within the region of interest (*circle*). (*B*) Axial opposed-phase image of the upper abdomen shows that the liver has a signal intensity (SI) of 71 within the region of interest (*circle*). Using the above signal intensities and the formula $\eta = (100\% * [SI_{In\text{-}phase} - SI_{Opposed\text{-}phase}]/[2* SI_{In\text{-}phase}])$, the fat fraction was calculated to be 26%. Subsequent liver biopsy showed steatohepatitis with fat in 80% of lobules.

Table 1
Protocol for proton density hepatic fat fractionation at 1.5T

Sequence	Plane	Approximate Scan Time (s)	TR (ms)	TE (ms)	Slice Thickness (mm)	Matrix Size
Opposed-phase	Axial	20 (total for both sequences)	7	2.2	3	320 × 192
In-phase	Axial	20 (total for both sequences)	7	4.4	3	320 × 192

echoes.[14,19–22] Although this technique allowed the images to be corrected for field inhomogeneity, scan acquisition times remained long. The introduction of fast gradient echo sequences led to a modified Dixon technique.[23–25] This method significantly reduces scan time to the point where both phases can be performed in a single breathhold.[14]

The modified Dixon technique using gradient recalled echo (GRE) images is widely used because of its simplicity; however, it has several limitations.[26] The dynamic range for the detection of fat is somewhat limited, ranging between 10% and 50%.[14,17] In addition, in patients with increased liver iron content (cirrhosis, hemochromatosis), the increased iron has a paramagnetic effect causing local field inhomogeneity and signal loss from T2* relaxation.[14] It is thus essential to make every effort to keep the TEs as short as possible to minimize the effects of T2* signal loss.

Complex chemical shift-based approaches, such as the iterative decomposition of water and fat with echo asymmetry and least-squares estimation technique, collect three images to separate fat and water signal.[27] Iterative decomposition of water and fat with echo asymmetry and least-squares estimation provides uniform and reliable fat suppression with rapid image acquisition times.[27] The addition of the third sequence helps account for field inhomogeneity and extends the range of fat quantification to 0% to 100%.[17]

Proton density fat fractionation has been developed to address the confounding factors that introduce error into fat quantification seen with other traditional techniques.[28] This method of hepatic fat quantification can be used on any MR imaging scanner, regardless of the vendor, and uses a spoiled gradient recalled echo sequence with the flip angle optimized to minimize T1 effects and multiple echoes to minimize T2* effects (**Fig. 1**).[28] With this technique, fat content can be measured throughout the entire dynamic range, 0% to 100% using the equation $\eta = (100\% * [SI_{\text{In-phase}} - SI_{\text{Opposed-phase}}]/[2* SI_{\text{In-phase}}])$ where η is the fat fraction, $SI_{\text{In-phase}}$ is the signal intensity of a region of interest from the liver on the in-phase images, and $SI_{\text{Opposed-phase}}$ is the signal

intensity of a region of interest from the liver on the opposed-phase images.[17] A recent study has shown that proton density fat fractionation significantly correlates with histologic steatosis grades.[28] For these reasons, the authors have decided to use proton density fat fractionation at their institution. An example protocol for pediatric fat fractionation is included in **Table 1** (**Box 2**).

HEPATIC IRON QUANTIFICATION

Hepatic iron overload is the abnormal and excessive intracellular accumulation of iron in liver cells.[29] Normally, excess iron is stored bound to the intracellular protein, ferritin. Increased and sustained systemic iron overwhelms the capacity of ferritin to collect and store iron, leading to accumulation of unbound iron in the cytoplasm of cells primarily in the liver, pancreas, spleen, and bone marrow.[29] This is problematic, because free intracellular iron can react with hydrogen and lipid-generating free radicals that cause cellular damage.[29] In the liver, this damage can lead to fibrosis and cirrhosis.

There are two basic mechanisms for iron overload: excess intestinal absorption or repeated blood transfusions.[29] Hereditary (primary) hemochromatosis is the characteristic disorder of iron overload caused by excess intestinal absorption. It is more common in whites and most prevalent in Ireland, where it affects up to 1 in 150 to 250

Box 2
Hepatic fat quantification key points

- Hepatic fat quantification is most commonly used for patients with NAFLD.
- MR spectroscopy is considered the imaging gold standard; however, it is a complex method and requires postprocessing software, limiting its general applicability.
- Because of its simplicity, chemical shift imaging has become the preferred method of performing hepatic fat quantification.
- There are multiple methods to determine the fat fraction using chemical shift imaging.

people.[30] Affected individuals are typically asymptomatic, particularly in early stages of the disease. If symptoms are present, they are vague and nonspecific and include weakness, lethargy, impotence, and arthralgias.[30] The disease is more commonly symptomatic in males, because females are protected by blood loss during menstruation. Patients typically present later in life, although presentation in infancy and childhood does occur.[31] In patients with hereditary hemochromatosis, iron deposition first occurs in the liver, heart, and pancreas.

Patients with syndromes that require repeated blood transfusions, such as thalassemia, are at risk to develop secondary hemochromatosis. Thalassemias are a group of hereditary blood

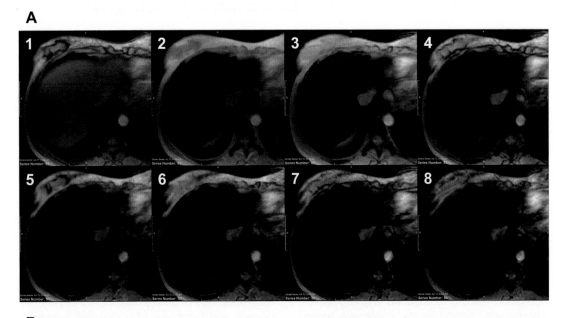

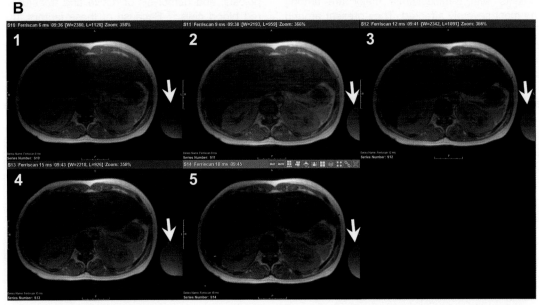

Fig. 2. (*A*) Eight successive echoes from a T2* weighted MR image of the liver in a 19-year-old woman with a history of sickle cell disease show progressive loss of signal in the liver with each echo. Using the R2* method, the liver iron concentration was determined to be 7300 μg/g. (*B*) Five successive echoes of the liver in the same patient show progressive loss of signal. Using the St. Pierre method, the liver iron content was determined to be 8100 μg/g. A proprietary phantom with a long T2 value is included in each image (*arrow*). (*C*) Report from Ferriscan showing the liver iron content for the images in (*B*). Note that the report is digitally modified to remove patient demographic information.

C

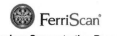

Liver Iron Concentration Report

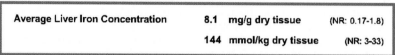

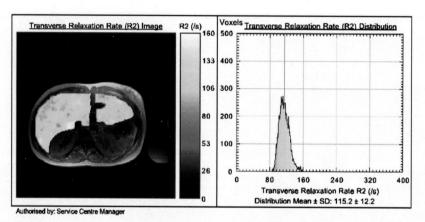

Fig. 2. (*continued*)

disorders caused by a defect in the genes that produce globin leading to impaired erythropoiesis.[32] Patients with β-thalassemia major are among the most severely affected. They present around 6 months of age with a severe microcytic hypochromatic anemia, irritability, poor growth, jaundice, hepatosplenomegaly, and high-output cardiac failure.[32] These patients are treated with repeated blood transfusions; however, the transfusional iron overload is exacerbated by increased intestinal iron absorption caused by tissue hypoxia, apoptosis of defective precursors of erythropoiesis, and hemolysis of native and transfused red blood cells.[29] Because of these factors, the iron overload can become severe in infancy or early childhood and lead to endocrine and cardiac dysfunction unless iron chelation therapy is provided.[29] As with other patients with secondary hemochromatosis, iron accumulates in the reticuloendothelial cells of the liver, spleen, bone

Table 2
Protocol for hepatic iron quantification

Sequence	Plane	Approximate Scan Time (s)	TR (ms)	TE (ms)	Slice Thickness (mm)	Matrix Size
T2*	Axial	20	180	Min (eight echoes)	8	256 × 224
St. Pierre method sequence 1	Axial	300 (total for five sequences)	1000	6	10	256 × 192
St. Pierre method sequence 2	Axial	300 (total for five sequences)	1000	9	10	256 × 192
St. Pierre method sequence 3	Axial	300 (total for five sequences)	1000	12	10	256 × 192
St. Pierre method sequence 4	Axial	300 (total for five sequences)	1000	15	10	256 × 192
St. Pierre method sequence 5	Axial	300 (total for five sequences)	1000	18	10	256 × 192

marrow, and lymph nodes.[29] Once the reticuloendothelial system is saturated, the iron begins to deposit in the hepatocytes themselves, and within the pancreas, myocardium, and endocrine glands.[29]

Technique

Liver iron quantification is an important technique used to help diagnose and manage patients with primary and secondary hemochromatosis. Although liver biopsy is the current gold standard for iron quantification, it shares the same limitations as liver biopsy for fat quantification and is not suitable for repeated measurements over time. Because of the limitations of biopsy, MR imaging has become the preferred method of determining liver iron content.

There are two main methods for determining liver iron content: signal intensity ratio and relaxometry.[29,33] The signal intensity ratio method compares the signal intensity of the liver on spin echo or gradient echo sequences with the signal intensity of a reference tissue that does not concentrate iron, such as skeletal muscle.[29] The most widely used method to determine the liver iron content by signal intensity ratio was developed by Gandon and colleagues.[34] In this method, five breathhold gradient echo sequences are obtained while the TE and flip angle are varied. On each series, the mean liver signal is obtained by drawing three regions of interest in the right lobe of the liver. The mean liver signal is compared with the mean muscle signal obtained by drawing a region of interest on the right and left paraspinal muscles. The mean liver signal intensity is then divided by the mean muscle signal intensity to give the liver/muscle ratio. Gandon and colleagues[35] have developed an online calculator to help estimate the liver iron content using the signal intensity values obtained from each region of interest on each sequence.

Gandon's method is in use throughout the world because of its simplicity, accuracy, and ability to be performed on any scanner.[33] However, there are limitations with this method. Perhaps the greatest limitation is that all of the sequences used to determine the liver iron content eventually saturate with very high iron content.[29,33] The maximum value that can be obtained using this method is 350 μmol/g. Values above this level are reported as greater than 350 μmol/g.[35] Another limitation is that biologic factors, such as steatosis or fatty infiltration of muscle, can change the mean signal intensity of liver and muscle. This is partially accounted for by fat saturation; however, fat saturation is often not homogeneous.[29] Finally, the technique requires several breathholds, which makes it difficult for younger children to complete.

Relaxometry methods for the assessment of liver iron content rely on decreases in the T2 relaxation times because of the paramagnetic properties of the iron in the liver.[33] In this approach, a series of spin echo or gradient echo images are obtained with increasing TE values. The signal intensity of the liver is then modeled across multiple TE values.[29] Depending on whether spin echo or gradient echo images are used, the signal decay constants T2 or T2* are calculated, respectively. Recent reports have favored using the reciprocal values of T2 or T2*, defined as R2 or R2*.[36–38] R2 or R2* values are preferred because they directly correlate with iron content; the larger the R2 or R2* value, the higher the iron content.[29]

R2 and R2* are not equivalent; each variable has theoretical advantages and disadvantages. R2 measurements are less sensitive to confounding factors, such as scanner, voxel size, magnetic inhomogeneities, and artifacts.[29] R2* measurements are more sensitive to detect low levels of iron content but they can become inaccurate in the setting of iron overload.[33] In addition, R2* measurements are less sensitive to variation in the size and distribution of iron particles and the complications of liver disease.[29] Perhaps the biggest advantage of using R2* is the significantly shorter acquisition time; R2* images can be performed in a single breathhold, whereas R2 measurements must be acquired over 2 to 20 minutes.

To address the complexity of performing and interpreting the data obtained in the relaxometry method, several commercial ventures have been created. FerriScan (Resonance Health, Claremont, Australia) is a US Food and Drug Administration–approved method used to measure liver iron content. This technique uses the St. Pierre method consisting of seven free-breathing spin echo sequences with increasing TE values to determine

---

Box 3
Hepatic iron quantification key points

- There are two basic mechanisms for iron overload: excess intestinal absorption and repeated blood transfusions.

- In patients with primary hemochromatosis, iron deposition first occurs in the liver, heart, and pancreas. In patients with secondary hemochromatosis, iron first accumulates in the reticuloendothelial cells of the liver, spleen, bone marrow, and lymph nodes.

- There are two main methods for determining liver iron content: signal intensity ratio and relaxometry.

the iron content.[29,37,39] A phantom with a long T2 value is placed in the field of view to help standardize values across sequences. Although this method is accurate and reproducible, it has several limitations, including a high cost; centralized image analysis; long image acquisition time (20 minutes); and 24–48 hours turnaround time for data analysis. Additionally, the method is insensitive to longitudinal changes in liver iron content in patients with severe iron overload.[29]

At the authors' institution, we use two different relaxometry methods to measure liver iron content: the R2* method and St. Pierre method (**Fig. 2**). The technique used for R2* relaxometry and the St. Pierre method are included in **Table 2**. The most common indication for iron quantification in the authors' institution is transfusional overload. Because of this, they often perform cardiac MR imaging and cardiac iron quantification in the same setting as they perform hepatic iron quantification (**Box 3**).

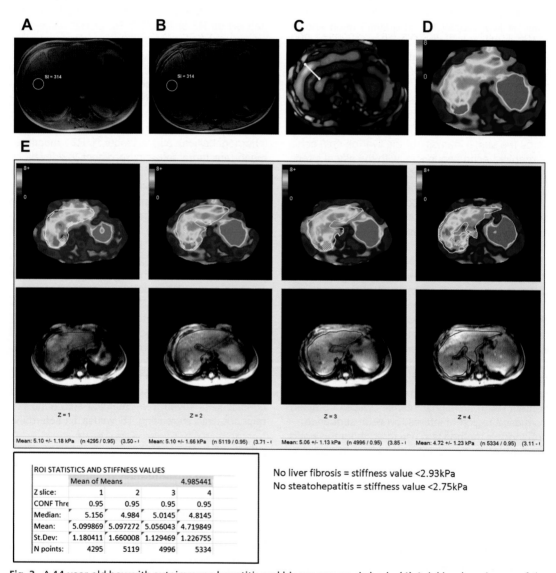

ROI STATISTICS AND STIFFNESS VALUES			
Mean of Means			4.985441
Z slice:	1	2	3	4
CONF Thre	0.95	0.95	0.95	0.95
Median:	5.156	4.984	5.0145	4.8145
Mean:	5.099869	5.097272	5.056043	4.719849
St.Dev:	1.180411	1.660008	1.129469	1.226755
N points:	4295	5119	4996	5334

No liver fibrosis = stiffness value <2.93kPa
No steatohepatitis = stiffness value <2.75kPa

Fig. 3. A 14-year-old boy with autoimmune hepatitis and biopsy-proven cirrhosis. (*A*) Axial in-phase image of the liver shows a mild nodular contour of the liver with prominence of the hepatic fissure. The liver has a signal intensity (SI) of 314 within the region of interest (*circle*). (*B*) Axial opposed-phase image of the upper abdomen shows the liver has a signal intensity (SI) of 314 within the region of interest (*circle*). Using the signal intensities, the liver fat content is 0. (*C*) MR elastography performed in the same patient shows marked elongation of the shear wave (*white line*). (*D*) MR elastogram shows increased liver stiffness represented by yellow, orange, and red colors in the expected region of the liver. (*E*) Report from MR elastography calculates the mean liver stiffness to be 4.99 kPa representing high-grade fibrosis.

MR ELASTOGRAPHY

The most common causes of chronic liver disease in the pediatric population are hepatitis; genetic and congenital disorders, such as α_1-antitrypsin deficiency; cystic fibrosis; biliary atresia; Wilson disease; glycogen storage disorders; NAFLD; and nonalcoholic steatohepatitis.[7] Each of these disorders has the potential to progress to hepatic fibrosis and eventually cirrhosis if untreated. However, if treated, the degree of fibrosis can be minimized or reversed; thus, early diagnosis of fibrosis is critical.[40–42]

Traditionally, liver fibrosis was diagnosed and monitored by biopsy. The limitations of liver biopsy highlight the need for an accurate, noninvasive method of detecting fibrosis. Several MR imaging techniques that have been developed to detect fibrosis include diffusion-weighted imaging, magnetization transfer, MR spectroscopy, and MRE.[15] There is little published describing fibrosis detection by MR imaging in pediatric patients.[7,43] At the authors' institution, we use MRE routinely in clinical practice to detect and quantify liver fibrosis in a wide variety of diseases, such as NAFLD, Gaucher disease, Turner syndrome, cardiac patients (especially those status post-Fontan procedure), and cystic fibrosis (**Fig. 3**).

Technique

MRE is able to assess the stiffness of the liver by measuring the propagation of shear waves through the hepatic parenchyma.[15] The technique is well described in adults and has been shown to detect hepatic fibrosis, distinguish low-grade from high-grade fibrosis, and distinguish steatosis from steatohepatitis.[44–50] Although the technique used in children is similar to that performed in adults, there are several important differences.[7]

Unlike the previously described techniques for iron and fat quantification, special hardware is required for MRE, consisting of an active driver and a passive driver. The active driver is similar to an audio subwoofer. It sits in the MR control room and generates 60-Hz vibrations as controlled by the MR pulse sequence. A pneumatic tube transmits the vibrations to the passive driver resting on the patient in the scanner (**Fig. 4**). Pediatric-sized passive drivers are currently in development. Child life specialists may use a vibrating passive driver simulator on the child before the MRE to help prepare patients for the light vibration sensation they feel during scanning.[7]

The MRE pulse sequences developed for adults by Ehman and colleagues[44,45,51] at the Mayo clinic were adapted and modified to fit pediatric

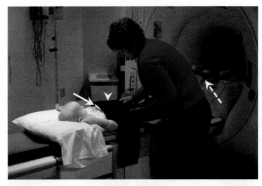

Fig. 4. Photograph of an MR technologist positioning a patient for liver MR elastography. The passive driver (*arrow*) is held in place with a snug wrap (*arrowhead*). A pneumatic tube (*dashed arrow*) connects the passive drive to the active driver (not shown), which is located in the MR control room.

patients. In addition to the standard changes to the specific absorption rate and the field of view, the driver power is reduced by 20% from adult levels in patients between 5 and 18 years of age and by 40% to 50% in patients younger than 2 years of age.[7] This is done to avoid abdominal wall discomfort/pain.[7] In addition, to maintain image quality and further reduce the risk of injury, a folded towel is placed between the passive driver and the child's abdominal wall.[7]

The imaging sequence used in the authors' department is included in **Table 3**. Four MRE sequences are obtained at different levels within the liver. For each level, four magnitude and four phase images are obtained (**Fig. 5**). These 16 images are then converted at the scanner into qualitative stiffness maps. To obtain quantitative values, the data are processed using dedicated software (MRE WAVE; Mayo Clinic, Rochester, MN). The resultant stiffness values can be used to determine the presence of fibrosis.

Normal and abnormal liver stiffness values have not yet been published for pediatric patients using MRE. Because ultrasound-based transient elastography has shown that liver stiffness values are independent of age, the authors use the cutoff values determined in adults to diagnose fibrosis (>2.93 kPa) and steatohepatitis (>2.74 kPa).[44,49,52,53]

There are several advantages of MRE compared with ultrasound-based transient elastography. The most notable is its higher degree of accuracy and higher rate of success.[50] Other advantages of MRE include its larger sample size, deeper penetration into the liver, and its ability to be performed in the presence of ascites and obesity.[43] Despite these advantages, there are still limitations of this

Table 3
Protocol for MR elastography sequence

Sequence	Plane	Approximate Scan Time (s)	TR (ms)	TE (ms)	Slice Thickness (mm)	Matrix Size
MR elastography FGRE	Axial	50	50	Min	10	256 × 64

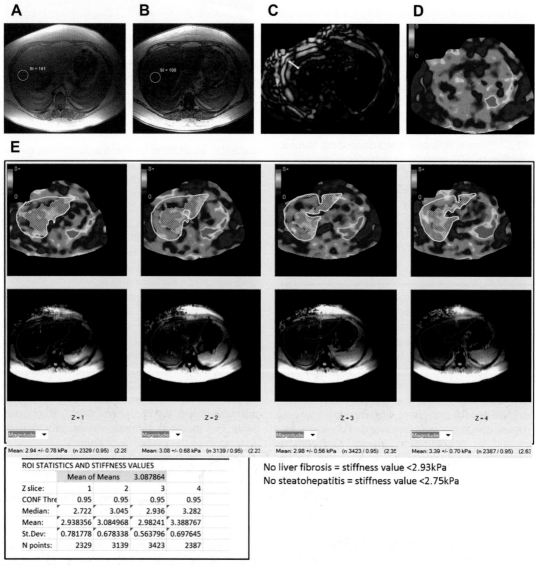

ROI STATISTICS AND STIFFNESS VALUES

	Mean of Means	3.087864		
Z slice:	1	2	3	4
CONF Thre	0.95	0.95	0.95	0.95
Median:	2.722	3.045	2.936	3.282
Mean:	2.938356	3.084968	2.98241	3.388767
St.Dev:	0.781778	0.678338	0.563796	0.697645
N points:	2329	3139	3423	2387

No liver fibrosis = stiffness value <2.93kPa
No steatohepatitis = stiffness value <2.75kPa

Mean: 2.94 +/- 0.78 kPa (n 2329 / 0.95) (2.28

Mean: 3.08 +/- 0.68 kPa (n 3139 / 0.95) (2.23

Mean: 2.98 +/- 0.56 kPa (n 3423 / 0.95) (2.35

Mean: 3.39 +/- 0.70 kPa (n 2387 / 0.95) (2.63

Fig. 5. A 17-year-old boy with obesity and elevated liver enzymes. (A) Axial in-phase image of the liver shows a normal contour of the liver. The liver has a signal intensity (SI) of 161 within the region of interest (*circle*). (B) Axial opposed-phase image of the upper abdomen shows the liver has a signal intensity (SI) of 100 within the region of interest (*circle*). Using the above signal intensities and the formula $\eta = (100\% * [SI_{In\text{-}phase} - SI_{Opposed\text{-}phase}]/[2* SI_{In\text{-}phase}])$, the fat fraction was calculated to be 19%. (C) MR elastography performed in the same patient shows mild elongation of the shear wave (*white line*). (D) MR elastogram shows increased liver stiffness represented by blue, green, and yellow colors in the expected region of the liver. (E) Report from MR elastography calculates the liver stiffness to be 3.09 kPa representing low-grade fibrosis. In a patient with a fatty liver, this represents steatohepatitis and possibly mild fibrosis.

Box 4
MRE key points

- Early detection and diagnosis of hepatic fibrosis is critical because, if treated, the changes can be minimized or reversed.
- MRE is able to assess the stiffness of the liver by measuring the propagation of shear waves through the hepatic parenchyma.
- There are several advantages of MRE compared with ultrasound-based transient elastography including a higher degree of accuracy, a higher rate of success, its ability to asses a larger portion of the liver, and its ability to be performed in the presence of ascites and obesity.

technique, including the cost of the hardware and an inability to detect the shear waves in the setting of iron overload (**Box 4**).

SUMMARY

Over the past decade, there have been significant advances made in liver imaging. These advances allow radiologists to offer noninvasive methods of quantifying the amount of fat and iron in the liver, and a method to quantify the degree of liver fibrosis. These capabilities have the potential to change the way liver disease is diagnosed and managed. At the authors' hospital, the techniques described previously have helped hepatologists to better determine which patients need a liver biopsy, and in many cases obviate biopsy. They rely on such techniques as fat quantification and MRE to manage their patients and determine if the therapies they are providing are having an effect on the patient's liver disease.

REFERENCES

1. Carter AJ, Greer ML, Gray SE, et al. Mock MRI: reducing the need for anaesthesia in children. Pediatr Radiol 2010;40:1368–74.
2. Hallowell LM, Stewart SE, de Amorim E Silva CT, et al. Reviewing the process of preparing children for MRI. Pediatr Radiol 2008;38:271–9.
3. Rosenberg DR, Sweeney JA, Gillen JS, et al. Magnetic resonance imaging of children without sedation: preparation with simulation. J Am Acad Child Adolesc Psychiatry 1997;36:853–9.
4. Pressdee D, May L, Eastman E, et al. The use of play therapy in the preparation of children undergoing MR imaging. Clin Radiol 1997;52:945–7.
5. Edwards AD, Arthurs OJ. Paediatric MRI under sedation: is it necessary? What is the evidence for the alternatives? Pediatr Radiol 2011;41:1353–64.
6. de Bie HM, Boersma M, Wattjes MP, et al. Preparing children with a mock scanner training protocol results in high quality structural and functional MRI scans. Eur J Pediatr 2010;169:1079–85.
7. Serai SD, Towbin AJ, Podberesky DJ. Pediatric liver MR elastography. Dig Dis Sci 2012;57:2713–9.
8. Koch BL. Avoiding sedation in pediatric radiology. Pediatr Radiol 2008;38(Suppl 2):S225–6.
9. Mitchell CL, Vasanawala SS. An approach to pediatric liver MRI. AJR Am J Roentgenol 2011;196: W519–26.
10. Vasanawala SS. MRI of the liver: how to do it. Pediatr Radiol 2010;40:431–7.
11. Lindbäck SM, Gabbert C, Johnson BL, et al. Pediatric nonalcoholic fatty liver disease: a comprehensive review. Adv Pediatr 2010;5:85–140.
12. Bravo AA, Sheth SG, Chopra S. Liver biopsy. N Engl J Med 2001;344:495–500.
13. Liu CY, McKenzie CA, Yu H, et al. Fat quantification with IDEAL gradient echo imaging: correction of bias from T1 and noise. Magn Reson Med 2007; 58:354–64.
14. Ma X, Holalkere NS, Kambadakone RA, et al. Imaging-based quantification of hepatic fat: methods and clinical applications. Radiographics 2009;29: 1253–77.
15. Talwalkar JA, Yin M, Fidler JL, et al. Magnetic resonance imaging of hepatic fibrosis: emerging clinical applications. Hepatology 2008;47:332–42.
16. Hu HH, Kim HW, Nayak KS, et al. Comparison of fat-water MRI and single-voxel MRS in the assessment of hepatic and pancreatic fat fractions in humans. Obesity (Silver Spring) 2010;18:841–7.
17. Reeder SB, Cruite I, Hamilton G, et al. Quantitative assessment of liver fat with magnetic resonance imaging and spectroscopy. J Magn Reson Imaging 2011;34:729–49.
18. Dixon WT. Simple proton spectroscopic imaging. Radiology 1984;153:189–94.
19. Glover GH, Schneider E. Three-point Dixon technique for true water/fat decomposition with B0 inhomogeneity correction. Magn Reson Med 1991; 18:371–83.
20. Levenson H, Greensite F, Hoefs J, et al. Fatty infiltration of the liver: quantification with phase-contrast MR imaging at 1.5 T vs biopsy. AJR Am J Roentgenol 1991;156:307–12.
21. Glover GH. Multipoint Dixon technique for water and fat proton and susceptibility imaging. J Magn Reson Imaging 1991;1:521–30.
22. Lodes CC, Felmlee JP, Ehman RL, et al. Proton MR chemical shift imaging using double and triple phase contrast acquisition methods. J Comput Assist Tomogr 1989;13:855–61.

23. Fishbein MH, Gardner KG, Potter CJ, et al. Introduction of fast MR imaging in the assessment of hepatic steatosis. Magn Reson Imaging 1997;15: 287–93.

24. Fishbein M, Castro F, Cheruku S, et al. Hepatic MRI for fat quantitation: its relationship to fat morphology, diagnosis, and ultrasound. J Clin Gastroenterol 2005;39:619–25.

25. Fishbein MH, Stevens WR. Rapid MRI using a modified Dixon technique: a non-invasive and effective method for detection and monitoring of fatty metamorphosis of the liver. Pediatr Radiol 2001;31:806–9.

26. Kim H, Taksali SE, Dufour S, et al. Comparative MR study of hepatic fat quantification using single-voxel proton spectroscopy, two-point Dixon and three-point IDEAL. Magn Reson Med 2008;59:521–7.

27. Costa DN, Pedrosa I, McKenzie C, et al. Body MRI using IDEAL. AJR Am J Roentgenol 2008;190: 1076–84.

28. Tang A, Tan J, Sun M, et al. Nonalcoholic fatty liver disease: MR imaging of liver proton density fat fraction to assess hepatic steatosis. Radiology 2013;267(2):422–31.

29. Sirlin CB, Reeder SB. Magnetic resonance imaging quantification of liver iron. Magn Reson Imaging Clin N Am 2010;18:359–81.

30. Crownover BK, Covey CJ. Hereditary hemochromatosis. Am Fam Physician 2013;87:183–90.

31. Camaschella C, Poggiali E. Inherited disorders of iron metabolism. Curr Opin Pediatr 2011;23:14–20.

32. Kelly N. Thalassemia. Pediatr Rev 2012;33:434–5.

33. Alústiza Echeverría JM, Castiella A, Emparanza JI. Quantification of iron concentration in the liver by MRI. Insights Imaging 2012;3:173–80.

34. Gandon Y, Olivié D, Guyader D, et al. Non-invasive assessment of hepatic iron stores by MRI. Lancet 2004;363:357–62.

35. Liver iron quantification by MRI (1.5 Tesla). Available at: http://radio.univ-rennes1.fr/Sources/EN/HemoCalc15.html. Accessed April 15, 2013.

36. Storey P, Thompson AA, Carqueville CL, et al. R2* imaging of transfusional iron burden at 3T and comparison with 1.5T. J Magn Reson Imaging 2007;25: 540–7.

37. St Pierre TG, Clark PR, Chua-anusorn W, et al. Noninvasive measurement and imaging of liver iron concentrations using proton magnetic resonance. Blood 2005;105:855–61.

38. Wood JC, Enriquez C, Ghugre N, et al. MRI R2 and R2* mapping accurately estimates hepatic iron concentration in transfusion-dependent thalassemia and sickle cell disease patients. Blood 2005;10:1460–5.

39. St Pierre TG, Clark PR, Chua-Anusorn W. Measurement and mapping of liver iron concentrations using magnetic resonance imaging. Ann N Y Acad Sci 2005;1054:379–85.

40. Friedman SL. Hepatic fibrosis—overview. Toxicology 2008;254:120–9.

41. Friedman SL. Evolving challenges in hepatic fibrosis. Nat Rev Gastroenterol Hepatol 2010;7: 425–36.

42. Bortolotti F, Guido M. Reversal of liver cirrhosis: a desirable clinical outcome and its pathogenic background. J Pediatr Gastroenterol Nutr 2007; 44:401–6.

43. Binkovitz LA, El-Youssef M, Glaser KJ, et al. Pediatric MR elastography of hepatic fibrosis: principles, technique and early clinical experience. Pediatr Radiol 2012;42:402–9.

44. Yin M, Talwalkar JA, Glaser KJ, et al. Assessment of hepatic fibrosis with magnetic resonance elastography. Clin Gastroenterol Hepatol 2007;5: 1207–13.

45. Yin M, Talwalkar JA, Glaser KJ, et al. Dynamic postprandial hepatic stiffness augmentation assessed with MR elastography in patients with chronic liver disease. AJR Am J Roentgenol 2011;197:64–70.

46. Rustogi R, Horowitz J, Harmath C, et al. Accuracy of MR elastography and anatomic MR imaging features in the diagnosis of severe hepatic fibrosis and cirrhosis. J Magn Reson Imaging 2012;35: 1356–64.

47. Wang Y, Ganger DR, Levitsky J, et al. Assessment of chronic hepatitis and fibrosis: comparison of MR elastography and diffusion-weighted imaging. AJR Am J Roentgenol 2011;196:553–651.

48. Kim BH, Lee JM, Lee YJ, et al. MR elastography for noninvasive assessment of hepatic fibrosis: experience from a tertiary center in Asia. J Magn Reson Imaging 2011;34:1110–6.

49. Chen J, Talwalkar JA, Yin M, et al. Early detection of nonalcoholic steatohepatitis in patients with nonalcoholic fatty liver disease by using MR elastography. Radiology 2011;259:749–56.

50. Huwart L, Sempoux C, Vicaut E, et al. Magnetic resonance elastography for the noninvasive staging of liver fibrosis. Gastroenterology 2008;135: 32–40.

51. Muthupillai R, Lomas DJ, Rossman PJ, et al. Magnetic resonance elastography by direct visualization of propagating acoustic strain waves. Science 1995;269:1854–7.

52. Menten R, Leonard A, Clapuyt P, et al. Transient elastography in patients with cystic fibrosis. Pediatr Radiol 2010;40:1231–5.

53. Nobili V, Vizzutti F, Arena U, et al. Accuracy and reproducibility of transient elastography for the diagnosis of fibrosis in pediatric nonalcoholic steatohepatitis. Hepatology 2008;48:442–8.

Magnetic Resonance Imaging of the Pediatric Pancreaticobiliary System

Nathan D. Egbert, MD[a],*, David A. Bloom, MD[b],
Jonathan R. Dillman, MD[c]

KEYWORDS

- Magnetic resonance cholangiopancreatography (MRCP) • Children • Pancreaticobiliary system
- Bile ducts • Pancreatic duct

KEY POINTS

- Magnetic resonance cholangiopancreatography (MRCP) uses heavily T2-weighted MR imaging pulse sequences to visualize fluid (pancreatic fluid and bile, respectively) within the pancreaticobiliary system. This technique is referred to as *MR hydrography*.
- MRCP has several distinct advantages over alternative imaging techniques, such as endoscopic retrograde cholangiopancreatography and percutaneous transhepatic cholangiography, including its noninvasive manner and lack of ionizing radiation.
- Three-dimensional (3D) MRCP has distinct advantages over traditional 2-dimensional (2D) MRCP techniques, including better signal-to-noise and contrast-to-noise ratios, improved spatial resolution, and the ability to create a variety of 2D multiplanar reformations and 3D reconstructions.

INTRODUCTION

Magnetic resonance cholangiopancreatography (MRCP) is an extremely useful tool for evaluating a wide variety of disorders of the pancreaticobiliary system in pediatric patients of all ages, including neonates/infants, children, and adolescents. MRCP has been shown to have good diagnostic accuracy in both children and adults[1–5]; it has distinct advantages over alternative imaging techniques, such as endoscopic retrograde cholangiopancreatography (ERCP) and percutaneous transhepatic cholangiography. The advantages include the lack of ionizing radiation, the ability to thoroughly image the hepatic and pancreatic parenchyma in addition to the pancreaticobiliary tree, and the capability for the generation of 2-dimensional (2D) multiplanar reformations and 3-dimensional (3D) reconstructions. MRCP is also noninvasive with no risk of causing acute pancreatitis, allergic-like reactions to iodinated contrast material, or bleeding. For all of these reasons, MRCP is now the preferred first-line advanced imaging test for assessing the pediatric pancreaticobiliary system, after ultrasonography.

The purpose of this article is to provide a contemporary review of pediatric MRCP, including techniques and indications. Additionally, the authors present the imaging appearance of numerous common and uncommon conditions affecting the pediatric pancreaticobiliary system, such as choledocholithiasis/cholelithiasis; choledochal cysts; stricturing disorders (eg, sclerosing cholangitis, anastomotic strictures, and ischemic strictures); biliary neoplasm; biliary congenital anatomic variants; and abnormalities of the pancreatic ducts (caused by congenital anatomic variants, pancreatitis, and trauma).

[a] Department of Radiology, University of Michigan Health System, 1500 East Medical Center Drive, Ann Arbor, MI 48109, USA; [b] Department of Radiology, Oakland University William Beaumont School of Medicine, Beaumont Children's Hospital, 3601 W. 13 Mile Road, Royal Oak, MI 48073, USA; [c] Section of Pediatric Radiology, Department of Radiology, University of Michigan Health System, 1540 East Hospital Drive, Ann Arbor, MI 48109, USA
* Corresponding author.
E-mail address: nathaneg@med.umich.edu

Magn Reson Imaging Clin N Am 21 (2013) 681–696
http://dx.doi.org/10.1016/j.mric.2013.04.009
1064-9689/13/$ – see front matter © 2013 Elsevier Inc. All rights reserved.

PEDIATRIC MRCP TECHNIQUES

MRCP most commonly uses a variety of heavily T2-weighted pulse sequences that allow visualization of fluid (pancreatic fluid and bile, respectively) within the pancreaticobiliary system (also known as *MR hydrography*). By using heavily T2-weighted fat-saturated pulse sequences, materials/tissues with longer T2 relaxation times appear markedly hyperintense (eg, fluid), whereas materials/tissues with shorter T2 relaxation times (eg, hepatic and pancreatic parenchyma) appear relatively hypointense.[6]

A variety of 2D and 3D techniques have been used to successfully image the pancreaticobiliary tree. Traditionally, MRCP protocols have been comprised of thin-section and/or thick-slab 2D single-shot fast spin-echo (SSFSE) pulse sequences. Coronal and axial thin-section images allow for cross-sectional assessment of the biliary and pancreatic ducts, with detailed assessment of the ducts themselves and the presence of filling defects (**Fig. 1**). Thick-slab images provide an overview of the pancreaticobiliary system and can be obtained in any projection. Commonly, multiple thick-slab coronal-oblique images are acquired

that are radially oriented around the pancreatic head. However, 2D SSFSE MRCP images are limited by

- Relatively poor spatial resolution
- Low signal-to-noise ratio
- Inability to create isotropic (or near-isotropic) 2D multiplanar reformations (in any plane) and 3D reconstructions (in any orientation) (**Box 1**).[6,7]

Three-dimensional T2-weighted fast spin-echo (FSE) MRCP imaging overcomes the 2D MRCP limitations mentioned earlier (See **Box 1**). Because these sequences typically take several minutes to acquire (even when parallel imaging is used), respiratory triggering or navigator (diaphragmatic) gating is required. The fast recovery FSE (FRFSE) technique is also commonly used when using 3D MRCP to provide high signal intensity from fluid and increased image contrast while reducing overall imaging time (FRFSE allows a shorter repetition time because of a negative 90° pulse that causes much faster recovery of tissues with long T2 time to the equilibrium). Three-dimensional MRCP allows for 2D multiplanar reformations in an infinite

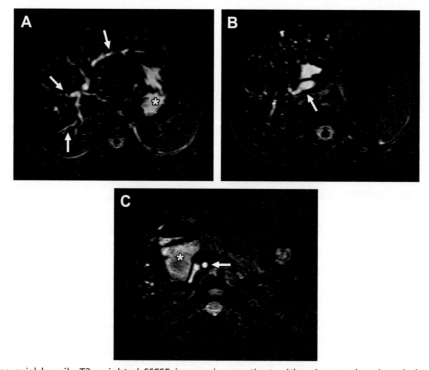

Fig. 1. Three axial heavily T2-weighted SSFSE images in a patient with primary sclerosing cholangitis. These images nicely highlight the long T2 relaxation of fluid-containing structures, such as the bile ducts, while suppressing the tissues with shorter T2 relaxation times. (*A*) Irregular intrahepatic bile ducts (*arrows*) with alternating areas of narrowing and dilatation. Stomach (*asterisk*). (*B, C*) Dilated, common hepatic and common bile ducts (*arrows*). Hepatic flexure of the colon (*asterisk*).

<table>
<tr><td>

Box 1
Advantages of 3D MRCP versus 2D MRCP

Higher signal-to-noise ratio

Higher contrast-to-noise ratio

Improved spatial resolution

Thin-section isotropic images

Ability to create

- 2D multiplanar reformations
- 3D reconstructions

</td></tr>
</table>

number of planes as well as a variety of 3D reconstructions (most commonly volume-rendered and maximum-intensity projection images) (**Fig. 2**).[7]

A standard pediatric MRCP protocol could include any of the following pulse sequences:

- Thin-section (3–6 mm) SSFSE with fat-saturation (coronal and/or axial)
  - Breath held or respiratory triggered
- Thick-slab (4–8 cm) SSFSE with fat saturation (any coronal-oblique plane)
  - Breath held

- Isotropic (near-isotropic) 3D T2-weighted FRFSE with fat saturation (coronal)
  - Respiratory triggered or navigator gated

Depending on the clinical indication, a variety of additional pulse sequences may prove complimentary. At the authors' institutions, they commonly include the following pulse sequences as part of the standard pediatric MRCP protocol:

- Coronal (5 mm) SSFSE
  - Respiratory triggered
- Axial (5 mm) T2-weighted FSE with fat-saturation
  - Respiratory triggered
- Axial (5 mm) T1-weighted gradient recalled echo (GRE) in and out of phase
  - Breath held
- Axial (2–3 mm) dynamic and delayed post-contrast 3D T1-weighted spoiled GRE (SPGR) with fat saturation

On occasion, delayed postcontrast T1-weighted 3D SPGR imaging using a hepatocyte-specific contrast material, such as gadoxetate disodium (Eovist), may prove useful for evaluating the biliary tree. For most patients, in the absence of biliary obstruction, excreted T1-weighted hyperintense

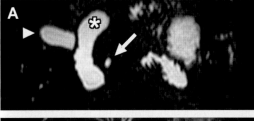

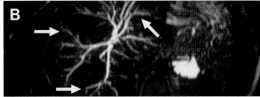

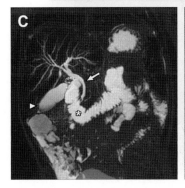

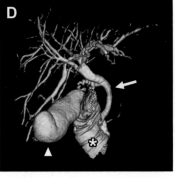

Fig. 2. Multiple 3D MRCP images in child with primary sclerosing cholangitis. (*A*) Axial reformatted and (*B*) axial subvolume maximum intensity projection 3D MRCP images nicely highlight the mildly dilated intrahepatic and extrahepatic bile ducts (*arrows*) as well as additional fluid-containing structures, including the gallbladder (*arrowhead*) and duodenum (*asterisk*). (*C*) Frontal maximum intensity projection and (*D*) volume-rendered 3D MRCP images illustrate the entire biliary system in a single image, allowing for a 3D visualization of the bile ducts (*arrow*) and their relationship to adjacent structures, such as the duodenum (*asterisk*) or gallbladder (*arrowhead*).

contrast material can be seen within the biliary system, including intrahepatic and extrahepatic bile ducts, the cystic duct, and the gallbladder, in about 10 to 30 minutes (**Fig. 3**). With time, excreted contrast material is eventually visualized in the duodenum and more distal small bowel. This form of MRCP may be particularly helpful when evaluating for bile duct injury (including traumatic/anastomotic leak or biloma), questionable biliary obstruction in the setting of mild bile duct dilatation, and when attempting to determine if cystic structures located within the liver or porta hepatis communicate with the biliary system (**Box 2**).[8–14]

In the authors' experience, for certain cases, more delayed imaging after several hours may prove useful to increase diagnostic accuracy (for example, when looking for contrast material in a perihepatic fluid collection suspected to be a biloma). A study by Ringe and colleagues[15] in adult patients concluded that this form of MRCP "adversely affects respiratory-triggered 3D MR cholangiography, both qualitatively and quantitatively," and they concluded that 3D T2-weighted MRCP imaging should be performed before injection of gadoxetate disodium. Another disadvantage of MRCP using a hepatocyte-specific contrast material is that this agent generally does not fill the pancreatic duct, thereby limiting its evaluation.

The intravenous injection of secretin immediately before MRCP has been described as a potentially beneficial adjunct maneuver.[16] Secretin stimulates secretion of bicarbonate-rich pancreatic fluid and, in theory, could improve visualization of the pancreatic duct. However, a recent study by Trout and colleagues[17] assessing the effect of secretin on pediatric patients undergoing MRCP imaging concluded that this medication "induces dilatation of the pancreatic duct but the

---

> **Box 2**
> **Potential uses of hepatocyte-specific contrast agents in patients with hepatobiliary disorders**
>
> Evaluation for bile duct injury
>
> - Trauma
> - Anastomotic leak
> - Biloma
>
> Evaluation for biliary obstruction in setting of mild bile duct dilatation
>
> Determining whether an intrahepatic or perihepatic cystic structure communicates with the biliary tree

---

value of that effect in pediatric MRCP is suspect given the small change in duct diameter and the lack of improvement in image quality and duct visibility."[17] At the authors' institutions, they do not routinely administer secretin when performing pediatric MRCP.

DISCUSSION
Cholelithiasis and Choledocholithiasis

The incidence of both cholelithiasis and choledocholithiasis is increasing in the pediatric population.[18] A variety of conditions that affect children of all ages are associated with gallstone formation, including the following:

- Obesity
- Hemolytic disorders
- Total parenteral nutrition
- Cystic fibrosis
- Terminal ileitis caused by Crohn disease[19]

Although ultrasound is the preferred test for diagnosing cholelithiasis, MRCP can also identify

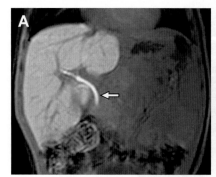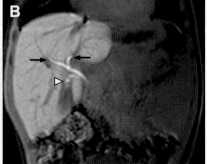

Fig. 3. A 1-year-old boy with history of hepatoblastoma status after resection of a portion of the left lobe. (*A, B*) Coronal T1-weighted 3D SPGR fat-saturated postcontrast images obtained 20 minutes after gadoxetic acid injection demonstrate contrast material filling central intrahepatic bile ducts (*black arrows*), cystic duct (*arrowhead*), and common bile duct (*white arrow*).

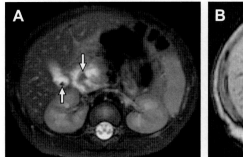 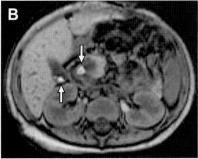 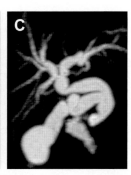

Fig. 4. A 1-year-old boy with jaundice and hyperbilirubinemia. (*A*) Axial T2-weighted FSE fat-saturated image demonstrates hypointense filling defects (*arrows*) in the gallbladder and distal common bile duct, consistent with calculi. (*B*) These calculi (*arrows*) are hyperintense on T1-weighted GRE imaging, suggesting pigmented calculi. (*C*) This 3D MRCP maximum intensity projection image shows diffuse intrahepatic and extrahepatic biliary dilatation to the level of the distal common bile duct, consistent with the presence of an obstructing calculus. Known calculi are difficult to appreciate on this 3D image.

the presence of gallstones and may be particularly helpful in cases in which sonographic evaluation of the gallbladder is limited. MRCP can also identify potential complications of cholelithiasis, such as cholecystitis or Mirizzi syndrome.[20,21] Gallstones on MRCP typically appear as low-signal filling defects within hyperintense bile on T2-weighted imaging. On T1-weighted imaging, gallstones may appear either hypointense or hyperintense depending on their composition[22] (pigmented stones are usually hyperintense, whereas cholesterol stones are hypointense) (**Fig. 4**). Careful attention should be paid to the gallbladder neck to avoid missing gallstones lodged in this region. In pediatric patients with cholelithiasis, the presence of pericholecystic fluid and/or gallbladder wall thickening on T2-weighted imaging should raise suspicion for cholecystitis (**Fig. 5**).[23]

Choledocholithiasis can arise either from calculi forming in situ within the biliary tree or from the passage of gallstones into the extrahepatic bile ducts from the gallbladder. Although the sensitivity of ultrasound for detecting cholelithiasis is high,

ultrasound is not as reliable for detecting choledocholithiasis because visualization of the common hepatic and common bile ducts can be limited (for example, because of shadowing from overlying bowel gas).[24] Fortunately, MRCP is generally sensitive for detecting choledocholithiasis, with a reported sensitivity in adults of 88% to 92% by Becker and colleagues[25] and 95% confidence interval by Nandalur and colleagues.[7] Potential complications of choledocholithiasis that MRCP can also identify include associated biliary obstruction, ascending cholangitis, and acute pancreatitis caused by obstruction of pancreatic drainage.[26,27] At MRCP, choledocholithiasis most often presents as a low-signal focal filling defect in the intrahepatic or extrahepatic bile ducts on T2-weighted imaging, best seen on thin-section axial or coronal SSFSE or 3D MRCP coronal source or axial reformatted images. Biliary calculi can be easily obscured on thick-slab SSFSE images or 3D MRCP volume-rendered or maximum intensity projection (MIP) reconstructions. Kim and colleagues[28] found that the addition of T1-weighted GRE imaging to

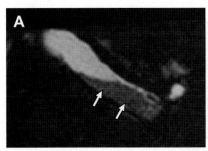 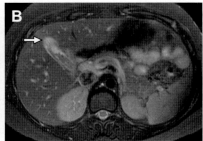

Fig. 5. A 15-year-old boy with acute right upper quadrant abdominal pain. (*A*) Axial reformatted 3D MRCP image reveals many tiny, dependent filling defects in the gallbladder, consistent with calculi (*arrows*). (*B*) Axial T2-weighted FSE fat-saturated image shows gallbladder wall thickening and pericholecystic fluid caused by cholecystitis (*arrow*).

standard MRCP pulse sequences increases detection of intrahepatic biliary calculi.

Choledochal Cysts

Choledochal cysts are a rare congenital anomaly of the biliary tree characterized by focal, abnormal dilatation of a bile duct (or ducts). Biliary involvement can be intrahepatic, extrahepatic, or both. Classically, choledochal cysts are characterized using the Todani classification system (types 1–5) (**Table 1**).[29] There are several potential complications associated with choledochal cysts, including choledocholithiasis, cholangitis, and rarely cholangiocarcinoma.[30] Although ultrasound readily detects many choledochal cysts, MRCP is often required for definitive characterization. Specifically, MRCP allows for the following:

- Precise Todani classification of the choledochal cyst (or cysts)
- Exact measurement of cyst size (including extent of intrahepatic/extrahepatic biliary tree involvement and relation to the cystic duct)
- Detection of intraluminal filling defects (most often debris or calculi and rarely neoplasm)

Choledochal cysts appear as either fusiform or saccular areas of cystic (T2-weighted hyperintense) biliary ectasia/dilatation and can be readily identified using both 2D and 3D MRCP techniques (**Figs. 6–8**).

Although often congenital, some choledochal cysts may be acquired, occurring in the setting of an anomalous junction of the main pancreatic duct with the common bile duct (CBD) and, thereby, the resultant reflux of pancreatic enzymes into the biliary tree.[31,32] MRCP allows for detailed evaluation of pancreaticobiliary junction anatomy.[33,34] An anomalous pancreaticobiliary junction (APBJ) is

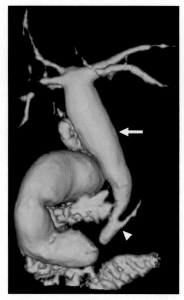

Fig. 6. A 17-year-old girl with recurrent epigastric pain. Volume-rendered 3D MRCP image demonstrates fusiform dilatation of the common hepatic duct and proximal common bile duct (*arrow*), consistent with a type 1c choledochal cyst. There is an anomalous pancreaticobiliary junction (*arrowhead*) with an abnormally elongated common channel measuring greater than 5 mm. The intrahepatic bile ducts are normal in caliber.

diagnosed when the pancreaticobiliary ductal union is located outside of the duodenal wall, typically when the junction is greater than 5 mm from the duodenum (See **Fig. 6**).[35–37] Three separate types of APBJ have been described (**Box 3**).[35,38]

Caroli syndrome, sometimes classified as a type 5 choledochal cyst, is a form of hepatorenal fibrocystic disease that is diagnosed when there are numerous areas of intrahepatic biliary ectasia/

Table 1
Todani classification of choledochal cysts

Type	Findings
Ia	Cystic dilatation of the extrahepatic bile duct
Ib	Focal cystic dilatation of the extrahepatic bile duct
Ic	Fusiform dilatation of the CBD
II	CBD diverticulum (saccular outpouching)
III	Cystic dilatation of the intraduodenal portion of the CBD (ie, choledochocele)
IVa	Dilatation of extrahepatic bile duct with involvement of intrahepatic bile ducts
IVb	Multiple cystic dilatations involving the extrahepatic bile duct
V	Dilatation involving only intrahepatic bile ducts (Caroli disease/syndrome)

Abbreviation: CBD, common bile duct.
Data from Todani T, Watanabe Y, Narusue M, et al. Congenital bile duct cysts: classification, operative procedures, and review of thirty-seven cases including cancer arising from choledochal cyst. Am J Surg 1977;134:263–9.

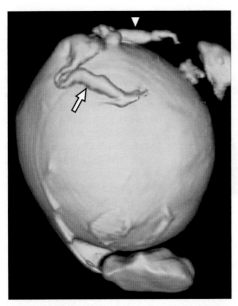

Fig. 7. A 5-day-old girl with palpable abdominal mass. Volume-rendered 3D MRCP image reveals marked cystic dilatation of the extrahepatic biliary tree, consistent with a type 1a choledochal cyst. Intrahepatic bile ducts (*arrowhead*) are mildly dilated, and the gallbladder is seen (*arrow*).

dilatation. This condition is an inheritable ciliopathy that can be found in association with autosomal recessive polycystic kidney disease, congenital hepatic fibrosis, and portal hypertension. On ultrasound, Caroli syndrome may be mistaken for multiple hepatic simple cysts. However, MRCP can be used to clearly depict the connection between these cysts and the biliary tree, which is a critical distinguishing factor in differentiating Caroli syndrome from polycystic liver disease (another form of hepatorenal fibrocystic disease) **(Fig. 9)**.[39] When this condition is sporadic and

Box 3
Types of anomalous pancreaticobiliary junction
Type A
• CBD joins main pancreatic duct at a right angle
Type B
• CBD joins main pancreatic duct at an acute angle
Type C
• Pancreaticobiliary ductal union is complex consisting of a network of ducts

limited to only biliary ductal ectasia/dilatation, the term *Caroli disease* may be used.[40]

Biliary Strictures

Sclerosing cholangitis

Sclerosing cholangitis is an idiopathic chronic inflammatory disorder that affects both intrahepatic and extrahepatic bile ducts, eventually leading to biliary stricture formation with variable obstruction and periductal fibrosis.[41,42] This condition is less common in children than in adults; when it does occur in children, it is commonly associated with a poor prognosis.[41] With time, advanced disease may lead to biliary cirrhosis and hepatic failure.[43] Although sclerosing cholangitis may be idiopathic (primary), it is commonly associated with inflammatory bowel disease (ulcerative colitis more commonly than Crohn disease), with a prevalence of primary sclerosing cholangitis (PSC) in patients with ulcerative colitis (UC) of approximately 2% to 7%.[44–46]

The diagnosis of sclerosing cholangitis in children can be challenging because the clinical

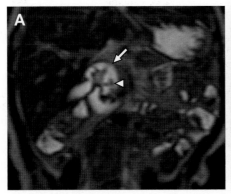
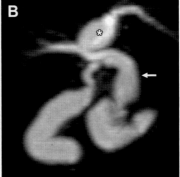

Fig. 8. A 2-month-old girl with trisomy 21 and direct hyperbilirubinemia. (*A*) Coronal SSFSE image shows dilatation of the common bile duct (*arrow*). Low-signal filling defects in the common bile duct are consistent with calculi (*arrowhead*). (*B*) This 3D MRCP MIP image reveals fusiform dilatation of the common bile duct (*arrow*) and central left intrahepatic bile duct (*asterisk*), consistent with a type 4A choledochal cyst.

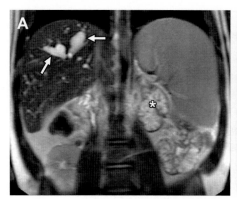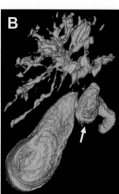

Fig. 9. A 9-year-old boy with autosomal recessive polycystic kidney disease and Caroli syndrome. (*A*) Coronal SSFSE image shows intrahepatic cystic structures in communication with the biliary tree (*arrows*). The left kidney is partially seen and contains innumerable tiny cysts (*asterisk*). The spleen is enlarged because of portal hypertension. (*B*) This 3D MRCP volume-rendered image confirms numerous focal areas of intrahepatic biliary ectasia/dilation. A large saccular choledochal cyst (type 2) (*arrow*) arises from the extrahepatic biliary tree.

features associated with PSC can be variable, ranging from a classic cholestatic picture to one indistinguishable from autoimmune hepatitis.[42] The diagnosis is most often made based on a combination of clinical, laboratory, and radiologic data, with or without pathologic confirmation.[47] MRCP is the preferred first-line radiologic test for diagnosing sclerosing cholangitis (**Figs. 10** and **11**). Common findings[41,48] include the following:

- Intrahepatic/extrahepatic biliary strictures with interposed segments of normal caliber or dilated ducts
- Irregular/beaded appearance of the biliary tree

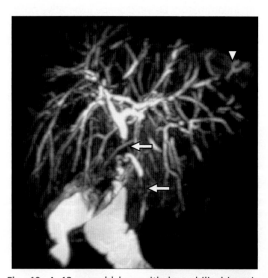

Fig. 10. A 13-year-old boy with hyperbilirubinemia. The 3D MRCP MIP image demonstrates multiple strictures of the intrahepatic and extrahepatic biliary tree (*arrows*), areas of alternating narrowing/dilatation of intrahepatic bile ducts, dilated peripheral floating intrahepatic bile ducts (*arrowhead*), and visualization of bile ducts too peripherally within the liver.

- Intrahepatic peripheral floating bile ducts

Based on a study by Chavhan and colleagues,[41] "an unequivocally positive MRCP study should not be followed by ERCP for diagnosing primary sclerosing cholangitis in children."

Anastomotic biliary strictures

Anastomotic stricture formation is a well-established complication following orthotopic liver transplant (OLT) and has been reported in up to 17.6% of adults following OLT.[49,50] A recent study by Chok and colleagues[51] demonstrated that 13 of 78 pediatric patients undergoing OLT developed a biliary anastomotic stricture. Anastomotic strictures most often present within the first year following surgery and are probably more often associated with duct-to-duct anastomoses (as opposed to hepaticojejunostomy).[51] Causes of anastomotic stricture formation may include the following:

- Inadequate mucosa-to-mucosa anastomotic contact
- Biliary ischemia (caused by hepatic artery narrowing or thrombosis)
- Inflammation and fibrosis related to anastomotic leak[52]

MRCP findings suggesting an anastomotic stricture include focal bile duct narrowing in the expected location of the surgical anastomosis and upstream ductal dilatation (**Figs. 12** and **13**).[53] The identification of anastomotic strictures can direct surgical revision of the anastomosis or a variety of percutaneous and endoscopic interventions, such as balloon dilatation and stent placement.[54]

Other biliary strictures

Nonanastomotic biliary strictures occur in 5% to 10% of patients following OLT and can be classified

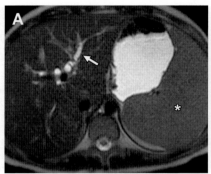
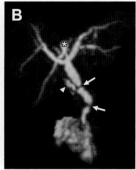

Fig. 11. A 13-year-old girl with ulcerative colitis and sclerosing cholangitis. (A) Axial SSFSE image demonstrates mild dilatation of central intrahepatic bile ducts (arrow). The spleen (asterisk) is enlarged because of portal hypertension. (B) This 3D MRCP MIP image shows 2 high-grade strictures involving the common bile duct (arrows) as well as upstream intrahepatic biliary dilatation. The bile duct draining the posterior inferior portion of the right hepatic lobe inserts in the central left hepatic duct (asterisk), a common congenital anatomic variant. The cystic duct (arrowhead) is blind ending because of surgical absence of the gallbladder.

as either ischemic (related to hemodynamically significant hepatic artery narrowing or thrombosis) or ischemic-type biliary lesions (related to infection or immunologic/graft preservation–related factors).[52,55] Nonanastomotic OLT strictures can involve both the intrahepatic and extrahepatic bile ducts, may be segmental or diffuse, and commonly affect the hepatic confluence.[52,55] In addition to bile duct irregularity and biliary narrowing with upstream dilation, other findings may be noted on MRCP, including the presence of intrahepatic bilomas or intraluminal filling defects caused by debris, stones, and/or sloughed mucosa.[52,55] Intrahepatic bilomas or bile lakes are intimately associated with the biliary tree, lack an epithelial lining, and may become secondarily infected because of bile stasis requiring percutaneous catheter drainage (Fig. 14).[56,57] Findings suggestive of intrahepatic biloma infection (or abscess

formation) include peripheral postcontrast hyperenhancement and internal gas.

Biliary pseudostrictures

Apparent isolated extrahepatic bile duct narrowing involving the proximal or midportion of the common hepatic duct is usually artifactual and caused by the loss of signal from pulsatile arterial compression (Fig. 15).[58] This well-known artifact most commonly occurs when the proximal right hepatic artery crosses the posterior aspect of the common hepatic duct, although it can also be secondary to compression by the gastroduodenal artery. The absence of upstream biliary ductal dilatation and identification of the offending artery as a flow void on noncontrast pulse sequences and/or as an enhancing structure on postcontrast imaging confirms the diagnosis of a pseudostricture.[58,59]

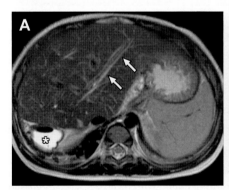
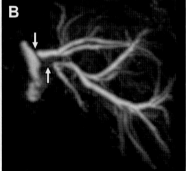

Fig. 12. A 2-year-old boy status after left lobe liver transplantation with biliary dilatation on ultrasound and hyperbilirubinemia. (A) Axial T2-weighted FSE image shows linear hyperintense structures in the transplant liver (arrows), consistent with dilated bile ducts. The jejunum is seen posterior to the allograft (asterisk). (B) This 3D MRCP MIP image confirms the presence of moderate intrahepatic biliary dilatation to near the level of the hepaticojejunostomy. High-grade anastomotic stricturing (arrows) causes abrupt cutoff of bile ducts as they approach the jejunum.

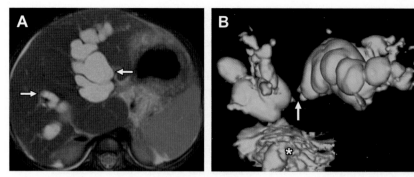

Fig. 13. A 1-year-old girl status after Kasai procedure for biliary atresia and new cystic liver lesions on ultrasound. (*A*) Axial T2-weighted FSE fat-saturated image shows numerous large cystic structures in both lobes of the liver that communicate (*arrows*), consistent with severe biliary dilatation. (*B*) This 3D MRCP volume-rendered image confirms the presence of severe intrahepatic biliary dilatation with abrupt bile duct narrowing (*arrow*) in the region of the hepatoportoenterostomy. Bowel (*asterisk*).

Susceptibility artifact caused by certain metallic surgical materials located in the region of the porta hepatis can also cause adjacent signal loss and give rise to apparent extrahepatic biliary narrowing (**Box 4**).[58]

Congenital Biliary Anatomic Variants

Although congenital anatomic variations of the biliary tree are most often asymptomatic,

knowledge of their existence is important because certain anomalies can be symptomatic or a source of potentially serious iatrogenic injury during surgery (eg, cholecystectomy) (**Fig. 16**). According to Filippo and colleagues,[60] anatomic variants involving either intrahepatic or extrahepatic bile ducts are commonly encountered in routine clinical practice and can be demonstrated in about 40% of patients who undergo MRCP imaging.

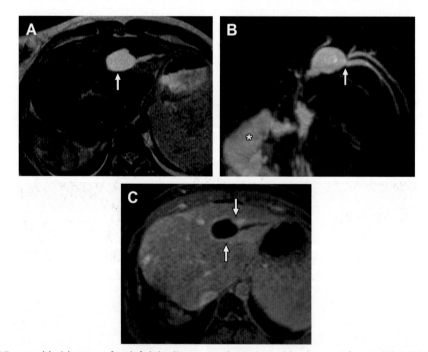

Fig. 14. A 17-year-old girl status after left lobe liver transplantation with recurrent fevers. (*A*) Axial T2-weighted FSE image reveals an oval-shaped fluid-filled structure in the liver (*arrow*) that seems to communicate with a bile duct. (*B*) This 3D MRCP MIP image confirms that the cystic structure communicates with the biliary tree (*arrow*) and is consistent with an intrahepatic biloma or bile lake. Bile ducts in the region of the hepaticojejunostomy are not well seen and are likely strictured, whereas more peripheral bile ducts are mildly dilated. Jejunum (*asterisk*). (*C*) Postcontrast axial T1-weighted image with fat-saturation shows that the bile lake peripherally hyperenhances (*arrows*). Percutaneous needle aspiration of this structure obtained purulent fluid.

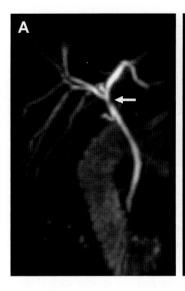
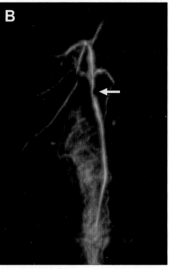

Fig. 15. A 15-year-old girl with abdominal pain following cholecystectomy. (*A*) Frontal MIP and (*B*) lateral volume-rendered 3D MRCP images demonstrate an apparent common hepatic duct stricture (*arrows*). This finding is an artifact caused by an adjacent pulsatile artery (not shown). Intrahepatic bile ducts are normal in caliber.

Common variants that are most often of no clinical importance to patients that are not undergoing hepatic resection include trifurcation of the central biliary tree and drainage of the right lobe dorsocaudal branch into the central left hepatic duct.[61] An important variant in the setting of cholecystectomy includes anomalous biliary drainage directly into the gallbladder, cystic duct, or common hepatic duct (see **Fig. 16**). If unrecognized, these variants can be a cause of postoperative bile leak or segmental biliary obstruction caused by inadvertent bile duct injury (inadvertent duct clipping or ischemia). MRCP can also be used to characterize more complex biliary anomalies, such as gallbladder interposition, a condition whereby the hepatic biliary drainage empties directly into the gallbladder and the cystic duct serves as the common bile duct (**Fig. 17**).[62,63]

Biliary Obstruction Caused by Masses and Masslike Lesions

MRCP can also be helpful when evaluating pediatric patients with suspected biliary obstruction caused by a mass or other masslike lesion. In the authors' experience, MRCP has aided in the diagnosis or evaluation of obstructing rhabdomyosarcoma of the biliary tree (**Fig. 18**), duodenal and ampullary neoplasms (**Fig. 19**), and Crohn disease (duodenitis). In the setting of a mass, MR imaging can be used to determine the exact level of obstruction, degree of obstruction, and presence of biliary intraluminal involvement. Cholangiocarcinoma, although common in adulthood, has been only very rarely reported in the pediatric population.[64]

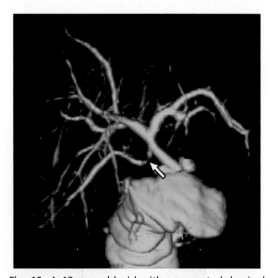

Fig. 16. A 12-year-old girl with recurrent abdominal pain following cholecystectomy. This 3D MRCP volume-rendered image shows aberrant drainage of the right posterior inferior intrahepatic duct into the common hepatic duct, with an apparent stricture near its insertion (*arrow*).

Box 4
Causes of pediatric biliary strictures on MRCP

Sclerosing cholangitis

Anastomotic strictures

Nonanastomotic strictures (orthotopic liver transplant setting)

- Ischemic
- Ischemic-type biliary lesions

Pseudostricture caused by adjacent artery or surgical material

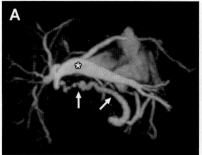
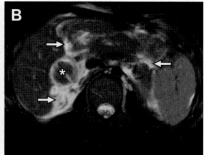

Fig. 17. A 17-year-old boy with VACTERL association and right upper quadrant abdominal pain. (*A*) This 3D MRCP MIP image reveals drainage of the common hepatic duct into the gallbladder (not seen because of low signal contents). The cystic duct (*arrows*) takes an anomalous course and drains through the major papilla. Intrahepatic bile ducts are dilated (*asterisk*). Imaging findings are consistent with interruption of the gallbladder. (*B*) Axial T2-weighted FSE fat-saturated image shows low-signal contents filling the gallbladder (*asterisk*). Extensive high-signal inflammatory changes and fluid within the upper abdomen (*arrows*) are caused by acute cholecystitis.

MR Pancreatography

Pancreatic ductal abnormalities in children may be caused by a variety of factors, including congenital variants (eg, pancreas divisum and annular pancreas), pancreatitis (including acute, chronic, and autoimmune pancreatitis), trauma, and neoplasms. MRCP is the preferred imaging test for evaluating suspected or known pediatric pancreatic ductal abnormalities because of its excellent contrast and spatial resolution and noninvasive nature.

Pancreas divisum

Pancreas divisum is the most common ductal congenital anatomic variant affecting the pancreas (occurring in up to 7% of patients) and occurs when the ventral and dorsal pancreatic buds fail to fuse.[65,66] Although this abnormality can be difficult to identify using ultrasound and computed tomography (CT), it is usually readily apparent at MRCP with the dorsal duct draining through the

smaller minor papilla and the shorter ventral duct draining through the larger major papilla.[67] There is often some degree of obstruction to the drainage of pancreatic secretions at the level of the minor papilla. MRCP can nicely demonstrate evidence of associated chronic pancreatitis, when present, including main pancreatic and side branch ductal dilatation (**Fig. 20**).

Pancreatitis

MRCP can suggest a variety of causes for acute and chronic pancreatitis in children, in addition to pancreas divisum. The presence of cholelithiasis or choledocholithiasis should raise suspicion for gallstone pancreatitis caused by an obstructing calculus. Findings suggestive of autoimmune pancreatitis include a diffusely enlarged, featureless pancreas (with or without peripheral capsule), focal narrowing or diffuse irregularity of the main pancreatic duct, and biliary strictures.[68] This condition occurs with increased frequency in patients with

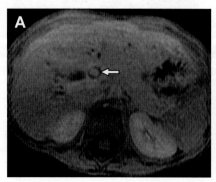
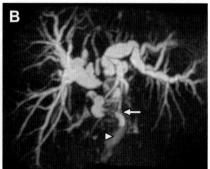

Fig. 18. A 23-month-old boy with hyperbilirubinemia due to biliary rhabdomyosarcoma. (*A*) Postcontrast axial T1-weighted fat-saturated image reveals an enhancing filling defect in the central biliary tree (*arrow*). (*B*) This 3D MRCP MIP image shows severe intrahepatic biliary ductal dilatation with high-grade hilar region obstruction. Irregularity (*arrow*) and filling defects (*arrowhead*) involving the extrahepatic biliary tree are caused by tumor.

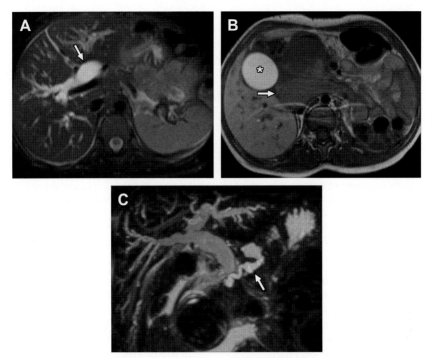

Fig. 19. A 17-year-old girl status after renal transplant with posttransplant lymphoproliferative disorder. (*A*) Axial T2-weighted fat-saturated image reveals intrahepatic biliary dilatation (*arrow*). (*B*) Axial T1-weighted FSE image shows a large heterogeneous abnormality in the expected location of the duodenum (*arrow*), found to be a combination of duodenal lymphoma and hemorrhage at endoscopy. T1-weighted hyperintense material is present in the gallbladder lumen (*asterisk*), possibly caused by obstruction or hemorrhage. (*C*) A 3D MRCP MIP image demonstrates markedly dilated, obstructed intrahepatic and extrahepatic biliary ducts to the level of the distal common bile duct. The main pancreatic duct (*arrow*) is also dilated and obstructed.

inflammatory bowel disease.[69] In the setting of suspected or known hereditary pancreatitis (commonly caused by a trypsin mutation that makes it difficult to deactivate), findings of chronic pancreatitis may be present, including pancreatic ductal irregularity and dilatation (including visualization of side ducts) and parenchymal calcifications (which can be difficult to appreciate on MR imaging).

Pancreatic Ductal Trauma

Pancreatic blunt trauma is a common cause of pediatric pancreatitis.[70] Although pancreatic trauma may be accidental (eg, bicycle handle injury), the possibility of nonaccidental trauma (child abuse) should be considered.[71] Pancreatic contusions present as focal or diffuse enlargement of the

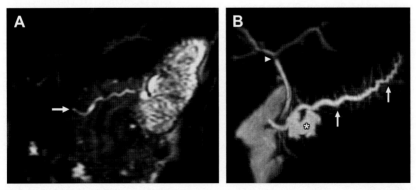

Fig. 20. A 17-year-old girl with chronic pancreatitis. (*A*) Coronal SSFSE demonstrates drainage of the main pancreatic (dorsal) duct through the minor papilla (*arrow*), consistent with pancreas divisum. (*B*) This 3D MRCP MIP image shows diffuse dilatation of the main pancreatic duct and side branches (*arrows*), consistent with changes from chronic pancreatitis. A small pseudocyst (*asterisk*) is also present. Apparent narrowing of the common hepatic duct (*arrowhead*) is an artifact caused by a crossing artery.

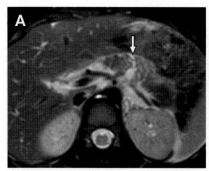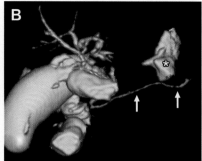

Fig. 21. A 6-year-old boy with epigastric pain after fall from his bicycle. (*A*) Axial T2-weighted FSE fat-saturated image shows focal linear signal abnormality within the pancreatic body (*arrow*), consistent with laceration. Increased signal within and surrounding the pancreas is caused by pancreatitis. (*B*) This 3D MRCP MIP image confirms that the main pancreatic duct is at least partly intact (*arrows*). A focal fluid collection (*asterisk*) abuts the main pancreatic duct and raises the possibility of ductal injury, however.

pancreas with associated increased glandular and periglandular T2-weighted signal hyperintensity caused by edema, fluid, and inflammation. MRCP is particularly valuable for evaluating the possibility of major pancreatic ductal injury (**Fig. 21**). If the main pancreatic duct appears at least partly intact, management is generally initially nonoperative with possible stent placement. If the main pancreatic duct appears completely transected, distal pancreatectomy is commonly performed.[72]

SUMMARY

MRCP is an incredibly valuable tool for evaluating pediatric patients of all ages with suspected or known disorders of the pancreaticobiliary system. The numerous advantages of MRCP over alternative diagnostic techniques make this imaging modality the preferred first-line advanced imaging test after ultrasound for dedicated assessment of the pediatric biliary tree and pancreatic ducts. Using a combination of 2D and 3D techniques, MRCP allows for the diagnosis and comprehensive characterization of a wide variety of pancreaticobiliary abnormalities and is playing an increasingly important role in guiding both medical and surgical management.

REFERENCES

1. Tipnis NA, Dua KS, Werlin SL. A retrospective assessment of magnetic resonance cholangiopancreatography in children. J Pediatr Gastroenterol Nutr 2008;46:59–64.
2. Taylor AC, Little AF, Hennessy OF, et al. Prospective assessment of magnetic resonance cholangiopancreatography for noninvasive imaging of the biliary tree. Gastrointest Endosc 2002;55:17–22.
3. Fulcher AS, Turner MA, Capps GW, et al. Half-Fourier RARE MRCP in 300 subjects. Radiology 1998; 207:21–32.
4. Albert JG, Riemann JF. ERCP and MRCP—when and why. Best Pract Res Clin Gastroenterol 2002; 16:399–419.
5. Arcement CM, Meza MP, Arumanla S, et al. MRCP in the evaluation of pancreaticobiliary disease in children. Pediatr Radiol 2001;31:92–7.
6. Sodickson A, Mortele KJ, Barish MA, et al. Three-dimensional fast-recovery fast spin-echo MRCP: comparison with two-dimensional single-shot fast spin-echo techniques. Radiology 2006;238:549–59.
7. Nandalur KR, Hussain HK, Weadock WJ, et al. Possible biliary disease: diagnostic performance of high-spatial-resolution isotropic 3D T2-wieigted MRCP. Radiology 2008;249:883–90.
8. Aduna M, Larena JA, Martín D, et al. Bile duct leaks after laparoscopic cholecystectomy: value of contrast-enhanced MRCP. Abdom Imaging 2005;30:480–7.
9. Lee NK, Kim S, Lee JW, et al. Biliary MR imaging with Gd-EOB-DTPA and its clinical applications. Radiographics 2009;29:1707–24.
10. Marin D, Bova V, Agnello F, et al. Gadoxetate disodium-enhanced magnetic resonance cholangiography for the noninvasive detection of an active bile duct leak after laparoscopic cholecystectomy. J Comput Assist Tomogr 2010;34:213–6.
11. Gupta RJ, Brady CM, Lotz J, et al. Dynamic MR imaging of the biliary system using hepatocyte-specific contrast agents. AJR Am J Roentgenol 2010;195:405–13.
12. An SK, Lee JM, Suh KS, et al. Gadobenate dimeglumine-enhanced liver MRI as the sole preoperative imaging technique: a prospective study of living liver donors. AJR Am J Roentgenol 2006; 187:1223–33.
13. Park MS, Yu JS, Lee JH, et al. Value of manganese-enhanced T1- and T2-weighted MR

cholangiography for differentiating cystic parenchymal lesions from cystic abnormalities which communicate with the bile ducts. Yonsei Med J 2007;48:1072–4.

14. Park M, Kim KW, Yu JS, et al. Early biliary complications of laparoscopic cholecystectomy: evaluation on T2-weighted MR cholangiography in conjunction with mangafodipir trisodium–enhanced 3D T1-weighted MR cholangiography. AJR Am J Roentgenol 2004;183:1559–66.

15. Ringe KI, Gupta RT, Brady CM, et al. Respiratory-triggered three-dimensional T2-weighted MR cholangiography after injection of gadoxetate disodium: is it still reliable? Radiology 2010;255:451–8.

16. Delaney L, Applegate KE, Karmazyn B. MR cholangiopancreatography in children: feasibility, safety, and initial experience. Pediatr Radiol 2008; 38:64–75.

17. Trout AT, Podbersky DJ, Serai SD, et al. Does secretin add value in pediatric magnetic resonance cholangiopancreatography? Pediatr Radiol 2012;43(4):479–86.

18. Poffenberger CM, Gausche-Hill M, Ngai S, et al. Cholelithiasis and its complications in children and adolescents: update and case discussion. Pediatr Emerg Care 2012;28:68–76.

19. Wesdorp I, Bosman D, Graaff A, et al. Clinical presentations and predisposing factors of cholelithiasis and sludge in children. J Pediatr Gastroenterol Nutr 2000;31:411–7.

20. Kim PN, Outwater EK, Mitchell DG. Mirizzi syndrome: evaluation by MR imaging. Am J Gastroenterol 1999;94:2546–50.

21. Smith EA, Dillman JR, Elsayes KM, et al. Cross-sectional imaging of acute and chronic gallbladder inflammatory disease. AJR Am J Roentgenol 2009; 192:188–96.

22. Tsai HM, Lin XZ, Chen CY, et al. MRI of gallstones with different compositions. AJR Am J Roentgenol 2004;182:1513–9.

23. Altun E, Semelka RC, Elias J, et al. Acute cholecystitis: MR findings and differentiation from chronic cholecystitis. Radiology 2007;244:174–83.

24. Laing FC. Ultrasound diagnosis of choledocholithiasis. Semin Ultrasound CT MR 1987;8:103–13.

25. Becker CD, Grossholz M, Becker M, et al. Choledocholithiasis and bile duct stenosis: diagnostic accuracy of MR cholangiopancreatography. Radiology 1997;205:523–30.

26. Hakansson K, Ekberg O, Hakansson HO, et al. MR characteristics of acute cholangitis. Acta Radiol 2002;43:175–9.

27. Darge K, Anupindi S. Pancreatitis and the role of US, MRCP and ERCP. Pediatr Radiol 2009;39: S153–7.

28. Kim YK, Kim CS, Lee JM, et al. Value of adding T1-weighted image to MR cholangiopancreatography for detecting intrahepatic biliary stones. AJR Am J Roentgenol 2006;187:W267–74.

29. Todani T, Watanabe Y, Narusue M, et al. Congenital bile duct cysts: classification, operative procedures, and review of thirty-seven cases including cancer arising from choledochal cyst. Am J Surg 1977;134:263–9.

30. Kim OH, Chung HJ, Choi BG. Imaging of the choledochal cyst. Radiographics 1995;15:69–88.

31. Song HK, Kim MH, Myung SJ, et al. Choledochal cyst associated with the anomalous union of pancreaticobiliary duct (AUPBD) has a more grave clinical course than choledochal cyst alone. Korean J Intern Med 1999;14:1–8.

32. Kamisawa T, Takuma K, Anjiki H, et al. Pancreaticobiliary maljunction. Clin Gastroenterol Hepatol 2009;7:S84–8.

33. Chavhan GB, Babyn PS, Manson D, et al. Pediatric MR cholangiopancreatography: principles, technique, and clinical applications. Radiographics 2008;28:1951–62.

34. Irie H, Honda H, Jimi M, et al. Value of MR cholangiopancreatography in evaluating choledochal cysts. AJR Am J Roentgenol 1998;171:1381–5.

35. Kim MJ, Han SJ, Yoon CS, et al. Using MR cholangiopancreatography to reveal anomalous pancreaticobiliary ductal union in infants and children with choledochal cysts. AJR Am J Roentgenol 2002; 179:209–14.

36. Jona JZ, Babbit DP, Starshak RJ, et al. Anatomic observations and etiologic and surgical considerations in choledochal cyst. J Pediatr Surg 1979; 14:315–20.

37. Okada T, Sasaki F, Honda S, et al. Usefulness of axial planes of helical computed tomography for diagnosis of pancreaticobiliary maljunction in early infants with negative findings on magnetic resonance cholangiopancreatography. J Pediatr Surg 2008;43:579–82.

38. Todani T, Watanabe Y, Fujii T, et al. Anomalous arrangement of the pancreatobiliary ductal system in patients with a choledochal cyst. Am J Surg 1984;147:672–6.

39. Fitoz S, Erden A, Boruban S. Magnetic resonance cholangiopancreatography of biliary system abnormalities in children. Clin Imaging 2007;31: 93–101.

40. Desmet VJ. Congenital diseases of intrahepatic bile ducts: variations on the theme "ductal plate malformation". Hepatology 1992;16:1069–83.

41. Chavhan GB, Roberts E, Moineddin R, et al. Primary sclerosing cholangitis in children: utility of magnetic resonance cholangiopancreatography. Pediatr Radiol 2008;38:868–73.

42. Lee WS, Saw CB, Sarji SA. Autoimmune hepatitis/ primary sclerosing cholangitis overlap syndrome in a child: diagnostic usefulness of magnetic

resonance cholangiopancreatography. J Paediatr Child Health 2005;41:225–7.

43. Ferrara C, Valeri G, Salvolini L, et al. Magnetic resonance cholangiopancreatography in primary sclerosing cholangitis in children. Pediatr Radiol 2002;32:413–7.

44. Bernstein CN, Blanchard JF, Rasthorne P, et al. The prevalence of extraintestinal diseases in inflammatory bowel disease: a population-based study. Am J Gastroenterol 2001;96:1116–22.

45. Alexopoulou E, Xenophontos PE, Economopoulos N, et al. Investigative MRI cholangiopancreatography for primary sclerosing cholangitis-type lesions in children with IBD. J Pediatr Gastroenterol Nutr 2012;55: 308–13.

46. Hyams J, Markowitz J, Treem W, et al. Characterization of hepatic abnormalities in children with inflammatory bowel disease. Inflamm Bowel Dis 1995;1:27–33.

47. Portincasa P, Vacca M, Moschetta A, et al. Primary sclerosing cholangitis: updates in diagnosis and therapy. World J Gastroenterol 2005;11:7–16.

48. Vitellas KM, Keogan MT, Freed KS, et al. Radiologic manifestations of sclerosing cholangitis with emphasis on MR cholangiopancreatography. Radiographics 2000;20:959–75.

49. Hintze RE, Adler A, Velzke W, et al. Endoscopic management of biliary complications after orthotopic liver transplantation. Hepatogastroenterology 1997;44:258–62.

50. St Peter S, Rodriguez-Davalos MI, Rodriguez-Luna HM, et al. Significance of proximal biliary dilatation in patients with anastomotic strictures after liver transplantation. Dig Dis Sci 2004;49:1207–11.

51. Chok KS, Chan SC, Chan KL, et al. Bile duct anastomotic stricture after pediatric living donor liver transplantation. J Pediatr Surg 2012;47:1399–403.

52. Girometti R, Cereser L, Como G, et al. Biliary complications after orthotopic liver transplantation: MRCP findings. Abdom Imaging 2008;33:542–54.

53. Ward J, Sheridan MB, Guthrie JA, et al. Bile duct strictures after hepatobiliary surgery: assessment with MR cholangiography. Radiology 2004;231:101–8.

54. Balderramo D, Navasa M, Cardenas A. Current management of biliary complications after liver transplantation: emphasis on endoscopic therapy. Gastroenterol Hepatol 2011;34:107–15.

55. Collettini F, Kroencke TJ, Heidenhain C, et al. Ischemic-type biliary lesions after orthotopic liver transplantation: diagnosis with magnetic resonance cholangiography. Transplant Proc 2011;43:2660–3.

56. Tainaka T, Kaneko K, Nakamura S, et al. Histological assessment of bile lake formation after hepatic portoenterostomy for biliary atresia. Pediatr Surg Int 2008;24:265–9.

57. Werlin SL, Sty JR, Starshak RJ, et al. Intrahepatic biliary tract abnormalities in children with corrected extrahepatic biliary atresia. J Pediatr Gastroenterol Nutr 1985;4:537–41.

58. Irie H, Honda H, Kuroiwa T, et al. Pitfalls in MR cholangiopancreatographic interpretation. Radiographics 2001;21:23–37.

59. Kondo H, Kanematsu M, Shiratori Y, et al. Potential pitfalls of MR cholangiopancreatography: right hepatic arterial impression of the common hepatic duct. J Comput Assist Tomogr 1999;23:60–2.

60. Filippo MD, Calabrese M, Quinto S, et al. Congenital anomalies and variations of the bile and pancreatic ducts: magnetic resonance cholangiopancreatography findings, epidemiology and clinical significance. Radiol Med 2008;113:841–59.

61. Yu J, Turner MA, Fulcher AS, et al. Congenital anomalies and normal variants of the pancreaticobiliary tract and the pancreas in adults: part 1, biliary tract. AJR Am J Roentgenol 2006;187:1536–43.

62. Phani Krishna R, Behari A. Interposition of gallbladder - a rare extrahepatic biliary anomaly. Indian J Surg 2011;73:453–4.

63. Rosato L, Ginardi A, Mondini G. Interposition of the gallbladder in the common hepatic duct: a rare dangerous anomaly. G Chir 2011;32:316–9.

64. Björnsson E, Angulo P. Cholangiocarcinoma in young individuals with and without primary sclerosing cholangitis. Am J Gastroenterol 2007;102: 1677–82.

65. Mosler P, Akisik F, Sandrasegaran K, et al. Accuracy of magnetic resonance cholangiopancreatography in the diagnosis of pancreas divisum. Dig Dis Sci 2012;57:170–4.

66. Yu J, Turner MA, Fulcher AS, et al. Congenital anomalies and normal variants of the pancreaticobiliary tract and the pancreas in adults: part 2, pancreatic duct and pancreas. AJR Am J Roentgenol 2006;187:1544–53.

67. Bret PM, Reinhold C, Taourel P, et al. Pancreas divisum: evaluation with MR cholangiopancreatography. Radiology 1996;199:99–103.

68. Yang DH, Kim KW, Kim TK, et al. Autoimmune pancreatitis: radiologic findings in 20 patients. Abdom Imaging 2006;31:94–102.

69. Børkje B, Vetvik K, Odegaard S, et al. Chronic pancreatitis in patients with sclerosing cholangitis and ulcerative colitis. Scand J Gastroenterol 1985;20:539–42.

70. Soergel K. Acute pancreatitis. In: Sleisenger MH, Fordtran JS, editors. Gastrointestinal disease: pathophysiology, diagnosis, management. 5th edition. Philadelphia: Saunders; 1993. p. 1628–53.

71. Lonergan GJ, Baker AM, Morey MK, et al. From the archives of the AFIP. Child abuse: radiologic-pathologic correlation. Radiographics 2003;23:811–45.

72. Canty TG Sr, Weinman D. Management of major pancreatic duct injuries in children. J Trauma 2001;50:1001–7.

Magnetic Resonance Imaging of the Pediatric Kidney
Benign and Malignant Masses

Michael S. Gee, MD, PhD[a], Mark Bittman, MD[b],
Monica Epelman, MD[c], Sara O. Vargas, MD[d],
Edward Y. Lee, MD, MPH[e],*

KEYWORDS

- Children • Pediatric • Kidney • Mass • Magnetic resonance imaging

KEY POINTS

- Children younger than 7 to 9 years may have difficulty undergoing renal magnetic resonance (MR) imaging because of anxiety and/or inability to lie still. Distraction techniques and sedation/general anesthesia are commonly used methods for helping young children cooperate with renal MR imaging.
- At present, renal MR imaging is performed at field strength of either 1.5 or 3-T. While the current trend is toward imaging at higher field strength, it is important for pediatric radiologists to understand the advantages and disadvantages of MR imaging at higher field strength as it applies to renal imaging.
- Angiomyolipoma is a benign renal mass that can often be diagnosed conclusively on MR imaging, owing to the presence of internal adipose tissue components. Fat-poor angiomyolipomas, however, pose a diagnostic dilemma and can be difficult to distinguish from malignancy.
- For malignant renal masses, MR imaging is very useful for detecting synchronous renal masses, abdominal metastasis, and extrarenal/vascular tumor invasion, all of which have important therapeutic implications.
- Patient age, clinical symptoms, and syndromic associations are important ancillary data for narrowing down the differential diagnosis of a pediatric renal mass.

INTRODUCTION

Imaging plays an important role in the detection and characterization of renal abnormalities in children. Noninvasive discrimination of benign from malignant renal masses is essential in avoiding unnecessary potential morbidity associated with invasive biopsy or surgical resection. Magnetic resonance imaging (MRI) plays an important role in renal lesion characterization because of its cross-sectional imaging capability, superior soft-tissue contrast resolution, and lack of ionizing radiation exposure. This article reviews the MR imaging features of benign and malignant renal masses that occur in the pediatric population.

[a] Pediatric Imaging and Abdominal Imaging & Intervention, Department of Radiology, Massachusetts General Hospital, Harvard Medical School, 55 Fruit Street, Ellison 237, Boston, MA 02114, USA; [b] Department of Radiology, Cohen Children's Medical Center of New York, North Shore-Long Island Jewish Medical Center, 270-05 76th Avenue, New Hyde Park, NY 11040, USA; [c] Department of Radiology, Nemours Children's Hospital, 13535 Nemours Parkway, Orlando, FL 32827, USA; [d] Department of Pathology, Boston Children's Hospital, 300 Longwood Avenue, Boston, MA 02115, USA; [e] Magnetic Resonance Imaging, Division of Thoracic Imaging, Department of Radiology, Boston Children's Hospital, Harvard Medical School, 300 Longwood Avenue, Boston, MA 02115, USA
* Corresponding author.
E-mail address: Edward.Lee@childrens.harvard.edu

Magn Reson Imaging Clin N Am 21 (2013) 697–715
http://dx.doi.org/10.1016/j.mric.2013.06.001

Imaging and clinical features that are helpful in distinguishing among these lesions are highlighted.

IMAGING TECHNIQUE

MR imaging evaluation of renal masses in pediatric patients is typically performed on a 1.5- or 3-Tesla (T) scanner using a phased-array receiver coil with the patient placed in supine position. Imaging at higher field strength (3-T) offers several benefits for pediatric imaging, including high signal-to-noise ratio (SNR), improved spatial resolution, and faster scan times.[1,2] However, 3-T MR imaging also has disadvantages that apply to pediatric renal imaging, including increased susceptibility artifacts from air within adjacent lungs and bowel loops as well as increased energy deposition, particularly for pediatric abdominal examinations, which can approach patient Specific absorption rate (SAR) limits. Overall, the current trend in United States academic medical centers is toward higher-field-strength pediatric abdominal MR imaging. The receiver coil for pediatric abdominal imaging should fit snugly around the patient to maximize spatial resolution and SNR while minimizing the risk of thermal injury from direct skin contact. However, this can be difficult, as typical adult MR coils need to be fitted to pediatric patients ranging from infants to young adults. A head or extremity or cardiac can often accommodate infants and small children, whereas a body coil is typically used for larger children and adolescents.[3,4] Whole-body coils that include coil elements embedded in the scan table have also been used with success.

Compared with adult imaging, patient motion is a more substantial problem with pediatric renal MR imaging. Sources include voluntary motion from patient muscular movements in the scanner, as well as involuntary motion predominantly caused by respiration in children unable to suspend breathing on command. To minimize scan times, parallel imaging and fast imaging techniques can be used (**Box 1**).[5]

Patient Preparation

Patients 7 to 9 years and older usually are able to cooperate with renal MR imaging after an explanation of the procedure and reassurance. Distraction techniques including the use of MR imaging–compatible music and video players as well as scanning during off-hours to minimize ambient noise and activity can also be helpful. Similarly, newborns and young infants may tolerate renal MR imaging without the need for sedation, if they are well fed and comfortably swaddled. For children younger than 7 years, sedation or general

---

Box 1
Pediatric renal MR imaging provides the following information

- Mass size, location, and number
- Postcontrast enhancement characteristics
- Tissue composition based on MR signal characteristics (eg, cystic, adipose, hemorrhagic/proteinaceous, ossified)
- Presence of additional lesions in ipsilateral and contralateral kidneys
- Presence of extrarenal extension
- Presence of vascular and lymphatic involvement
- Presence of intra-abdominal metastasis

---

anesthesia often is essential to relieve patient anxiety and minimize patient motion during imaging.

Sedation

Several sedation medications are currently used for pediatric MR imaging, including chloral hydrate, pentobarbital, propofol, midazolam, and dexmedetomidine.[6,7] The level of sedation required can be as little as anxiolysis in an awake patient, but typically involves either moderate/deep sedation or general anesthesia in young children undergoing MR imaging. Advantages of sedation include minimization of total scan time and improvement in image quality from reduced motion artifact. In general, the least amount of sedation necessary for the patient to tolerate MR imaging is administered, both to minimize post–MR imaging side effects and to facilitate patient induction and emergence from sedation. Airway protection via endotracheal intubation may be necessary if high-quality imaging with respiratory suspension is required or if the child has a several breath holds significant risk of aspiration while under sedation. Good communication between the radiologist and the anesthesiologist or other health care provider administering sedation is of paramount importance. As always, the proper balance should be struck between adequate sedation for patient comfort and scan performance, and minimization of potential neurologic and cognitive effects associated with prolonged anesthesia.[8]

Administration of intravenous contrast material

Contrast agents used for clinical pediatric renal MR imaging are gadolinium chelate extracellular contrast agents that cause T1 shortening of blood vessels and perfused tissues. The typical dose for intravenous administration is 0.1 mmol/kg.[9] These contrast agents are generally avoided in the setting of acute kidney injury or severe chronic kidney disease (estimated glomerular filtration rate <30 mL/min) owing to the risk of nephrogenic systemic fibrosis.

Imaging Sequences

In general, the main MRI sequences for evaluation of renal masses in pediatric patients include coronal half-Fourier (or single-shot) fast spin-echo (HASTE or SSFSE) T2-weighted, axial dual-echo (in- and opposed-phase) gradient-recalled echo (GRE) T1-weighted, axial fast spin-echo (FSE) fat-suppressed T2-weighted, and 3-dimensional GRE fat-suppressed T1-weighted pre- and post-contrast administration in multiple planes.[10] There has also been increasing use of diffusion-weighted (DW) imaging for renal mass characterization, based on the premise that densely cellular masses are associated with restriction in the molecular motion of water. In older children and adolescents, most of these MR imaging sequences can be performed as a 15- to 25-second breath-hold acquisition. However, in younger children and sedated patients, these sequences often need to be modified to account for respiratory motion and longer scan-acquisition times. Such modifications include increased use of SSFSE sequences, respiratory triggering/navigator echoes, T2-weighted sequences with motion correction, and signal averaging to reduce respiratory artifact.[3]

SPECTRUM OF IMAGING FINDINGS
Primary Neoplasms

Benign neoplasms
A principal role of MR imaging is to confirm and characterize that a suspected renal lesion seen on another imaging modality (often ultrasonography in children) represents a solid renal mass and not a benign cyst or normal anatomic structure (eg, prominent column of Bertin). Because of the substantial overlap in imaging appearance between benign and malignant renal neoplasms in children, the MR appearance of a solid renal mass often is indeterminate, and histologic sampling is usually required for definitive diagnosis. Among benign renal neoplasms that occur in children, angiomyolipoma is the one type that often can be definitively diagnosed by MR imaging. Patient age, as well as the location and imaging appearance, can be helpful in narrowing the differential diagnosis (**Table 1**).

Congenital mesoblastic nephroma
Congenital mesoblastic nephroma is the most common solid renal tumor presenting in the neonatal period. Typically this mass presents in utero or within the first 3 months of life, and almost all cases occur within the first year.[11] The tumor consists of spindle-shaped cells showing fibroblastic/myofibroblastic differentiation (**Fig. 1**). It may occur as (1) the classic type, which resembles infantile fibromatosis, (2) the cellular type, which histologically and genetically resembles infantile fibrosarcoma, or (3) a mixed histologic pattern with areas of both.[12] The most common clinical presentation is a palpable abdominal mass, with hematuria being less frequent.[13]

On imaging (**Fig. 2**), mesoblastic nephroma usually appears as a large solid mass occupying a significant portion of the kidney; associated renal sinus involvement is frequent. Because of the large size of the mass, there may be associated hemorrhagic or cystic internal areas, although the margins of the mass are typically smooth.[11] Mesoblastic nephroma typically exhibits benign behavior, and complete cure is often achieved by nephrectomy alone. Recurrences and metastasis, occurring only in tumors with cellular histology, are seen in approximately 5% to 10% of patients.[14,15] For this reason, patients are typically followed for a short time after excision to exclude residual/recurrent disease.

Angiomyolipoma Angiomyolipoma (AML) is a hamartomatous mass composed of multiple benign tissue elements, including vascular, smooth-muscle, and adipose components. It is currently viewed as a neoplastic proliferation of perivascular epithelioid cells (PEC), and is thus a member of the "PEComa" family. Sporadic AMLs typically occur as single lesions and most often occur in adults. By contrast, AMLs occurring in children are most often multiple, bilateral, and associated with tuberous sclerosis complex (TSC).[13] Eighty percent of patients with TSC develop AMLs by 10 years of age.[16] AMLs in children are often asymptomatic and are discovered incidentally on imaging studies or as part of TSC workup. AMLs greater than 4 cm in diameter are associated with an increased risk of spontaneous hemorrhage because of the formation of aneurysms within the vascular components of the tumor.[17] AML associated hemorrhage bleeding can produce symptoms ranging from flank/abdominal pain or hematuria to life-threatening hypotension and volume loss. Severe spontaneous renal hemorrhage into the subcapsular and retroperitoneal space has been termed Wunderlich syndrome.[18]

The characteristic imaging feature of AML (**Fig. 3**) is the presence of bulk fatty elements, which on MR imaging appear as T1-/T2-weighted

Table 1
Characteristic clinical and imaging features of malignant renal masses in children

Tumor Type	Typical Age at Presentation	Associated Conditions	Imaging Features
Wilms tumor	<7 y (mean 3–4 y)	WAGR, Beckwith-Wiedemann, hemihypertrophy, sporadic aniridia	Large solid mass compressing normal kidney, "claw sign" of normal renal solid +/− cystic areas, +/− renal vein/IVC invasion
Renal cell carcinoma	Older children and adolescents (mean 9–10 y)	VHL, possibly TSC	Small or large solid or cystic renal mass; +/− calcification, hemorrhage
Medullary carcinoma	Adolescents and young adults	Sickle cell trait, hemoglobin SC disease	Large central renal mass causing hydronephrosis, usually metastatic at time of presentation
Rhabdoid tumor	<2 y (median 11 mo)	Synchronous or metachronous intracranial tumors	Large renal mass extending to hilum, often with calcifications or necrosis, frequently metastatic
Clear cell sarcoma	Young children (1–4 y)	None	Solid mass with well-circumscribed borders, associated with bone metastasis
Lymphoma	Children and adolescents >5 y	Non-Hodgkin lymphoma	One or more solid hypoenhancing masses, often exhibiting restricted diffusion on DW imaging
Leukemia	Young children (3–5 y)	Acute lymphoblastic leukemia	Diffuse renal parenchymal infiltration with reniform enlargement, or multiple renal masses

Abbreviations: DW, diffusion-weighted; IVC, inferior vena cava; TSC, tuberous sclerosis complex; VHL, von Hippel-Lindau syndrome; WAGR, WAGR syndrome (Wilms tumor, aniridia, genitourinary anomalies, mental retardation).

hyperintense internal foci that display signal loss on fat-suppressed sequences.[10] However, AMLs with scant fat can be difficult to distinguish from malignant renal masses. MR imaging features such as T2-weighted signal hypointensity, as well as homogeneous signal loss on T1-weighted GRE opposed-phase chemical shift imaging, have been proposed as MR features suggestive of lipid-poor AML.[10,19] T1-weighted opposed-phase images can also be useful for visualizing

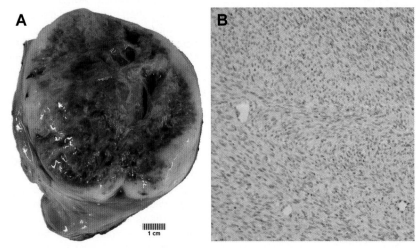

Fig. 1. Pathologic features of congenital mesoblastic nephroma. (*A*) Gross appearance of a cellular congenital mesoblastic nephroma (primary renal infantile fibrosarcoma), occurring as a well-circumscribed tan mass with central hemorrhage and necrosis. (*B*) Microscopic examination shows characteristic spindle-shaped cells arranged in fascicles (hematoxylin-eosin, original magnification ×20).

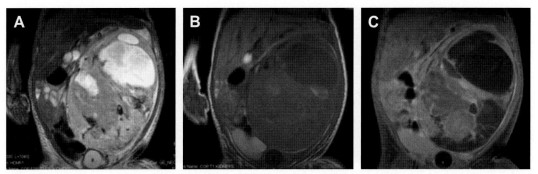

Fig. 2. Imaging appearance of congenital mesoblastic nephroma in a 2-day-old female infant. (*A*) Coronal T2-weighted image demonstrates a large mixed solid-cystic mass occupying almost the entire left abdomen. Coronal T1 fat-suppressed precontrast (*B*) and postcontrast (*C*) images demonstrate enhancement of the solid portions of the mass with absence of enhancement in the cystic component. This mass was excised and found on pathology to be congenital mesoblastic nephroma. (*Courtesy of* Ethan Smith, MD, Section of Pediatric Radiology, Department of Radiology, C.S. Mott Children's Hospital, University of Michigan, Ann Arbor, MI.)

areas of signal loss (so-called India ink artifact) at the interface of fat-containing AMLs and normal renal parenchyma (**Fig. 4**). For lesions smaller than 4 cm, serial imaging surveillance is recommended to document growth rate. For rapidly growing lesions with no obvious adipose elements, biopsy or surgical excision may be performed to exclude malignancy (typically renal cell carcinoma). For AMLs larger than 4 cm, catheter embolization or surgical excision are commonly performed to prevent catastrophic hemorrhage.[20]

In TSC patients with large AMLs, surgery is avoided whenever possible to preserve renal parenchyma, as these patients typically undergo premature loss of renal function from renal replacement by cysts and AMLs.[13]

Cystic nephroma and cystic partially differentiated nephroblastoma: These terms encompass uncommon, benign, loculated cystic renal neoplasms that vary with respect to the histologic composition of the internal septa.[13] Cystic

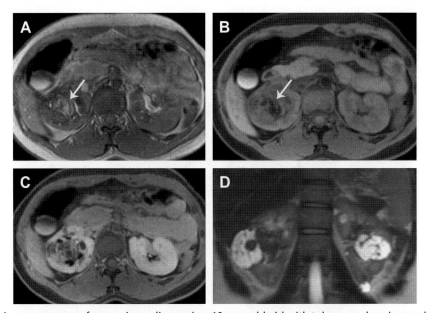

Fig. 3. Imaging appearance of an angiomyolipoma in a 10-year-old girl with tuberous sclerosis complex. Axial T1-weighted MR images without (*A*) and with (*B*) fat suppression demonstrate a right renal mass containing adipose tissue evidenced as T1-weighted hyperintense foci exhibiting signal loss on fat-suppressed imaging (*arrows*). T1-weighted fat-suppressed postcontrast image (*C*) demonstrates lesion enhancement, consistent with an angiomyolipoma. Coronal T2-weighted image (*D*) shows multiple additional cysts and angiomyolipomas in both kidneys, consistent with tuberous sclerosis complex.

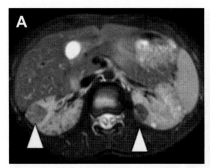
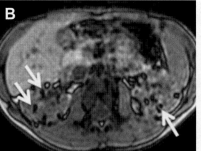
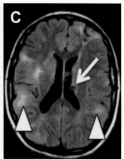

Fig. 4. MR imaging of TSC. Axial T2-weighted fat-suppressed image (*A*) shows bilateral T2-hypointense renal masses (*arrowheads*). Axial T1-weighted gradient-recalled echo opposed-phase image (*B*) shows numerous areas of chemical shift artifact within the kidneys at the interface of the masses and normal renal parenchyma (*arrows*), confirming these lesions are AMLs. Axial fluid-attenuated inversion recovery image (*C*) through the lateral ventricles shows numerous geographic areas of cortical/subcortical hyperintensity (*arrowheads*), consistent with tubers in this patient with TSC. A calcified subependymal nodule (*arrow*) is also noted. (*Courtesy of* Jonathan R. Dillman, MD, Section of Pediatric Radiology, Department of Radiology, C.S. Mott Children's Hospital, University of Michigan, Ann Arbor, MI.)

nephroma has septations composed of fibrous tissue and may contain mature renal elements (**Fig. 5**), whereas cystic partially differentiated nephroblastoma has septa containing immature/blastemal elements.[12,21,22] The lesions have traditionally been considered a part of a histologic spectrum that at the more malignant end encompasses Wilms tumor. Cystic nephroma and cystic partially differentiated nephroblastoma are, however, distinct as cystic renal tumors that may be associated with pleuropulmonary blastoma family cancer syndrome, recently found to occur in patients with mutations in the gene *DICER1*.[23] Cystic nephroma and cystic partially differentiating nephroblastoma demonstrate a bimodal age distribution, with an initial peak in children younger than

4 years (predominantly boys with cystic partially differentiated nephroblastoma). A second peak in adulthood is accounted for predominantly by women with multilocular adult cystic nephroma, thought to represent a different entity from the pediatric cystic nephroma.[22] The typical clinical presentation is a palpable abdominal mass.

On imaging, cystic nephroma and cystic partially differentiating nephroblastoma appear as discrete cystic masses (**Fig. 6**) with multiple thin internal septations that can enhance.[11] Classically, extension of the mass into the renal pelvis has been considered a specific feature. Cystic nephroma and cystic partially differentiated nephroblastoma cannot be reliably distinguished by imaging from each other or from other primary renal

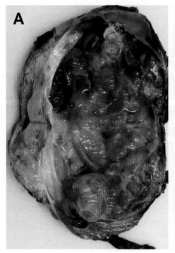
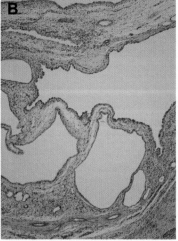

Fig. 5. Pathologic features of cystic nephroma. (*A*) Gross appearance, showing multiple thin-walled cysts filled with clear fluid. (*B*) Microscopically, the cysts show hobnailed epithelium-lined septa containing benign stromal elements (hematoxylin-eosin, original magnification ×20).

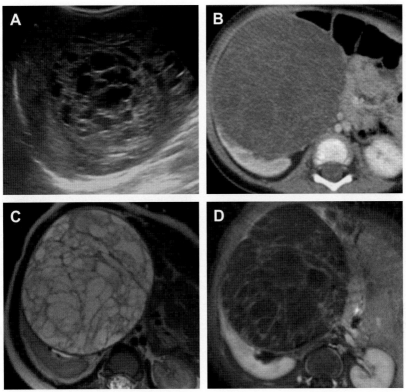

Fig. 6. Imaging features of a cystic partially differentiated nephroblastoma in an 8-year-old boy. (*A*) Ultrasonography shows a complex cystic mass in the right abdomen. (*B*) Axial contrast-enhanced CT shows the mass to be renal in origin. Axial T2-weighted (*C*) and T1-weighted fat-suppressed postcontrast (*D*) MR images show the mass to be predominantly composed of innumerable cysts (*C*) separated by thin enhancing septations (*D*).

neoplasms that can have a markedly cystic growth pattern, such as Wilms tumor, renal cell carcinoma. Surgical excision is considered the mainstay of treatment, with local tumor recurrence being rare.

Ossifying renal tumor of infancy Ossifying renal tumor of infancy (ORTI) is a rare benign renal tumor that was first identified in 1980, with only a small number of cases reported in the literature.[24,25] Ossifying renal tumors are thought to be urothelial in origin and attached to the papillae of the renal medullary pyramids, from which they extend centrally into the renal collecting system.[13] These lesions consist of spindle cells and osteoid matrix, and exhibit clonal cytogenetic aberrations. The reported age range for ORTI is 6 days to 14 months.[11] Hematuria is the most commonly reported clinical presentation.

On imaging, ORTI most commonly appears as a calcified soft-tissue mass in the renal collecting system, with no significant contrast enhancement.[11] On MR imaging, the calcifications typically appear T1-/T2-weighted hypointense and can exhibit susceptibility artifact. The mass is typically

less than 3 cm in diameter.[26] It can be associated with hydronephrosis and be mistaken for a stag-horn calculus. This tumor exhibits benign behavior, with no cases of metastasis or tumor recurrence following surgical resection.[13]

Malignant neoplasms
As mentioned earlier, it is often difficult to differentiate benign from malignant renal lesions by MRI. One of the most important roles of MRI is local staging of a suspected renal malignancy, with MR imaging being helpful for the detection of extracapsular and vascular invasion because of its superior soft-tissue contrast and the availability of multiple MR image acquisitions following intravenous administration of contrast material. Local staging by MR imaging is often performed in tandem with systemic staging (eg, thoracic computed tomography).

Nephrogenic rests and nephroblastomatosis Nephrogenic rests are persistent collections of embryonic cells within the kidneys after 36 weeks' gestational age (**Fig. 7**). These cells are considered to represent a kidney malformation, but in reality

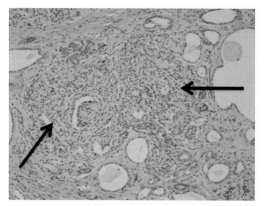

Fig. 7. Histologic appearance of nephrogenic rest. An intralobar nephrogenic rest (*arrows*) from the kidney of a 4-year-old with Wilms tumor shows primitive abortive tubules and glomerular structures, sclerotic stroma, and calcifications (hematoxylin-eosin, original magnification ×20).

they occupy a spectrum between malformation and neoplasm, because they may proliferate, at times becoming larger than the kidney itself, and may give rise to Wilms tumors. When diffuse or multifocal, they are referred to as nephroblastomatosis. Nephroblastomatosis is a benign but premalignant condition that carries an increased risk of malignant degeneration to Wilms tumor. Nephrogenic rests are classified by location into perilobar and intralobar rests, which have different syndromic associations and malignant potential.[13,27] Perilobar rests are the more common form and are confined to the renal cortex. These rests have relatively lower malignant potential (1%–2% risk) and are associated with Beckwith-Wiedemann (omphalocele, macroglossia, gigantism, genitourinary anomalies) and Perlman (polyhydramnios, cryptorchidism, gigantism, characteristic facies) syndromes, as well as trisomy 18.[3] By contrast, intralobar rests are less

common, can be located anywhere in the renal parenchyma, have a higher rate of Wilms degeneration (4%–5% risk), and are associated with Drash (renal failure and ambiguous genitalia in genotypic males) and WAGR (Wilms tumor, aniridia, growth retardation) syndromes (**Fig. 8**) as well as sporadic aniridia.[28] Nephrogenic rests occur in approximately 1% of all infants and are seen in the kidneys of approximately 30% to 40% of patients with Wilms tumor.[27] Virtually all patients with bilateral Wilms tumor have nephroblastomatosis.[29]

On MR imaging, macroscopic nephrogenic rests typically appear as multiple T1-weighted hypointense, T2-weighted isointense or hyperintense, minimally enhancing nodules (**Fig. 9**) distributed along the periphery of the kidneys.[3,11,13] Confluent diffuse nephroblastomatosis can also manifest as diffuse renal enlargement associated with a heterogeneously enhancing peripheral rind.[27] Management of nephroblastomatosis is controversial and consists of either prophylactic chemotherapy or close imaging surveillance for enlarging nodules (**Fig. 10**) suggestive of malignant transformation to Wilms tumor.[3]

Wilms tumor Wilms tumor is the most common pediatric renal mass, with an annual incidence of 1 in 10,000 children younger than 15 years worldwide.[3,13] Similar to nephroblastomatosis, Wilms tumor is thought to arise from rests of embryonic nephrogenic cells that persist in the kidney after birth. Most cases occur before 5 years of age, with a mean age between 3 and 4 years.[30,31] Grossly, Wilms tumor consists of a fleshy pale mass, usually quite large, often with foci of hemorrhage, necrosis, and cyst formation. Microscopically, it is composed of 3 elements ("triphasic"): blastema, stroma, and epithelial elements in varying proportions (**Fig. 11**). Although the vast majority of Wilms tumors arise sporadically, there are 2 genes on chromosome 11, known as *WT1* and

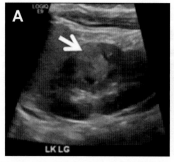
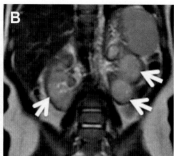
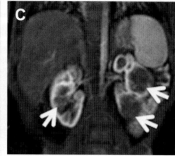

Fig. 8. A 7-month-old boy with WAGR syndrome. Screening ultrasonography (*A*) shows an echogenic mass in mid left kidney (*arrow*). Coronal T2-weighted MR image (*B*) shows multiple hyperintense masses in left kidney (*arrows*). Similar abnormal signal is noted in the right kidney lower pole. Postcontrast fat-suppressed T1-weighted images (*C*) show bilateral areas of hypoenhancement (*arrows*), consistent with nephroblastomatosis.

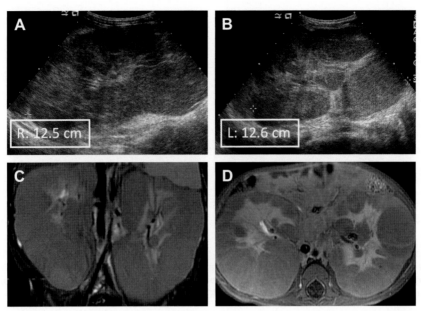

Fig. 9. Imaging appearance of nephroblastomatosis in a 14-month-old boy. Renal ultrasonography (*A, B*) demonstrates marked enlargement and heterogeneous echotexture of both kidneys. Coronal T2-weighted fat-suppressed (*C*) and axial T1-weighted fat-suppressed postcontrast (*D*) MR images demonstrate innumerable, conglomerate peripheral hypoenhancing nodules in both kidneys, consistent with nephroblastomatosis.

WT2, associated with congenital Wilms tumor formation.[13] *WT1* (on 11p13) is associated with WAGR syndrome and Drash syndrome, whereas *WT2* (on 11p1) is associated with Beckwith-Wiedemann syndrome and hemihypertrophy.[3,32] Inherited Wilms tumor without other syndromic manifestations is rare and is not associated with mutations in either gene.[30] Wilms tumor has been reported to be associated with a variety of genitourinary tract anomalies including horseshoe kidney, cryptorchidism, renal hypoplasia, ectopic renal positioning, and ureteropelvic duplication.[33] The typical presentation is a palpable abdominal mass. Up to 25% of patients have hypertension at presentation because of tumor renin production.[27] Hematuria and pain are uncommon clinical manifestations of Wilms tumor.

On imaging, Wilms tumor frequently appears as a solid renal mass that distorts the surrounding renal parenchyma and collecting system (**Fig. 12**). Wilms tumors are often quite large at presentation and can be difficult to distinguish from extrarenal tumors such as neuroblastoma. The presence of a "claw sign," whereby a semicircular rim of normal renal parenchyma can be seen surrounding the mass, is considered a helpful imaging sign of Wilms tumor. Wilms tumors on MR imaging are typically T1-weighted hypointense and T2-weighted hyperintense, with initial hypoenhancement relative to normal renal parenchyma followed by delayed washout on dynamic postgadolinium imaging. Imaging staging of Wilms tumor involves evaluation of both kidneys for tumor involvement, the renal veins and inferior vena cava for vascular

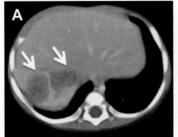
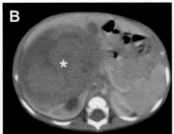
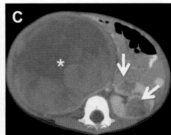

Fig. 10. Imaging appearance of a Wilms tumor arising in a 10-month-old boy with a history of nephroblastomatosis. Serial (*A–C*) axial contrast-enhanced CT images demonstrate numerous hypoenhancing nodules in both kidneys (*arrows*), consistent with nephroblastomatosis. In the right kidney mid pole there is a dominant, partially cystic mass (*asterisk*), consistent with Wilms tumor.

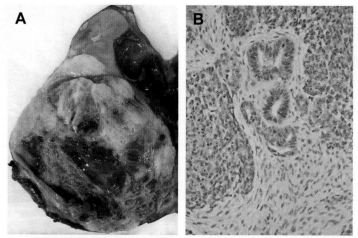

Fig. 11. Pathologic features of Wilms tumor in an 8-year-old girl. (*A*) Grossly, the tumor was a large (10.5 cm) mass replacing the lower pole and hilum; with a tan appearance containing internal areas of hemorrhage, necrosis, and cystic degeneration. (*B*) Microscopically, the tumor was "triphasic," showing blastema, stroma, and epithelial elements (hematoxylin-eosin, original magnification ×40).

invasion, perinephric and lymphatic involvement, and distant sites of metastasis.[3,11] MR is considered the imaging modality of choice to assess multifocal disease and venous invasion, both of which have treatment implications.[13] Renal vein extension is present in 15% to 20% of cases while bilateral disease is present in 5% to 10%.[3] The most common sites of distant metastasis are the lungs (15%–20%) and liver (10%–15%).[34] Wilms tumor is typically treated with a combination of nephrectomy/tumor resection and neoadjuvant/adjuvant chemotherapy depending on tumor size and stage, with radiation therapy added in cases of residual disease suspected at surgery.[13] In bilateral Wilms tumor, the goal of treatment is preservation of as much normal renal parenchyma as possible.

Imaging also plays an important role in screening children with syndromes that carry increased risk of development of Wilms tumor. For these patients, serial ultrasonographic evaluation every 3 to 4 months until at least the age of 7 years is recommended.[31,35] Among children with Beckwith-Wiedemann syndrome or idiopathic hemihypertrophy, one study suggested that frequent ultrasonography screening led to earlier detection of Wilms tumor, with a significantly higher percentage of early-stage tumors identified.[35]

Renal cell carcinoma Renal cell carcinoma (RCC) is predominantly an adult disease, with less than 2% of cases occurring in the pediatric population. It accounts for less than 10% of all pediatric primary renal malignancies and may occur in older children (mean age 9–10 years).[11,36,37] Patients with von Hippel–Lindau syndrome (VHL; hemangioblastoma, pheochromocytoma, pancreatic cysts) are at increased risk of developing multiple RCCs at an early age, and all pediatric patients who develop RCC should be screened for VHL.[38] Pediatric patients are particularly subject to the

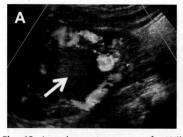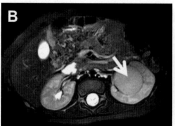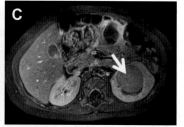

Fig. 12. Imaging appearance of a Wilms tumor in a 6-month-old girl with hemihypertrophy syndrome. Surveillance ultrasonography with color Doppler (*A*) demonstrates a near-isoechoic mass in the left kidney (*arrow*). MR T2-weighted fat-suppressed (*B*) and T1-weighted fat-suppressed postcontrast (*C*) imaging confirms the presence of a T2 hyperintense (*B*; *arrow*), hypoenhancing (*C*; *arrow*) mass in the central left kidney that was resected and confirmed to be a Wilms tumor by histology.

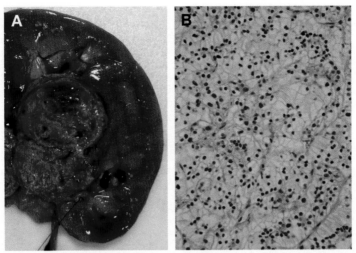

Fig. 13. Pathologic features of a renal cell carcinoma harboring an Xp11 chromosomal translocation in an 11-year-old girl. Grossly (*A*), the tumor is a 5-cm well-circumscribed tan-red mass. Microscopically (*B*), it showed nested epithelial cells with abundant clear cytoplasm (hematoxylin-eosin, original magnification ×40).

development of specific subtypes of RCC, namely translocation-associated RCC (eg, Xp11 RCC), papillary RCC, renal medullary carcinoma (see later discussion), and neuroblastoma-associated oncocytic RCC.[39] Microscopically, RCC consists of epithelial cells, often in nests or acini separated by a rich vascular network (**Fig. 13**). RCC in children typically presents with gross hematuria, flank pain, and a palpable mass, similar to its presentation in adults. Compared with Wilms tumor, hematuria is more frequently observed children with RCC.[36]

The imaging features of RCC are often similar to those of Wilms tumor (**Figs. 14** and **15**).[13,40] RCC is a T1-weighted hypointense, T2-weighted hyperintense, enhancing renal mass that distorts the surrounding parenchyma and has variable degrees of necrosis, calcification, and hemorrhage. Imaging by MR imaging or computed tomography (CT) plays an important role in locoregional staging of

RCC, including assessment of tumor size, and extracapsular and vascular extension. Nodal spread to adjacent retroperitoneal lymph nodes can also be assessed by imaging. Twenty percent of pediatric RCC patients present with metastatic disease, predominantly to lungs, bones, liver, or brain.[13,40] Surgical resection is a standard part of treatment, with prognosis being related to tumor staging.

Renal medullary carcinoma Renal medullary carcinoma, which is considered histologically to be a subset of RCC, is an extremely aggressive renal malignancy that occurs almost exclusively in adolescent and adult patients with sickle cell trait or hemoglobin SC disease.[41] The age range for renal medullary carcinoma is 10 to 39 years, with a mean age of 20 years.[13] Renal medullary carcinoma is believed to arise within the renal medullary tissue at the pelvic-mucosal interface. The tumor

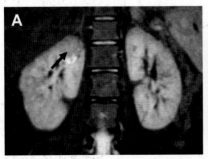
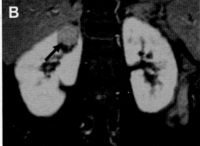

Fig. 14. Imaging appearance of a renal cell carcinoma in a 14-year-old girl. Coronal T2-weighted fat-suppressed (*A*) and T1-weighted fat-suppressed postcontrast nephrographic phase (*B*) MR images demonstrate a small, well-circumscribed, hypoenhancing mass (*arrows*), which was excised and diagnosed as renal cell carcinoma.

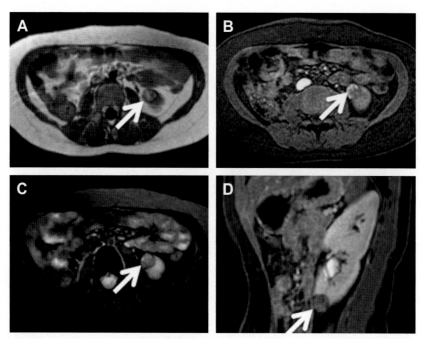

Fig. 15. A 10-year-old girl with prior right nephrectomy for Wilms tumor. Follow-up surveillance MR imaging demonstrates a left lower pole renal mass (*arrows*) exhibiting hyperintensity on T1-weighted images (*A*) that persists on T1-weighted fat-suppressed imaging (*B*), and is due to lesional hemorrhage. The lesion is predominantly hypointense on T2-weighted fat-suppressed images (*C; arrow*), and demonstrates hypoenhancement compared with normal kidney parenchyma (*D; arrow*) on postcontrast T1-weighted fat-suppressed imaging. Pathology on the surgically excised mass diagnosed a translocation renal cell carcinoma. (*Courtesy of* Jonathan R. Dillman, MD, Section of Pediatric Radiology, Department of Radiology, C.S. Mott Children's Hospital, University of Michigan, Ann Arbor, MI.)

then grows quickly to occupy the renal pelvis, where it is then free to disseminate via hilar vessels and lymphatics.[13] The most common presenting symptom is painless gross hematuria, but abdominal pain, weight loss, and fever are other clinical signs.[42,43]

On imaging, renal medullary carcinoma appears as a central T1-weighted hypointense, T2-weighted hyperintense renal mass that involves the renal sinus (**Fig. 16**) and produces hydronephrosis as well as renal enlargement. The mass usually exhibits diminished enhancement in comparison with normal renal parenchyma, and contains central nonenhancing necrotic areas.[3] Renal medullary carcinoma may be sonographically occult due its central location, which may not alter the global renal contour.[43] As a result, MR imaging plays an important role in the workup of patients suspected of having this rare and rapidly progressive disease. Typically the mass has undergone metastasis at the time of presentation and prognosis is poor, with mean survival of less than 6 months.[13]

Rhabdoid tumor Rhabdoid tumor is a rare, highly aggressive renal malignancy of young children. It

comprises 2% of total renal malignancies in children, with a median age at diagnosis of 11 months, and 80% of cases occur in patients younger than 2 years.[30] The term rhabdoid refers to the histologic resemblance of the tumor to skeletal muscle, although the tumor is not of myogenic origin.[13] Rhabdoid tumors of infancy are associated with abnormalities in the *hSNF5/INI1* gene, sometimes as a germline mutation. There is an association between rhabdoid tumor and the presence of additional synchronous or metachronous primary intracranial tumors, including primitive neuroendocrine tumor, ependymoma, and astrocytoma, as well as atypical teratoid rhabdoid tumors.[44] The brain tumors associated with rhabdoid tumor usually occur near the midline and involve the posterior fossa.[3] Clinical manifestations of rhabdoid tumor vary, but include hematuria related to the primary tumor, or hypercalcemia from tumor-associated parathyroid-related hormone production.[20] Because of the aggressive nature of rhabdoid tumors, presenting symptoms are often related to metastatic lesions or associated intracranial lesions.

On imaging, rhabdoid tumors often appear as central renal masses extending to the renal hilum,

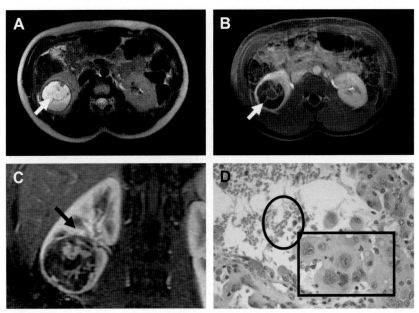

Fig. 16. Renal medullary carcinoma in a 17-year-old girl with sickle cell trait. Axial T2-weighted (*A*), and axial (*B*) and coronal (*C*) T1-weighted fat-suppressed postcontrast MR images demonstrate a mixed cystic-solid mass in the right kidney (*B; arrow*) that is centered in the renal medulla (*C; arrow*) and contains multiple internal cystic or necrotic areas (*A; arrow*). Hematoxylin-eosin staining of histologic specimen (*D; original magnification ×40*) from the excised mass demonstrates sickle-shaped erythrocytes (*ellipse*) adjacent to tumor cells (*rectangle*).

with indistinct margination (**Fig. 17**). Specific imaging features suggestive of rhabdoid tumor include subcapsular fluid, linear calcifications, and soft-tissue lobules interspersed with areas of hemorrhage/necrosis.[13] The crescentic subcapsular fluid collection is not pathognomonic for rhabdoid tumor, and has been reported be present in approximately half of cases. Rhabdoid tumors are extremely aggressive and frequently are metastatic at the time of clinical presentation, with pulmonary metastases most common. Prognosis is uniformly poor, with an 18-month survival rate of 20%.[45]

Clear cell sarcoma Clear cell sarcoma of the kidney is another rare malignancy, accounting for less than 5% of all pediatric primary renal tumors.[30] It is a tumor of young children, with a peak age of incidence between 1 and 4 years of age.[13] The tumor is composed of undifferentiated cells separated into cords and nests by a fine vascular network (**Fig. 18**). The clinical presentation is nonspecific, with the most common presenting symptom being a palpable abdominal mass.

Imaging most frequently demonstrates a solid T1-weighted hypointense/T2-weighted hyperintense, enhancing renal mass with well-circumscribed

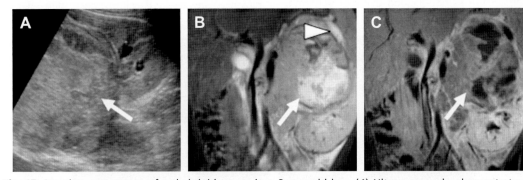

Fig. 17. Imaging appearance of a rhabdoid tumor in a 3-year-old boy. (*A*) Ultrasonography demonstrates the presence of a large, heterogeneous, ill-defined mass associated with the left kidney (*arrow*). Coronal T2-weighted (*B*) and T1-weighted fat-suppressed postcontrast (*C*) MR images show a large renal mass extending to the renal hilum (*arrows*) with internal necrotic regions, consistent with rhabdoid tumor. A small crescentic subcapsular fluid collection is also present (*arrowhead*).

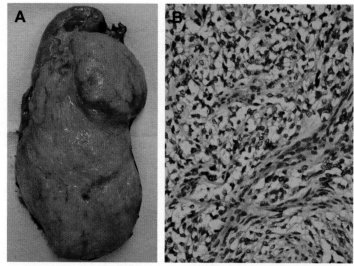

Fig. 18. Pathologic features of clear cell sarcoma. Grossly (*A*), the tumor appears as a tan, well-circumscribed mass. Microscopically (*B*), the tumor is composed of spindle-shaped cells separated into cords and nests by a fine vascular network (hematoxylin-eosin, original magnification ×20).

borders that is difficult to distinguish from Wilms tumor.[11] Compared with Wilms tumor, clear cell sarcoma of the kidney is a more aggressive tumor and carries increased rates of disease relapse and mortality. Therapy usually consists of nephrectomy plus chemotherapy; however, metastases can develop years later. The most common sites of metastasis are osseous (hence the tumor's former name of bone-metastasizing tumor of infancy); the presence of osseous metastasis from a renal primary malignancy is rare in Wilms tumor and should suggest alternative diagnoses, such as clear cell sarcoma. Spread to lymph nodes, brain, liver, and lungs is also seen.[13] Long-term survival rates range from 60% to 70%.[30]

Other sarcomas Other malignant tumors of childhood that occur with some regularity as primary tumors in the kidney include synovial sarcoma, Ewing sarcoma/primitive neuroectodermal tumor (**Fig. 19**), and desmoplastic round cell tumor.[12,46] These tumors typically contain characteristic genetic translocations, which have aided in their increasing recognition as primary renal occurrences. Radiologic features of this emerging category of pediatric disease have yet to be well characterized, although they are often indistinguishable from more common pediatric primary renal malignancies.

Secondary Neoplasms/Metastatic Disease

Lymphoma and leukemia
Lymphoma in children is most commonly non-Hodgkin lymphoma, which invades the kidney through either hematogenous or retroperitoneal spread. Lymphomatous involvement of the kidneys typically involves B-cell rather than T-cell

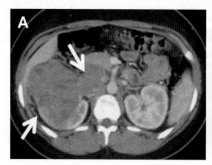
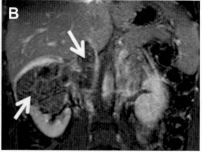

Fig. 19. A 14-year-old girl with right flank pain caused by renal Ewing sarcoma/primitive neuroectodermal tumor. Axial contrast-enhanced CT (*A*) shows a large right infiltrative renal mass with renal vein and inferior vena cava (IVC) extension (*arrows*). Coronal postcontrast fat-suppressed T1-weighted MR image (*B*) shows that the mass is hypoenhancing compared with normal kidney, and extends into the IVC (*arrows*).

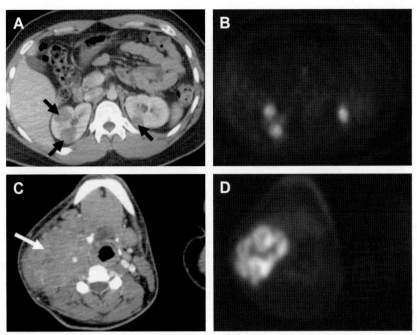

Fig. 20. Imaging appearance of renal lymphoma in an 18-year-old male with non-Hodgkin lymphoma. Positron emission tomography/CT demonstrates soft-tissue masses in both kidneys (*A; black arrows*) that demonstrate high ^{18}F-fluorodeoxyglucose (FDG) avidity (*B*). The same scan demonstrates confluent right cervical lymphadenopathy (*C; white arrow*) that exhibits a level of FDG uptake (*D*) similar to that of the renal lesions.

processes.[11] Primary renal lymphoma is extremely rare because of the absence of lymphatic vessels in the kidneys,[13] but has been reported in the literature.[47] Leukemic involvement of the kidneys in children most often arises from acute lymphoblastic leukemia (ALL),[48,49] which is the most common childhood malignancy. Clinical features of renal lymphoma or leukemia include abdominal pain, hematuria, weight loss, anemia, and a palpable mass,[13] although renal involvement by leukemia is more often clinically occult. Lymphoma most often affects children older than 5 years, whereas the typical age of presentation of ALL is 3 to 5 years.[3]

Renal lymphoma has multiple imaging manifestations.[50] Most commonly it appears as 1 or multiple renal masses that exert mass effect on the surrounding parenchyma and are hypoenhancing in comparison with normal kidney (**Fig. 20**).[13] There can also be diffuse infiltrative involvement of the kidney with reniform enlargement (**Fig. 21**).

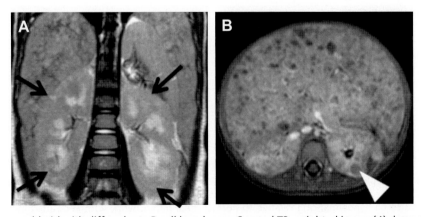

Fig. 21. A 3-year-old girl with diffuse large B-cell lymphoma. Coronal T2-weighted image (*A*) demonstrates innumerable liver masses and diffuse reniform enlargement of the kidneys (*arrows*). Axial T1-weighted fat-suppressed postcontrast image (*B*) shows that the enlarged kidneys contain many small hypoenhancing masses replacing most of the renal cortex (*arrowhead*).

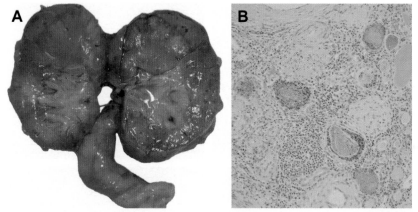

Fig. 22. Pathologic features of pyelonephritis occurring in the setting of a chronically obstructed dysplastic kidney with megaureter. Grossly (*A*), the bisected kidney demonstrates patchy areas of inflammatory infiltration corresponding to hypoenhancing regions seen on imaging. (*B*) Microscopic examination shows neutrophils within renal tubules and a lymphocytic interstitial inflammatory infiltrate, as well as underlying dysplastic features (hematoxylin-eosin, original magnification ×20).

These 2 imaging appearances are also commonly observed with renal leukemia.[11,49] The third and least common imaging appearance is a rind of perinephric soft tissue surrounding the kidney from tumor extension from either the retroperitoneum or the kidney,[51] with associated hydronephrosis if the tumor encases the renal pelvis. Lymphomatous masses frequently exhibit

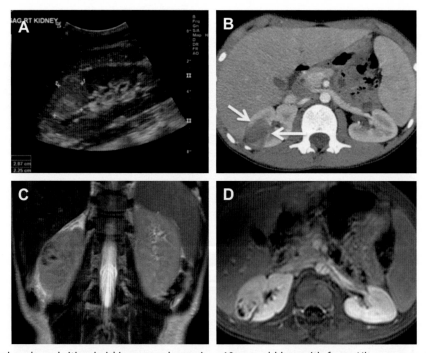

Fig. 23. Focal pyelonephritis mimicking a renal mass in a 10-year-old boy with fever. Ultrasonography (*A*) demonstrates a mass-like echogenic lesion in the upper pole of the right kidney. Contrast-enhanced CT (*B*) demonstrates the mass to be hypoenhancing relative to normal renal parenchyma, with ill-defined margins (*arrows*). Coronal T2-weighted MR image (*C*) demonstrates heterogeneous signal intensity with areas of focal signal hypointensity, which do not enhance on T1-weighted fat-suppressed postcontrast imaging (*D*). The lesion resolved following antibiotic treatment. (*Courtesy of* Jonathan R. Dillman, MD, Section of Pediatric Radiology, Department of Radiology, C.S. Mott Children's Hospital, University of Michigan, Ann Arbor, MI.)

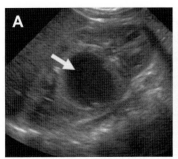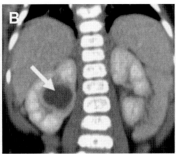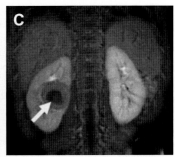

Fig. 24. Imaging appearance of a renal abscess in a 6-year-old boy. (*A*) Ultrasonography demonstrates the presence of a thick-walled fluid collection in the central right kidney (*arrow*). (*B*) On coronal contrast-enhanced CT, the central portion of the collection demonstrates fluid attenuation (*arrow*). (*C*) Coronal T1-weighted fat-suppressed postcontrast MR image confirms that only the peripheral wall of the collection enhances (*arrow*), consistent with an abscess.

restricted diffusion on MR DW imaging, and demonstrate increased ^{18}F-fluorodeoxyglucose avidity on positron emission tomography.

Infection

Pyelonephritis/renal abscess

Both acute and chronic bacterial infection of the kidney can result in a focal mass–like appearance that may mimic a tumor.[52] Acute pyelonephritis is associated with renal interstitial edema and vasospasm, which lead to compression of renal tubules[11] and focal mass–like areas of diminished contrast enhancement on imaging. It is characterized histologically by neutrophilic inflammation (**Fig. 22**). The term acute lobar nephronia has been used to describe this mass-like appearance of acute pyelonephritis.[53] Clinical symptoms of acute pyelonephritis in adolescents are similar to those in adults, including fever, chills, and flank pain. In infants and young children, however, symptoms may be vague and nonspecific.

On imaging, renal tubular compression related to infection leads to reduced cortical clearance of intravenous contrast and the appearance of either a focal hypoenhancing mass (**Fig. 23**) or a striated nephrogram on T1-weighted fat-suppressed postcontrast imaging. This area can exhibit mild T2-weighted signal hyperintensity. Although the presence of a superimposed renal parenchymal abscess is rare, it can arise as a result of incomplete treatment of acute pyelonephritis.[11] A renal (or perirenal) abscess would appear as a focal T1-weighted hypointense/T2-weighted hyperintense, peripherally enhancing parenchymal collection that often requires drainage (**Fig. 24**). There are numerous risk factors for acute pyelonephritis, including renal dysplasia or other anatomic abnormality, vesicoureteral reflux,

and nephrolithiasis. Imaging evaluation at the time of presentation typically starts with ultrasonography to help establish the diagnosis, followed by cross-sectional imaging (CT or MR imaging) to assess for associated anatomic risk factors or abscess. Following treatment, voiding cystoureterography and renal cortical scintigraphy may be performed to assess for vesicoureteral reflux and parenchymal scarring, respectively.

Chronic renal infection in the form of xanthogranulomatous pyelonephritis (XGP) can also mimic malignancy, appearing mass-like. Chronic urinary tract obstruction, usually due to a large obstructing calculus in the renal pelvis, causes renal enlargement, hydronephrosis, and parenchymal necrosis. XGP can be either a focal or diffuse process and can cause extensive surrounding inflammation within the retroperitoneum and even the body wall.[52]

SUMMARY

MR imaging is valuable in the confirmation and characterization of pediatric renal masses by providing information on tissue composition and number of lesions, as well as detecting extracapsular invasion, vascular involvement, and metastasis. In combination with clinical data, including age, genetic history, and presenting symptom(s) of patients, MR imaging can often suggest the diagnosis of renal masses arising in children, which in turn leads to optimal patient care.

REFERENCES

1. Chavhan GB, Babyn PS, Singh M, et al. MR imaging at 3.0 T in children: technical differences, safety issues, and initial experience. Radiographics 2009; 29:1451–66.

2. Chang KJ, Kamel IR, Macura KJ, et al. 3.0-T MR imaging of the abdomen: comparison with 1.5 T. Radiographics 2008;28:1983–98.

3. Siegel MJ, Chung EM. Wilms' tumor and other pediatric renal masses. Magn Reson Imaging Clin N Am 2008;16:479–97, vi.

4. Anupindi S, Jaramillo D. Pediatric magnetic resonance imaging techniques. Magn Reson Imaging Clin N Am 2002;10:189–207.

5. Pruessmann KP. Parallel imaging at high field strength: synergies and joint potential. Top Magn Reson Imaging 2004;15:237–44.

6. Slovis TL. Sedation and anesthesia issues in pediatric imaging. Pediatr Radiol 2011;41(Suppl 2):S14–6.

7. Cravero JP, Blike GT. Pediatric sedation. Curr Opin Anaesthesiol 2004;17:247–51.

8. Rappaport B, Mellon RD, Simone A, et al. Defining safe use of anesthesia in children. N Engl J Med 2011;364:1387–90.

9. Haliloglu M, Hoffer FA, Gronemeyer SA, et al. Applications of 3D contrast-enhanced MR angiography in pediatric oncology. Pediatr Radiol 1999; 29:863–8.

10. Pedrosa I, Sun MR, Spencer M, et al. MR imaging of renal masses: correlation with findings at surgery and pathologic analysis. Radiographics 2008;28: 985–1003.

11. Lee EY. CT imaging of mass-like renal lesions in children. Pediatr Radiol 2007;37:896–907.

12. Murphy WM, Grignon DJ, Perlman EJ. Tumors of the kidney, bladder, and related urinary structures. Washington, DC: American Registry of Pathology; 2004.

13. Lowe LH, Isuani BH, Heller RM, et al. Pediatric renal masses: Wilms tumor and beyond. Radiographics 2000;20:1585–603.

14. Schlesinger AE, Rosenfield NS, Castle VP, et al. Congenital mesoblastic nephroma metastatic to the brain: a report of two cases. Pediatr Radiol 1995;25(Suppl 1):S73–5.

15. Furtwaengler R, Reinhard H, Leuschner I, et al. Mesoblastic nephroma—a report from the Gesellschaft fur Padiatrische Onkologie und Hamatologie (GPOH). Cancer 2006;106:2275–83.

16. Ewalt DH, Sheffield E, Sparagana SP, et al. Renal lesion growth in children with tuberous sclerosis complex. J Urol 1998;160:141–5.

17. Kennelly MJ, Grossman HB, Cho KJ. Outcome analysis of 42 cases of renal angiomyolipoma. J Urol 1994;152:1988–91.

18. Eble JN. Angiomyolipoma of kidney. Semin Diagn Pathol 1998;15:21–40.

19. Hindman N, Ngo L, Genega EM, et al. Angiomyolipoma with minimal fat: can it be differentiated from clear cell renal cell carcinoma by using standard MR techniques? Radiology 2012;265: 468–77.

20. Geller E, Smergel EM, Lowry PA. Renal neoplasms of childhood. Radiol Clin North Am 1997;35:1391–413.

21. Sacher P, Willi UV, Niggli F, et al. Cystic nephroma: a rare benign renal tumor. Pediatr Surg Int 1998;13: 197–9.

22. Eble JN, Bonsib SM. Extensively cystic renal neoplasms: cystic nephroma, cystic partially differentiated nephroblastoma, multilocular cystic renal cell carcinoma, and cystic hamartoma of renal pelvis. Semin Diagn Pathol 1998;15:2–20.

23. Hill DA, Ivanovich J, Priest JR, et al. DICER1 mutations in familial pleuropulmonary blastoma. Science 2009;325:965.

24. Chatten J, Cromie WJ, Duckett JW. Ossifying tumor of infantile kidney: report of two cases. Cancer 1980;45:609–12.

25. Vazquez JL, Barnewolt CE, Shamberger RC, et al. Ossifying renal tumor of infancy presenting as a palpable abdominal mass. Pediatr Radiol 1998; 28:454–7.

26. Sotelo-Avila C, Beckwith JB, Johnson JE. Ossifying renal tumor of infancy: a clinicopathologic study of nine cases. Pediatr Pathol Lab Med 1995;15: 745–62.

27. Lonergan GJ, Martinez-Leon MI, Agrons GA, et al. Nephrogenic rests, nephroblastomatosis, and associated lesions of the kidney. Radiographics 1998;18:947–68.

28. Beckwith JB. Precursor lesions of Wilms tumor: clinical and biological implications. Med Pediatr Oncol 1993;21:158–68.

29. White KS, Grossman H. Wilms' and associated renal tumors of childhood. Pediatr Radiol 1991; 21:81–8.

30. Charles AK, Vujanic GM, Berry PJ. Renal tumours of childhood. Histopathology 1998;32:293–309.

31. Brodeur AE, Brodeur GM. Abdominal masses in children: neuroblastoma, Wilms tumor, and other considerations. Pediatr Rev 1991;12:196–207.

32. Coppes MJ, Pritchard-Jones K. Principles of Wilms' tumor biology. Urol Clin North Am 2000;27: 423–33, viii.

33. Neville H, Ritchey ML, Shamberger RC, et al. The occurrence of Wilms tumor in horseshoe kidneys: a report from the National Wilms Tumor Study Group (NWTSG). J Pediatr Surg 2002;37:1134–7.

34. Owens CM, Veys PA, Pritchard J, et al. Role of chest computed tomography at diagnosis in the management of Wilms' tumor: a study by the United Kingdom Children's Cancer Study Group. J Clin Oncol 2002;20:2768–73.

35. Choyke PL, Siegel MJ, Craft AW, et al. Screening for Wilms tumor in children with Beckwith-Wiedemann syndrome or idiopathic hemihypertrophy. Med Pediatr Oncol 1999;32:196–200.

36. Lack EE, Cassady JR, Sallan SE. Renal cell carcinoma in childhood and adolescence: a clinical

and pathological study of 17 cases. J Urol 1985;
133:822–8.

37. Selle B, Furtwängler R, Graf N, et al. Population-based study of renal cell carcinoma in children in Germany, 1980-2005: more frequently localized tumors and underlying disorders compared with adult counterparts. Cancer 2006;107:2906–14.

38. Hartman DS, Davis CJ Jr, Madewell JE, et al. Primary malignant renal tumors in the second decade of life: Wilms tumor versus renal cell carcinoma. J Urol 1982;127:888–91.

39. Perlman EJ. Pediatric renal cell carcinoma. In: Parham DR, editor. Current concepts in pediatric pathology. Philadelphia: Saunders; 2010. p. 641–51.

40. Downey RT, Dillman JR, Ladino-Torres MF, et al. CT and MRI appearances and radiologic staging of pediatric renal cell carcinoma. Pediatr Radiol 2012;42:410–7 [quiz: 513–4].

41. Davidson AJ, Choyke PL, Hartman DS, et al. Renal medullary carcinoma associated with sickle cell trait: radiologic findings. Radiology 1995;195:83–5.

42. Davis CJ Jr, Mostofi FK, Sesterhenn IA. Renal medullary carcinoma. The seventh sickle cell nephropathy. Am J Surg Pathol 1995;19:1–11.

43. Blitman NM, Berkenblit RG, Rozenblit AM, et al. Renal medullary carcinoma: CT and MRI features. AJR Am J Roentgenol 2005;185:268–72.

44. Agrons GA, Kingsman KD, Wagner BJ, et al. Rhabdoid tumor of the kidney in children: a comparative study of 21 cases. AJR Am J Roentgenol 1997;168: 447–51.

45. Chung CJ, Lorenzo R, Rayder S, et al. Rhabdoid tumors of the kidney in children: CT findings. AJR Am J Roentgenol 1995;164:697–700.

46. Wang LL, Perlman EJ, Vujanic GM, et al. Desmoplastic small round cell tumor of the kidney in childhood. Am J Surg Pathol 2007;31:576–84.

47. Dyer RB, Lowe LH, Zagoria RJ, et al. Mass effect in the renal sinus: an anatomic classification. Curr Probl Diagn Radiol 1994;23:1–27.

48. Son J, Lee EY, Restrepo R, et al. Focal renal lesions in pediatric patients. AJR Am J Roentgenol 2012; 199:W668–82.

49. Hilmes MA, Dillman JR, Mody RJ, et al. Pediatric renal leukemia: spectrum of CT imaging findings. Pediatr Radiol 2008;38:424–30.

50. Chepuri NB, Strouse PJ, Yanik GA. CT of renal lymphoma in children. AJR Am J Roentgenol 2003; 180:429–31.

51. Reznek RH, Mootoosamy I, Webb JA, et al. CT in renal and perirenal lymphoma: a further look. Clin Radiol 1990;42:233–8.

52. Smith EA, Styn N, Wan J, et al. Xanthogranulomatous pyelonephritis: an uncommon pediatric renal mass. Pediatr Radiol 2010;40(8):1421–5.

53. Rosenfield AT, Glickman MG, Taylor KJ, et al. Acute focal bacterial nephritis (acute lobar nephronia). Radiology 1979;132:553–61.

Magnetic Resonance Urography in Evaluation of Duplicated Renal Collecting Systems

Melkamu Adeb, MD[a],*, Kassa Darge, MD, PhD[a,b],
Jonathan R. Dillman, MD[c], Michael Carr, MD, PhD[b,d],
Monica Epelman, MD[e]

KEYWORDS

- MR urography • Children • Duplex kidney • Duplicated renal collecting system • Ureterocele
- Ectopic ureter

KEY POINTS

- Duplex renal collecting systems are common congenital anomalies of the upper urinary tract.
- Complicated duplex renal systems may require further evaluation using cross-sectional imaging and/or functional imaging after an ultrasound (US) and voiding cystourethrography (VCUG).
- Functional magnetic resonance urography (fMRU) provides comprehensive morphologic and functional evaluation of duplex kidneys.
- Magnetic resonance urography (MRU) can demonstrate barely or nonfunctioning renal poles as well as ectopic ureters.
- fMRU allows better delineation of each pole of a duplex kidney, leading to improved calculation of differential renal function.

Duplex renal collecting systems are one of the most common congenital anomalies of the urinary tract.[1,2] The exact prevalence of this anomaly is difficult to ascertain because most patients are asymptomatic, and the abnormality is frequently detected incidentally on imaging studies performed for other reasons. In general, it is estimated that ureteral duplication occurs in 1 in 125 (0.8%) of the autopsy population.[1] Hartman and Hodson[3] reported a higher incidence of 2% to 4% in a clinical series of patients with urinary symptoms. In a large study of 700 children presenting with urinary tract infection, ureteral duplication was identified in 8% of the patients.[4] The right and left kidneys are affected equally.

Bilateral duplication occurs in approximately 20% to 40% of the affected individuals.[2–5] Girls are affected 2 times more often than boys.[4–7] Duplication may be transmitted as an autosomal dominant trait with incomplete penetrance, with an incidence of approximately 8% among members of affected families.[6,8–10]

TERMINOLOGY

A standard set of terminologies is used in describing duplex systems based on the recommendation by the Committee on Terminology, Nomenclature and Classification of the Section on Urology of the American Academy of Pediatrics.[11]

[a] Division of Body Imaging, Department of Radiology, The Children's Hospital of Philadelphia, 34th Street and Civic Center Boulevard, Philadelphia, PA 19104, USA; [b] Perelman School of Medicine, University of Pennsylvania, 34th Street and Civic Center Boulevard, Philadelphia, PA 19104, USA; [c] Section of Pediatric Radiology, Department of Radiology, C.S. Mott Children's Hospital, University of Michigan Health System, Ann Arbor, MI 48109, USA; [d] Division of Urology, Department of Surgery, The Children's Hospital of Philadelphia, Philadelphia, PA 19104, USA; [e] Department of Medical Imaging, Nemours Children's Hospital, 13535 Nemours Parkway, Orlando, FL 32827, USA
* Corresponding author.
E-mail address: melkdm@gmail.com

Magn Reson Imaging Clin N Am 21 (2013) 717–730
http://dx.doi.org/10.1016/j.mric.2013.04.002
1064-9689/13/$ – see front matter © 2013 Elsevier Inc. All rights reserved.

- Duplex kidney refers to a single renal parenchymal unit that is drained by 2 pyelocaliceal (pelvicalyceal) systems.
- Upper poles or lower poles represent 1 of the components of a duplex kidney.
- Duplex system refers to a kidney that has 2 pyelocaliceal systems and is associated with a single or bifid ureter (partial/incomplete ureteric duplication) or, in cases of a complete duplication, 2 ureters (double ureters) that drain separately into the urinary bladder.
- Bifid system refers to 2 pyelocaliceal systems that join at the ureteropelvic junction (bifid pelvis) or 2 ureters that join before draining into the urinary bladder (bifid ureters).
- Double ureters are 2 independent ureters that drain separate pyelocaliceal systems and open separately intravesical or extravesical.
- Upper pole ureter (UPU) and lower pole ureter (LPU) drain the upper pole and lower pole, respectively, of a duplex kidney.
- Upper pole or lower pole orifice refers to the orifice in the bladder associated with the ureter draining the upper pole or lower pole.
- Ectopic ureter refers to either a medially (caudal) ectopic ureter, where the ureter (most often upper pole) inserts medial and distal (inferior) to the normal position of the trigone, or a laterally (cranial) ectopic ureter, where the ureteral orifice is situated lateral to the normal position. Ureteral ectopy can be intravesical or extravesical.
- Ureterocele refers to cystic dilation of the intravesical submucosal distal ureter. Ureteroceles contained entirely within the bladder are classified as intravesical ureteroceles, whereas ectopic (extravesical) ureteroceles contain a portion permanently situated at the bladder neck or in the urethra. A single-system ureterocele is associated with a kidney with only 1 ureter. A duplex system ureterocele is associated with the upper pole of a kidney with a complete ureteral duplication.

EMBRYOLOGY

Basic understanding of the embryology of urinary tract development is important to describe duplicated renal collecting systems and associated abnormalities.[6,12,13] The ureter forms from the ureteral bud, which arises as a diverticulum from a ventral bend or elbow in the mesonephric (wolffian) duct, at the end of the 4th week of gestation. This is the point at which the mesonephric duct bends to enter the cloaca. The ventral cloaca develops into the urogenital sinus and ultimately the urinary bladder and urethra. The portion of the mesonephric duct between the cloaca and the origin of the ureteral bud forms the common excretory duct. This duct gradually expands to be incorporated onto the urogenital sinus and forms a portion of the trigone and the underlying detrusor musculature.[6,12] The growing ureteral bud penetrates the metanephric blastemal ridge, the kidney progenitor, late in the 5th week. The ureteral bud subsequently forms the ureter, renal pelvis, calyces, papillary ducts, and collecting tubules. The metanephros differentiates into the more proximal portions of the nephron. The process of branching of the ureteric bud is complete by approximately 14 weeks, but new nephrons are produced throughout gestation.

Incomplete ureteral duplication results from a ureteral bud that bifurcates shortly after its origin from the mesonephric duct. If the division occurs after the ureteral bud penetrates into the metanephric blastema (5th week of gestation), a bifid pelvis results. If the division occurs before the 5th week of gestation, varying degrees of ureteral duplication result with fusion distally as a single ureter entering the urinary bladder.

A duplex kidney with complete double ureters requires 2 ureteral buds arising from the mesonephric duct. The bud that arises more cranial on the mesonephric duct extends to the upper pole of the kidney, and the caudally positioned bud drains the lower pole. During the process of incorporation of the buds onto the urogenital sinus, the lower pole orifice makes first contact with the urogenital sinus, rendering it affected more by the rotation and migration forces affecting the ureters and mesonephric duct. As a consequence, its final position is lateral and cranial to the ultimate position of the upper pole orifice. This relationship of the orifices of the UPU and LPU is described in the Weigert-Meyer rule, which states that the UPU is medial and caudal in relation to the lateral and cranially positioned lower pole orifice.[12,14,15] Exceptions to this rule occur but are rare.

Typically, the ureteric orifice draining the upper pole develops caudal to the normal location and is often ectopic, somewhere along the pathway of the mesonephric system. In boys, ectopic ureteral orifices always terminate into a suprasphincteric structure, usually into the posterior urethra but also into the ejaculatory ducts, vas deferens, seminal vesicle, or epididymis. In girls, ectopic ureters may be suprasphincteric (anywhere between the trigone and striated sphincter) or infrasphincteric—in the lower urethra, at the introitus, or in the vagina.[6,12,16–18] This explains why urinary dribbling, daytime-nighttime wetness, and incontinence are common presentations in girls but not boys.[6,19–21] Other uncommon sites for ectopic ureteral insertion include the uterus, Gartner duct cyst, cervix, perineum, and, rarely, rectum.[22,23] Varying degrees of renal hypoplasia or dysplasia are frequently associated with ectopically inserting ureters. In general, the more ectopic the ureter is, the more dysplastic the associated renal parenchyma. Severe ectopy with an orifice in the genital system is almost always associated with nonfunctioning renal tissue.[20,24]

CLINICAL PRESENTATION

Most cases of duplex kidneys are diagnosed in asymptomatic children as incidental findings during imaging for other reasons.[21] Other common clinical presentations, however, include urinary tract infection (**Fig. 1**), flank/abdominal pain from intermittent ureteropelvic junction obstruction (UPJO) (**Figs. 2** and **3**), urinary incontinence/dribbling from ectopic ureteral insertion (**Figs. 4** and **5**), intravaginal/extravaginal mass from a prolapsing ureterocele, *epididymo*-orchitis in boys with ectopic UPU insertion to the *epididymis*, and, rarely, a bladder outlet obstruction from a ureterocele. The latter may mimic posterior urethral valves in boys.[25]

Ectopic ureter can be associated with significant urinary tract obstruction, rarely with vesicoureteric reflux (VUR), or both. Currently, many duplex renal systems are identified by prenatal US, particularly if one pole is dilated.[26–30] It is even possible to differentiate between ectopic ureter and uretroceles in utero using US.[28–32] In these children, the anomaly is confirmed by US after birth and further work-up includes VCUG and sometimes MRU.[32] The impact of prenatal detection of duplex systems remains uncertain, and prenatal diagnosis at present does not distinguish between those who eventually present clinically with complications and those who remain asymptomatic.[33–35] It is generally thought that prenatal diagnosis may not reduce the need for surgery but does result in earlier, less complex, and more definitive surgery, with a consequent small reduction in long-term bladder dysfunction.[36]

The natural history of prenatally diagnosed duplex kidneys remains uncertain. For simple, nondilated duplex systems that are not complicated by vesicoureteral reflux or obstruction, there is no need for treatment or intervention. Treatment of complex duplex systems depends on the pathology and presence of dilatation in the renal poles. The goal in medical and surgical treatment options is to conserve as much renal function as possible, by correcting the underlying pathology. Consideration of a surgical procedure is indicated based on the presence of associated abnormalities like VUR, ureterocele, ectopic ureter, obstruction, or nonfunctional moiety.[19,37] Some pathologic cases may evolve unrecognized up to late childhood,

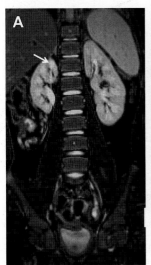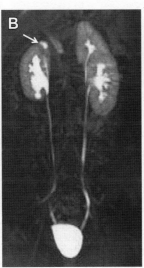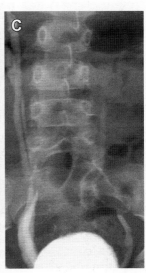

Fig. 1. Coronal fat-saturated T2-weighted fast spin-echo (*A*) and postcontrast T1-weighted MIP (*B*) images from MRU examination of a 7-year-old girl who presented with repeated episodes of urinary tract infections. Bilateral duplicated renal collecting systems are noted with a small eccentrically located right upper pole (*arrows*) that is dysplastic with reduced and delayed function. The right side is completely duplicated, with both ureters inserting separately into the bladder, whereas left side ureters join distally to form a common ureter. Low grade bilateral vesicoureteral reflux was noted on VCUG (*C*).

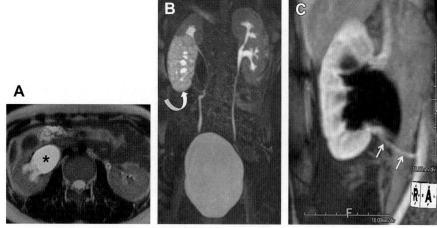

Fig. 2. Axial T2-weighted fast spin-echo image without fat saturation (*A*) and delayed postcontrast MIP (*B*) MRU images in a 10-year-old boy who had intermittent right-sided flank pain. Prior imaging with US revealed that the patient had a right UPJO. Evaluation with MRU demonstrated, however, that the child also had a right duplex kidney with pelvicaliectasis of the right lower moiety (*asterisk*). A hyperintense nephrogram is noted on the post-contrast scan (*curved arrow*) as a result of ureteropelvic junction obstruction. There is normal right upper moiety and left kidney function and contrast material excretion. A crossing artery (*arrows*) was noted on oblique post-contrast T1-weighted MIP image (*C*), which was confirmed at surgery.

such as ectopically draining upper poles with poor function.[38]

DIAGNOSTIC IMAGING

Duplex kidneys are most often noted as incidental findings on imaging for non-urologic indications, or during the work-up of urologic complaints such as urinary tract infection or incontinence, especially in girls. The uncomplicated duplex kidney is most often detected during an US examination and presents with 2 distinct renal hila separated by a bridge of normal renal parenchyma, namely a hypertrophied column of Bertin. This is excellently

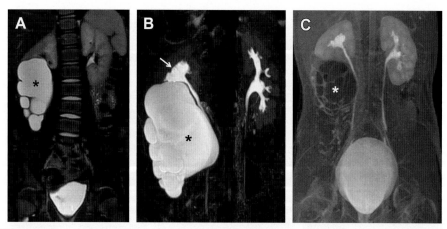

Fig. 3. MRU in an 8-year-old boy with recent onset of right flank pain. The patient was diagnosed with right-sided UPJO on renal US and no evidence of duplex kidney was noted. Further evaluation with MRU, however, revealed a right-side duplicated renal collecting system with severe lower pole UPJO. Coronal fat-saturated T2-weighted fast spin-echo (*A*) and fat-saturated 3-D T2-weighted MIP (*B*) MRU images depict detailed renal collecting system anatomy, including marked dilatation of the right lower moiety pelvicalyceal system (*asterisk*). No fluid is seen in the right lower moiety ureter. The right upper moiety collecting system (*arrow*) appears only mildly dilated and is associated with a normal caliber ureter. The left renal collecting system is unremarkable. Delayed postcontrast T1-weighted MIP image confirms that the obstructed right lower pole (*asterisk*) has only minimal enhancing parenchyma and no significant function (*C*). The right upper moiety and left kidney show normal parenchymal enhancement and contrast material excretion.

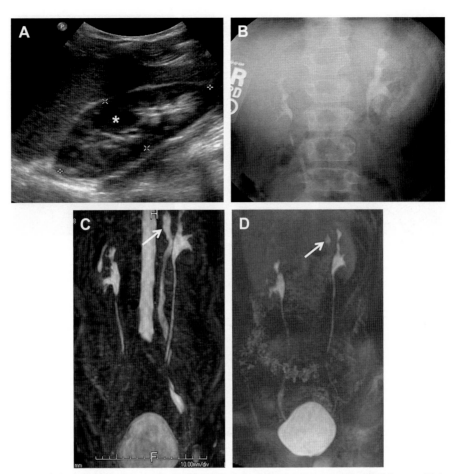

Fig. 4. US image of the left kidney in sagittal plane (*A*) and intravenous urography (IVU) image (*B*) in a 17-year-old adolescent girl with repeated negative investigations for urinary incontinence. A hypetrophied column of Bertin noted in the midpole of left kidney (*asterisk*) without visualization of definite duplicated renal collecting systems (*A*). No definite abnormality is also detected on the IVU (*B*). MRU reveals a left duplex kidney with a small dysplastic left upper moiety (*arrow*) on fat-saturated 3-D T2-weighted (*C*) and delayed postcontrast T1-weighted MIP (*D*) MRU images. This dysplastic moiety has a markedly reduced function with delayed excretion (calyceal transit time, renal transit time) that was thoroughly assessed with fMRU. The ectatic left upper pole ureter was found to insert ectopically into the vagina (not shown) explaining the cause for urinary incontinence. The patient had a complete resolution of symptoms after surgical correction.

demonstrated on US by depicting in transverse plane 3 distinct levels (ie, an upper hilum, a mid-kidney area of hilar separation [faceless kidney], and a lower hilum). Unless there is a clinical indication, no further examination is necessary for a noncomplicated duplex system.[21]

Prenatal diagnosis of duplex systems and associated anomalies is frequently made on antenatal US and possibly MR imaging (**Fig. 6**), particularly if there is dilatation of the collecting system.[28–32] Suggestive antenatal sonographic and MR imaging features of complicated duplex systems include hydroureteronephrosis of upper pole or lower pole (or both), an apparent cystic structure within 1 pole, intravesical ureteroceles, and, rarely, ectopic ureters.[28] These findings need to be

confirmed using postnatal imaging, starting with US. Further evaluation with VCUG may be performed to assess for VUR, particularly in the setting of lower pole renal collecting system dilatation.[21] MRU further provides valuable diagnostic information, particularly in complicated duplex systems. Evaluation of ectopic ureteral insertion can be difficult with US. MRU is able to demonstrate the ectopic extravesical insertion, even in cases where the upper pole parenchyma is small or functions poorly (see **Figs. 4** and **5**).[38–41] Moreover, MRU provides surgical planning for complicated duplex renal systems and thoroughly assesses the quality of parenchyma and function in complex anatomic cases, particularly during early infancy.

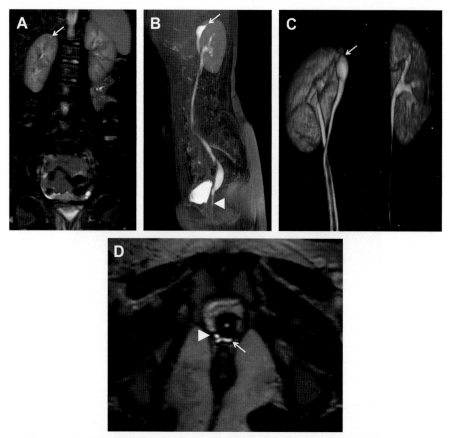

Fig. 5. Coronal fat-saturated T2-weighted fast spin-echo (*A*), sagittal postcontrast T1-weighted MIP (*B*), and post-contrast T1-weighted volume-rendered (*C*) MRU images in a 7-year-old girl with daytime-nighttime wetness. US and VCUG examinations (not shown) were normal. A right duplex kidney, however, with a very small contrast-excreting dysplastic upper pole (*arrow*) is noted on the MRU examination. The right upper pole ureter was found to have an ectopic vaginal insertion (*arrowhead*) (*B, D*). Fluid is present in the vagina near the insertion of the ectopic ureter on axial 3-D T2-weighted fast spin-echo image.

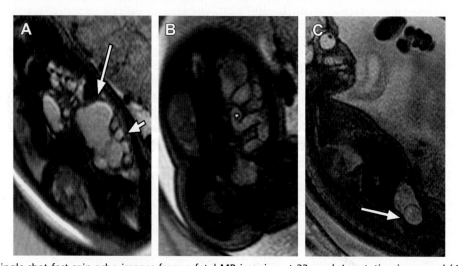

Fig. 6. Single-shot fast spin-echo images from a fetal MR imaging at 33 weeks' gestation in coronal (*A, B*) and sagittal (*C*) planes performed to assess large congenital diaphragmatic hernia. Images also demonstrate complete duplication of the left renal collecting system with hydroureteronephrosis of both the upper (*long arrow*) and lower (*short arrow*) poles. The upper pole ureter (*asterisk*) is also noted as dilated and tortuous (*B*), and it terminates as an intravesical ureterocele (*C*) (*arrow*).

Magnetic Resonance Urography

MRU provides a comprehensive morphologic and functional evaluation of the urinary tract in a single examination.[42–46] Several studies have demonstrated the clinical utility of MRU in evaluating the kidneys and the urinary tract.[41,47–55] The absence of ionizing radiation makes it a suitable method for use in children. MRU provides excellent spatial and contrast resolution and rapid temporal resolution, thereby providing exceptional anatomic detail of the urinary tract, with the use of T2-weighted (MR hydrography) and contrast-enhanced images.[42] Dynamic scanning after intravenous injection of a gadolinium chelate contrast agent yields important functional information related to the perfusion, concentration, and excretion of the contrast agent in the renal cortex and the medulla. Comparative functional studies with scintigraphy have shown high concordance of the 2 methods.[46,52–55]

Technique

The preparation for an MRU typically entails the use of intravenous hydration, administration of furosemide (Lasix, Sanofi-Aventis, Paris, France), and in most cases urinary bladder catheterization.[42,56,57] For optimal distention of the urinary tract and thus improved visualization, it is recommended to inject furosemide approximately 15 minutes before intravenous contrast agent administration.[56,57] Additional advantages of furosemide include evaluation of excretory function under diuresis, minimization of T2* artifacts on postcontrast MRU, and shortened examination time.[56] The placement of a urinary bladder catheter may be important for the following reasons[57]:

- It reduces the potential negative effect of a distended bladder on renal contrast material excretion.
- It decreases confounding effects from possible high-grade VUR.
- It avoids disruption of the examination from increased urgency of voiding due to hydration and furosemide.
- It helps improve the delineation of the urethra in case of an extravesical ectopic ureter.

The imaging protocols commonly used for clinical MRU studies consist of fat-saturated T2-weighted sequences before and dynamic T1-weighted 3-D rapid gradient-recalled echo sequences after intravenous contrast agent administration.[43–45,56] Maximum intensity projection (MIP) and volume-rendered images are generated for further evaluation of the urinary tract.[42,56] fMRU analysis is based on the evaluation of the dynamic postcontrast images. Routinely obtained functional parameters include calyceal transit time, renal transit time, time-to-peak, differential renal functions (based on renal parenchymal volume or on the estimation of individual kidney Patlak number, which is used to calculate the Patlak DRF), and, lastly, both renal parenchymal enhancement and excretion curves.[42,56,57] Several fMRU freewares are available that provide functional analysis based on these parameters, including the CHOP fMRU software (www.chop-fmru.com) that the authors currently use.[57]

For accurate functional analysis of duplex kidneys, each pole of a duplex kidney needs to be segmented separately. This is best achieved when there is a distinct parenchymal bridge, dilated renal pelvis, or different enhancement patterns. When 1 pole is very small, the separation may become difficult.

Role of MRU in Evaluating Duplex Renal Systems

Most of the literature on MR imaging of duplex renal systems is limited to case reports and case series.[39,58–61] Avni and colleagues[58] reported on the use of MRU in 20 cases of duplex kidneys:

- MR imaging provided satisfactory and precise assessment of complications associated with duplex renal systems.
- MRU was found particularly useful in evaluation of duplex kidneys with upper pole dilation, extravesical ureteral insertions, and evaluation of occult or dysplastic upper poles.
- An ectopic ureter extending from a poorly functioning moiety of a duplex kidney, invisible on other imaging, may be depicted with MRU (see **Fig. 3**).[58–61]
- An important advantage of MRU is its ability to demonstrate dysplastic/hypoplastic poles with no or little function, partly as a result of the natural contrast provided by urine on precontrast T2-weighted images.[42,56,58,60–62]

The typical imaging features associated with a dysplastic pole/kidney include small size, disorganized architecture with loss of normal corticomedullary differentiation, small subcortical cysts, decrease in signal intensity on T2-weighted images, poor perfusion, a dim and patchy nephrogram with minimal excretion on dynamic contrast-enhanced images, and dysmorphic calyces (**Fig. 7**).[21,42] In the past, many severely dysplastic kidneys were identified only at time of surgery.[19] With the advent of fMRU, it is possible to determine the remaining function of the dysplastic parenchyma (see **Fig. 3**).[39,42,56] This

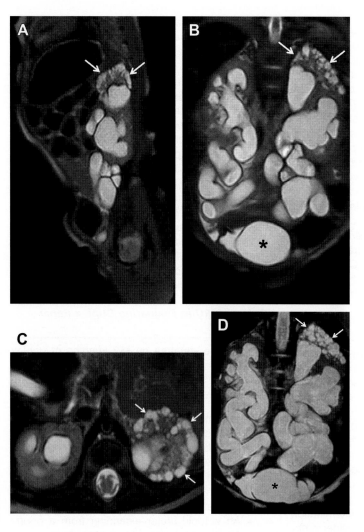

Fig. 7. T2-weighted single-shot fast spin-echo MRU images in sagittal (*A*), coronal (*B*), and axial (*C*) planes in a 3-week-old girl with left duplicated renal collecting systems and right megaureter (nonduplicated). Left upper pole and lower pole pelvicalyces and ureters are markedly dilated. The left upper pole has a severely dysplastic renal parenchyma, containing many cortical cysts (*arrows*). Finding is likely due to severe in utero upper pole obstruction. The lower pole has no evidence of dysplasia. A very large ureterocele is present in the urinary bladder (*asterisk*) (*B*). Precontrast coronal fat-saturated 3-D T2-weighted fast spin-echo MIP image (*D*) demonstrates all of these imaging findings on a single image with excellent morphologic detail.

is achieved with better delineation of the 2 poles than expected on scintigraphic studies, with likely improved calculation of the differential renal function. Upper pole heminephrectomy may be required to stop the urinary dribbling or recurrent urinary tract infection when the dysplastic upper pole is still functioning. The distal part of the ureter is usually left in place and atrophies or may contain fluid due to vesicoureteral reflux. Additional advantages of MRU include evaluation of ectopic and supernumerary kidneys, particularly in the setting of a poorly functioning parenchyma.

DUPLEX TYPES, ASSOCIATED ABNORMALITIES, AND COMPLICATIONS
Incomplete Ureteral Duplication

As discussed previously, incomplete ureteral duplication occurs when the ureteral bud bifurcates early. The most proximal bifurcation results in bifid,

trifid, or multifid pelves (**Fig. 8**) and is thought to occur in approximately 10% of cases.[19] The other types of incomplete duplication are bifid ureters that drain a duplex kidney and join distally to form a single ureter that usually empties into the bladder or rarely inserts ectopically.[63,64] Most commonly, the ureters may join outside the bladder (extravesical [or Y junction or fork junction]) but they can also join intravesically (V junction). Most extravesical junctions occur in the lower third of the distance from the kidney to the bladder (**Fig. 9**). Partial duplications are usually discovered incidentally. Uretrouretral reflux can occur in Y junction ureters (referred to as "yo-yo reflux"). This is usually a functional problem, although obstruction caused by stenosis or ureterocele may exist.[65,66] The resting pressure in the common chamber is always higher than the pressure in either of the 2 ureters above it. Urine, flowing to the site of the lowest pressure, easily progresses up the other ureter. At irregular

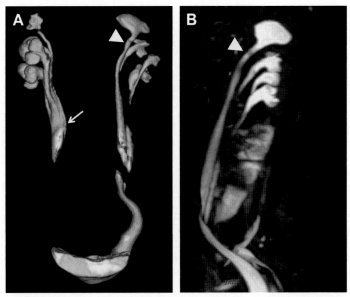

Fig. 8. Frontal 3-D T2-weighted fast spin-echo volume-rendered (*A*) and sagittal MIP (*B*) MRU images in a 6-year-old boy demonstrate bilateral quadruplicate ureters. The right side exhibits incomplete quadruplication with the proximal 4 ureters joining distally to form a single common ureteral trunk (*arrow*) that inserts orthotopically into the urinary bladder (the distal right ureter is not seen on this 3-D image due to decompressed state). The left side, however, demonstrates a completely separate uppermost ureter (*arrowhead*) that courses distally to insert ectopically into the bladder neck (not shown). The uppermost moiety calyx and distal ureter are dilated due to stenosis at the ureteral orifice. The remaining 3 lower ureters join together to form a common distal ureter that inserts into the urinary bladder (not shown).

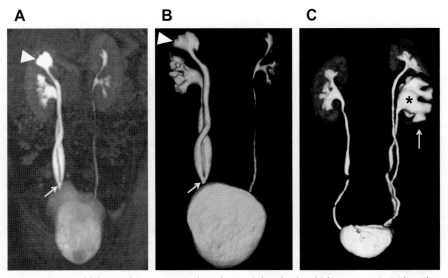

Fig. 9. MRU in a 9-year-old boy who was noted to have right duplex kidney on US. Delayed postcontrast T1-weighted MIP (*A*) and volume-rendered (*B*) images demonstrate an incomplete right-sided duplication with distal union of the ureters (Y or fork junction) (*arrow*). There is also caliectasis and focal parenchymal thinning affecting the right upper pole (*arrowhead*). Postcontrast T1-weighted volume-rendered MRU image in a 6-year-old girl demonstrates complete duplication of the left renal collecting systems and ureters (*C*). Left lower pole pelvicaliectasis (*asterisk*) is due to vesicoureteral reflux (the left ureteropelvic junction is shown widely patent). Left lower moiety parenchymal thinning is due to scarring (*arrow*).

intervals, the peristalsis proceeds down to the distal common ureter, propelling urine to the bladder. Because these ureters can serve as sites of persistent infection, surgery has sometimes been performed to alleviate the abnormal situation and usually involves anastomosing the upper to the lower pole renal pelvis.[67,68] Intravesical (V junctions) do not manifest a yo-yo reflux because pressure in the common systems is low owing to the muscle surrounding the intramural ureter.

Approximately 50% of bifid ureters with extravesical junctions have some associated anomaly. Those involving the common sheath include VUR, ureterocele, stenosis, and atresia causing multicystic dysplastic kidney. Anomalies of the bifid ureters include ureteropelvic junction obstruction (UPJO), usually of the lower pelvis, and stenosis of 1 of the 2 ureters. There may be associated urinary stasis, infection, ureteral dilation, and flank discomfort, but these findings are rare.[64] MRU provides excellent depiction of incomplete duplex ureters (see **Fig. 9**; **Fig. 10**). Visualization of the ureteral reflux usually requires fluoroscopic or dynamic radionuclide cystogram.[64] The role of dynamic contrast-enhanced MRU to evaluate this phenomenon has yet to be determined. A VCUG is essential to exclude ureteral dilation owing to VUR.

Complete Duplication

Complete duplication occurs when 2 separate ureteral buds develop, and the ureters almost always

follow the Weigert-Meyer rule of distal insertion.[14,15,19] In approximately 15% of cases, the UPU can open anywhere along the so-called ectopic pathway, either intravesically or extravesically.[69] This area extends from the superior and medial aspect of the lateral angle of the trigone and then extends across the trigone down the urethra. The LPU is usually affected by VUR, although the UPU or both ureters may reflux.[4,70] In general, VUR occurs 2 times more often in the LPU than in UPU because the LPU usually inserts lateral and cephalad than the UPU, rendering it as having a smaller subepithelial tunnel and thus a higher incidence of reflux.[71]

UPJO is more prevalent in patients with complete duplication than in the general population and it almost always involves the lower pole. When a dilated lower pole collecting system is identified in the absence of a VUR, evaluation with fMRU is helpful to assess the presence and severity of obstruction. In children who present with UTI and are found to have ureteral duplication, associated ectopic ureteroceles are present in 6% to 20% of children.[4,72] The ureters that terminate ectopically or with a ureterocele have an increased incidence of renal hypoplasia or dysplasia.[19] In summary, the ureter draining the upper pole is usually complicated by ectopia (see **Figs. 4** and **5**) (either intravesical/extravesical), obstruction, and/or ureterocele (See **Figs. 6** and **7**; **Fig. 11**), whereas the lower pole is usually complicated by UPJO (See **Figs. 2** and **3**) and/or VUR.

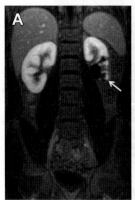 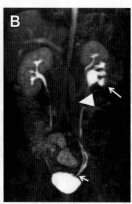 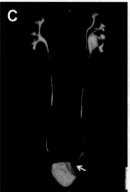 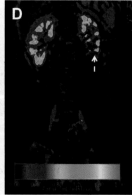

Fig. 10. MRU in an 8-year-old girl with history of frequent urinary tract infections. Coronal postcontrast fat-saturated T1-weighted nephrographic phase (*A*), delayed postcontrast T1-weighted MIP (*B*), and precontrast 3-D T2-weighted fast spin-echo volume-rendered (*C*) images demonstrate a left duplex kidney with marked thinning of lower pole renal parenchyma (*long arrows*) (*A, B*). The left lower pole ureter joins the upper pole ureter distally (*short arrows*) (*B, C*). Grade III left lower pole VUR was found on VCUG (not shown). fMRU evaluation revealed decreased function of this pole on the Patlak map (*dashed arrow*) (*D*). Incidental note is made of a duplicated inferior vena cava (*arrowhead*).

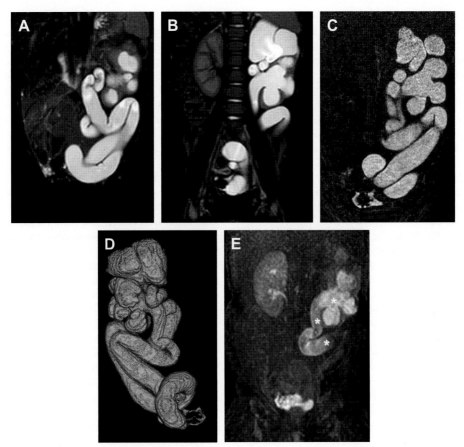

Fig. 11. A 1-year-old girl with marked left hydroureteronephrosis on US and anatomy unclear. Coronal fat-saturated T2-weighted fast spin-echo (*A, B*) and coronal fat-saturated 3-D T2-weighted fast spin-echo (*C*) MRU images demonstrate completely duplicated left renal collecting systems and ureters with severe upper pole and lower pole hydroureteronephrosis. There is severe left upper pole and lower pole renal parenchymal thinning. 3-D T2-weighted fast spin-echo volume-rendered image (posterior view) (*D*) shows the relationship between UPU and LPU clearly. Postcontrast T1-weighted MIP image confirms nearly completely absent function of the left upper moiety (*E*). Excreted contrast material is noted in the left lower moiety pelvicalyceal system and proximal ureter. The right kidney is normal.

SUMMARY

MRU allows for excellent morphologic and functional evaluation of the kidneys and urinary tract. This imaging technique is particularly useful for assessing complex duplicated renal collecting systems and demonstrating barely or nonfunctioning renal poles and associated ectopic ureters. Thus, MRU is the imaging choice in girls with urinary dribbling when an infrasphincteric ectopic ureter is suspected. Additionally, because of its exceptional anatomic resolution, fMRU allows better separation of the renal poles than renal scintigraphy and likely allows improved calculation of the differential renal functions.

What the referring physician needs to know:

- Most duplicated renal collecting systems are asymptomatic and are undetected.

- A majority of duplicated renal collecting systems diagnosed by imaging (eg, US) are uncomplicated and incidental.
- MRU excellently depicts complex anatomy related to complicated duplex renal collecting systems without ionizing radiation.
- MRU is the imaging study of choice for identifying ectopic ureters and characterizing dysplastic renal poles.
- fMRU allows better separation of the renal poles than renal scintigraphy and likely allows improved calculation of differential renal function.

REFERENCES

1. Nation EF. Duplication of the kidney and ureter: a statistical study of 230 new cases. J Urol 1944; 51:456.

2. Peters CA, Schlussel RN, Mendelsohn C. Ectopic ureter, ureterocele, and ureteral anomalies. In: Wein AJ, editor. Campbell-walsh urology. 10th edition. Philadelphia: Saunders Elsevier; 2011. p. 3236–66.

3. Hartman GW, Hodson CJ. The duplex kidney and related abnormalities. Clin Radiol 1969;20(4):387–400.

4. Siomou E, Papadopoulou F, Kollios KD, et al. Duplex collecting system diagnosed during the first 6 years of life after a first urinary tract infection: a study of 63 children. J Urol 2006;175(2):678–81 [discussion: 681–2].

5. Timothy RP, Decter A, Perlmutter AD. Ureteral duplication: clinical findings and therapy in 46 children. J Urol 1971;105(3):445–51.

6. Decter RM. Renal duplication and fusion anomalies. Pediatr Clin North Am 1997;44(5):1323–41.

7. Privett JT, Jeans WD, Roylance J. The incidence and importance of renal duplication. Clin Radiol 1976;27(4):521–30.

8. Whitaker J, Danks DM. A study of the inheritance of duplication of the kidneys and ureters. J Urol 1966; 95(2):176–8.

9. Babcock JR Jr, Belman AB, Shkolnik A, et al. Familial ureteral duplication and ureterocele. Urology 1977;9(3):345–9.

10. Atwell JD, Cook PL, Howell CJ, et al. Familial incidence of bifid and double ureters. Arch Dis Child 1974;49(10):825–6.

11. Glassberg KI, Braren V, Duckett JW, et al. Suggested terminology for duplex systems, ectopic ureters and ureteroceles. J Urol 1984;132(6):1153–4.

12. Tanagho EA. Embryologic basis for lower ureteral anomalies: a hypothesis. Urology 1976;7:451.

13. Stephens FD. Caecoureterocele and concepts on the embryology and aetiology of ureteroceles. Aust N Z J Surg 1971;40:239.

14. Meyer R. Zur Anatomie und Entwicklungsgeschichte der Ureterverdoppelung. Virchows Arch [Pathol Anat] 1907;187:408.

15. Weigert C. Ueber einige Bildungsfehler der Ureteren. Virchows Arch [Pathol Anat] 1877;70:490.

16. Ambrose SS, Nicolson WP III. The causes of vesicoureteral reflux in children. J Urol 1962;87:688.

17. Mackie GG, Stephens FD. Duplex kidneys: a correlation of renal dysplasia with position of the ureteral orifice. J Urol 1975;114:274.

18. Ellerker AG. The extravesical ectopic ureter. Br J Surg 1958;45:344–53.

19. Stephens FD, Smith ED, Huston JM. Congenital anomalies of the kidney, urinary and genital tracts. London: Martin Dunitz; 2002.

20. Nepple KG, Cooper CS, Snyder HM III. Ureteral duplication, ectopy, and ureteroceles. In: Gearhart JP, Rink RC, Mouriquand PD, editors. Pediatric urology. 2nd edition. Philadelphia: WB Saunders; 2003. p. 337–40.

21. Avni EF, Hall M, Collier F, et al. Anomalies of the Renal Pelvis and Ureter. In: Fotter R, editor. Pediatric uroradiology. 2nd edition. Heidelberg, Germany: Springer, Verlag; 2008. p. 89–118.

22. Vanhoutte JJ. Ureteral ectopia into a Wolffian duct remnant (Gartner's ducts or cysts) presenting as a urethral diverticulum in two girls. AJR Am J Roentgenol 1970;110:540.

23. Uson AC, Schulman CC. Ectopic ureter emptying into the rectum: report of a case. J Urol 1972;108: 156.

24. Schlecker BA, Snyder HM, Duckett JW. Ectopic ureters in children [abstract 153]. J Urol 1986; 135:142A.

25. Nussbaum AR, Lebowitz RL. Interlabial masses in little girls. AJR Am J Roentgenol 1983;141:65–71.

26. Adiego B, Martinez-Ten P, Perez-Pedregosa J, et al. Antenatally diagnosed renal duplex anomalies: sonographic features and long-term postnatal outcome. J Ultrasound Med 2011;30(6):809–15.

27. Whitten SM, Wilcox DT, McHoney M, et al. Accuracy of antenatal fetal ultrasound in the diagnosis of duplex kidneys. Ultrasound Obstet Gynecol 2003;21:342–6.

28. Abuhamad AZ, Horton CE, Horton SH, et al. Renal duplication anomalies in the fetus: clues for prenatal diagnosis. Ultrasound Obstet Gynecol 1996;7: 174–7.

29. Vergani P, Ceruti P, Locatelli A, et al. Accuracy of prenatal US diagnosis of duplex kidney. J Ultrasound Med 1999;18:463–7.

30. Jee LD, Rickwood AM, Williams MP, et al. Experience with duplex system anomalies detected by prenatal ultrasonography. J Urol 1993;149:808–10.

31. Joseph DB, Bauer SB, Colodny AH, et al. Lower pole UPJ obstruction and incomplete duplication. J Urol 1989;141:896–9.

32. Avni EF, Dacher JN, Stallenberg B, et al. Renal duplica-tions: the impact of perinatal US on diagnosis and management. Eur Radiol 1991;20:43–8.

33. Hulbert WC, Rabinowitz R. Prenatal diagnosis of duplex system hydronephrosis: effect on renal salvage. Urology 1998;51(5A):23–6.

34. Van Savage JG, Mesrobian HG. The impact of prenatal sonography on the morbidity and outcome of patients with renal duplication anomalies. J Urol 1995;153:768–70.

35. Shankar KR, Vishwanath N, Rickwood AM. Outcome of patients with prenatally detected duplex system ureterocoele: natural history of those managed expectantly. J Urol 2001;165: 1226–8.

36. Whitten SM, Wilcox DT, Chitty LS. Prenatal diagnosis of duplex kidneys—does it make a difference? Ultrasound Obstet Gynecol 2007;30:370.

37. Merguerian PA, Taenzer A, Knoerlein K, et al. Variation in management of duplex system intravesical

ureteroceles: a survey of pediatric urologists. J Urol 2010;184(Suppl 4):1625–30.

38. Share JC, Lebowitz RL. The unsuspected duplex collecting system. AJR Am J Roentgenol 1990; 155:561–4.

39. Avni EF, Matos C, Rypens F, et al. Ectopic vaginal insertion of an upperpole ureter. J Urol 1997;158: 1931–2.

40. Avni EF, Bali M, Regnault M, et al. MR urography in children. Eur J Radiol 2000;43:154–66.

41. Braveman RM, Lebowitz RL. Occult ectopic ureter in girls: diagnosis with CT. AJR Am J Roentgenol 1991;156:365–6.

42. Grattan-Smith JD, Jones RA. MR urography in children. Pediatr Radiol 2006;36:1119–32.

43. Jones RA, Perez-Brayfield MR, Kirsch AJ, et al. Renal transit time With MR urography in children. Radiology 2004;233:41–50.

44. Jones RA, Easley K, Little SB, et al. Dynamic contrast-enhanced MR urography in the evaluation of pediatric hydronephro- sis: part 1, functional assessment. AJR Am J Roentgenol 2005;185:1598–607.

45. Perez-Brayfield MR, Kirsch AJ, Jones RA, et al. A prospective study comparing ultrasound, nuclear scintigraphy and dynamic contrast enhanced magnetic resonance imaging in the evaluation of hydro- nephrosis. J Urol 2003;170(Pt 1):1330–4.

46. McDaniel BB, Jones RA, Scherz H, et al. Dynamic contrast-enhanced MR urography in the evaluation of pediatric hydrone- phrosis: part 2, anatomic and functional assessment of uteropelvic junction obstruction. AJR Am J Roentgenol 2005;185:1608–14.

47. Borthne A, Nordshus T, Reiseter T, et al. MR urography: the future gold standard in paediatric urogenital imaging? Pediatr Radiol 1999;29:694–701.

48. Borthne A, Pierre-Jerome C, Nordshus T, et al. MR Urography in children: current status and future development. Eur Radiol 2000;10:503–11.

49. Riccabona M. Pediatric MRU–Its potential and its role in the diagnostic work-up of upper urinary tract dilatation in infants and children. World J Urol 2004; 22:79–87.

50. Riccabona M, Koen M, Beckers G, et al. Magnetic resonance urography: a new gold standard for the evaluation of solitary kidneys and renal buds? J Urol 2004;171:1642–6.

51. Nolte-Ernsting CC, Adam GB, Gunther RW. MR urography: examination techniques and clinical applications. Eur Radiol 2001;11:355–72.

52. Rohrschneider WK, Hoffend J, Becker K, et al. Combined static-dynamic MR urography for the simultaneous evaluation of morphology and function in urinary tract obstruction. I. Evaluation of the normal status in an animal model. Pediatr Radiol 2000;30:511–22.

53. Rohrschneider WK, Becker K, Hoffend J, et al. Combined static-dynamic MR urography for the simultaneous evaluation of morphology and function in urinary tract obstruction. II. Findings in experimentally induced ureteric stenosis. Pediatr Radiol 2000;30:523–32.

54. Rohrschneider WK, Haufe S, Wiesel M, et al. Functional and morphologic evaluation of congenital urinary tract dilatation by using combined static-dynamic MR urography: findings in kidneys with a single collecting system. Radiology 2002;224: 683–94.

55. Rohrschneider WK, Haufe S, Clorius JH, et al. MR to assess renal function in children. Eur Radiol 2003;13:1033–45.

56. Grattan-Smith JD, Perez-Bayfield MR, Jones RA, et al. MR imaging of kidneys: functional evaluation using F-15 perfusion imaging. Pediatr Radiol 2003; 33:293–304.

57. Khrichenko D, Darge K. Functional analysis in MR urography—made simple. Pediatr Radiol 2010; 40(2):182–99.

58. Avni FE, Nicaise N, Hall M, et al. The role of MR imaging for the assessment of complicated duplex kidneys in children: preliminary report. Pediatr Radiol 2001;31(4):215–23.

59. Yanagisawa N, Yajima M, Takahara T, et al. Diagnostic magnetic resonance-urography in an infant girl with an ectopic ureter associated with a poorly functioning segment of a duplicated collecting system. Int J Urol 1997;4(3):314–7.

60. Engin G, Esen T, Rozanes I. MR urography findings of a duplicated ectopic ureter in an adult man. Eur Radiol 2000;10(8):1253–6.

61. Jain KA. Ectopic vaginal insertion of an obstructed duplicated ureter in an adult female: demonstration by magnetic resonance imaging. Clin Imaging 2007;31(1):54–6.

62. Riccabona M, Simbrunner J, Ring E. Feasibility of MR urography in neonates and infants with anomalies of the upper urinary tract. Eur Radiol 2002;12: 1442–50.

63. Lenaghan D. Bifid ureters in children: an anatomical, physiological and clinical study. J Urol 1962; 87:808.

64. Kaplan N, Elkin M. Bifid renal pelves and ureters: radiographic and cinefluorographic observations. Br J Urol 1968;40:235.

65. Campbell JE. Ureteral peristalsis in duplex renal collecting systems. AJR Am J Roentgenol 1967; 99:577.

66. Tresidder GC, Blandy JP, Murray RS. Pyelopelvic and uretero-ureteric reflux. Br J Urol 1970;42:728.

67. Amar AD. Treatment of reflux in bifid ureters by conversion to complete duplication. J Urol 1972; 108:77.

68. Amar AD. Ureteropyelostomy for relief of single ureteral obstruction in cases of ureteral duplication. Arch Surg 1970;101:379.

69. Friedland GW, Cunningham J. The elusive ectopic ureteroceles. AJR Am J Roentgenol 1972;116: 792–811.
70. Fehrenbaker LG, Kelalis PP, Stickler GB. Vesicoureteral reflux and ureteral duplication in children. J Urol 1972;107:862.
71. Ambrose SS, Nicolson WP. Ureteral reflux in duplicated ureters. J Urol 1964;92:439.
72. Bisset GS, Strife JL. The duplex collecting system in girls with urinary tract infection: prevalence and significance. AJR Am J Roentgenol 1987; 148:497.

Magnetic Resonance Enterography
Inflammatory Bowel Disease and Beyond

Sudha A. Anupindi, MD[a],*,
Owens Terreblanche, MD (FC Rad)[b], Jesse Courtier, MD[b]

KEYWORDS

- MR enterography • Inflammatory bowel disease (IBD) • Children • Polyps • Masses
- Crohn disease • Ulcerative colitis • Small bowel

KEY POINTS

- Magnetic resonance (MR) enterography is the preferred imaging examination for the evaluation of inflammatory bowel disease (IBD) in children and adolescents, as it provides a comprehensive look at intraluminal and extraluminal pathology without the use of ionizing radiation.
- Bowel distention is one of the important challenges in achieving diagnostic imaging; however, post-contrast imaging, diffusion-weighted imaging (DWI) and cine imaging also play significant roles and provide complementary information, making them important parts of the MR enterography protocol.
- Attempts should be made to identify and subjectively quantify active bowel wall inflammation; active inflammation and fibrosis can coexist in the same narrowed bowel segment.
- MR enterography is useful to evaluate for diagnoses outside of IBD including infections, polyps, tumors, and vascular lesions in the setting of occult gastrointestinal (GI) bleeding.
- It is critical to interpret MR enterographic studies systematically, including evaluation of both normal and abnormal bowel segments. This evaluation is especially important when assessing jejunal disease, as this is an area of many pitfalls and false-positive results.

INTRODUCTION

MR enterography has gained momentum during the last decade and has become a standard imaging technique in the evaluation of children with IBD. The sensitivity and specificity of MR enterography have been validated in both adults and children.[1,2] There has been an emphasis on advancing MR enterography because of the concerns of the effects of cumulative ionizing radiation exposure in this population due to repeated imaging, especially in children. The risks of irradiation and importance of radiation safety in children are well recognized and extensively addressed in the medical literature, Web sites (www.imagegently. org, www.imagewisely.org), and other media available to the general public. In many places in North America, MR enterography has replaced conventional GI fluoroscopy and computed tomographic (CT) enterography and has become the first-line imaging test for known or suspected IBD. With the advent of faster MR imaging sequences, improvement in oral contrast agents and patient compliance, and optimization of DWI and functional cine sequences, radiologists are able to provide valuable, accurate information about disease activity and progression to guide medical versus surgical treatment in children with IBD.

Disclosures: None.
[a] Department of Radiology, The Children's Hospital of Philadelphia, Perelman School of Medicine, University of Pennsylvania, 34th Street and Civic Center Boulevard, Philadelphia, PA 19104, USA; [b] Department of Radiology, UCSF Benioff Children's Hospital & San Francisco General Hospital, UCSF School of Medicine, 505 Parnassus Avenue, M396, San Francisco, CA 94143, USA
* Corresponding author.
E-mail address: anupindi@email.chop.edu

mri.theclinics.com

Several years ago, authors first described using MR enterography for applications beyond IBD[3,4]; however, there are limited data in the literature on the use of MR enterography for non-IBD diseases. One factor driving the expansion of the role of MR enterography among pediatric imagers is the use of MR imaging for appendicitis in children.[5] However, ultrasonography (US) is still the first-line of imaging for assessing appendicitis, and MR imaging protocols for evaluation of appendicitis commonly do not warrant oral or intravenous contrast. In the setting of acute or chronic abdominal pain, US is often the initial examination ordered and may be followed by CT if the clinical question has not been answered. Yet, the multiplanar capability, lack of ionizing radiation, inherent high soft-tissue contrast, and capacity to examine extramural findings make MR enterography an excellent tool for assessing causes of generalized abdominal pain, particularly if thought to relate to the bowel. MR enterography is at present used to assess gastrointestinal tract diagnoses including infections, polyps, masses (tumors), sources of occult GI bleeding such as vascular lesions, and graft-versus-host disease.

In this article, the authors (1) describe the latest techniques, challenges, and tips for performing high-quality MR enterographic examinations; (2) describe the spectrum of findings in IBD, including Crohn disease (CD) and ulcerative colitis (UC); and (3) discuss techniques and applications of MR enterography for non-IBD entities.

NOMENCLATURE OF MR BOWEL IMAGING

There are several MR imaging techniques for the bowel: MR enterography (MR imaging after oral contrast ingestion), MR enteroclysis (MR imaging after instilling a large volume of enteric contrast via a nasojejunal tube), and MR colonography (MR imaging performed after rectal and colonic administration of contrast or saline enema). Of these, MR enterography is the most common, practical, and acceptable imaging examination performed in pediatric patients.

PATIENT PREPARATION

All patients should be given nothing by mouth between 4 and 6 hours before the study. Adequate hydration up to 4 hours before the MR imaging study is recommended to reduce vasovagal reactions, reduce side effects of administered medications and contrast agents (both oral and intravenous [IV]), and facilitate IV line placement. Most patients having an MR enterography examination are adolescents; therefore, sedation is not usually required. However, use of sedation for MR enterography depends on institutional sedation policies, and alternatives to sedation may need to be considered (**Box 1**).

Box 1
Considerations before scanning

These are important points to address in conjunction with nursing, technologists, and clinicians

Bowel preparation: No routine bowel cleansing protocol is needed, except in cases for evaluation of colonic polyps

Sedation: Most cases (especially adolescents) do not require sedation. Follow sedation guidelines per institution. Consider (1) patients alternative examination, (2) MR enterography under general anesthesia with airway protection because oral contrast is required, (3) child life involvement, and (4) use of video goggles

Oral contrast type and delivery: Biphasic contrast is ideal and recommended. Continuous drinking during a 45-minute period. Can be given through G-tube if required or nasogastric tube if patient refuses by mouth

Antispasmolytics: Helps improve image quality. May still perform MR enterography without but recommended.

    Options outside of the United States: Buscopan (butylscopolamine)

    Options in the United States: Glucagon (IV or intramuscular) or hyoscyamine (Levsin) IV or sublingual

    For IV glucagon: Slowly inject with adequate saline flush to reduce side effects

Intravenous contrast: Recommended for all MR enterographic examinations. If IV contrast is contraindicated, DWI and fat-saturated T2-weighted imaging can provide valuable information about disease activity

If MR imaging is contraindicated: Alternative examinations such as bowel US or CT enterography should be considered (the former is preferred by the authors)

CONTRAST: ORAL, RECTAL, AND INTRAVENOUS

Although there is no consensus on the optimal oral contrast regimen, the most favorable contrast agents used for MR enterography are biphasic agents (hypointense on T1-weighted and hyperintense on T2-weighted sequences). The literature on pediatric MR enterographic imaging describes use of mannitol, polyethylene glycol, low-concentration barium solution (0.1% weight/volume) with sorbitol (VoLumen [Bracco Diagnostics, Inc.]), and sorbitol alone with flavoring (**Box 2**). In general, these agents prevent the absorption of water and allow for bowel distention. Patients are encouraged to drink continuously and steadily during a period of 45 to 60 min, with total oral contrast volumes varying from 600 to 1000 mL. Some institutional protocols also include 200 to 240 mL of water in the last 10 to 15 minutes before placing patient on the scanner. One way to improve duodenal and jejunal distention is to ask the patient to lay right side down the last 10 to 15 min before scanning. A study in adult patients performed a head-to-head comparison of oral contrast agents and reported that volumes greater than 1000 mL led to increased cathartic side effects.[6] MR imaging scanning ideally begins within 1 hour from the beginning of contrast ingestion. Rectal contrast in the form of saline enema could be considered in certain cases, including (1) concern of a rectal or colonic stricture and (2) incomplete or inadequate colonic endoscopy. IV contrast is also given for every MR enterography, unless there is a contraindication.

Helpful tips to improve patient compliance with MR enterography

1. Provide patient and family education
2. Have nursing staff supervise and encourage oral contrast ingestion
3. Chill and flavor contrast
4. Offer a nasogastric tube for contrast administration early on in a child who is reluctant to drink

---

ANTIPERISTALTICS AND OTHER MEDICATIONS

Antiperistaltics have the advantage of improving the quality of MR enterography examinations by reducing motion from bowel peristalsis. These agents do have significant side effects, most notably nausea and vomiting. These side effects

---

Box 2
Common oral contrast agents for pediatric MR enterographic studies

VoLumen (Bracco Diagnostics, Inc.), alone or mixed with ferumoxsil iron oxide suspension

Mannitol

Polyethylene glycol (mixed with juice, flavoring)

Sorbitol (mixed with flavoring)

---

can be limited by slow administration, hydration, and administration of antiemetics. Butylscopamine (Buscopan) is approved for use outside the United States. In the United States, glucagon and hyoscyamine are approved for use. Glucagon, the more common of the 2 medications used in pediatrics, can be given IV or intramuscular, 0.5 to 1.0 mg total. Glucagon can be given in a split dose, half at the beginning of the MR enterographic study and half just before the contrast-enhanced images are acquired. Patients should be thoroughly screened for glucagon by the nursing staff as outlined in the article by Darge and colleagues.[7] Other medications advocated by some anecdotally in adults include metoclopramide and erythromycin, which accelerate gastric emptying, promoting adequate proximal small-bowel filling in the early part of the examination. These are not used in children for MR enterography. Some centers chose not to give antiperistaltic agents, and researchers have described that in these situations the MR enterographic studies can still be diagnostic.[8] However, a recent pediatric study has shown benefits in using IV glucagon, as there was significant improvement in visualization of the bowel wall after IV glucagon was administered in comparison to the same sequence without glucagon.[9]

TECHNIQUE: POSITIONING, COILS, AND SEQUENCES

Patients can be scanned in the prone or supine position using a multichannel torso or body phased array coil on a 1.5- or 3-Tesla (T) magnet. Anatomic coverage should always include the pelvis but need not include the lung bases or top of the liver. Although not always possible, prone imaging may be useful to separate the bowel loops and help reduce bowel motion.[7,10] Exceptions to the prone position include presence of an ostomy, recent abdominal surgery, abdominal wall fistula, severe nausea, or if the study is being done under anesthesia. In these exceptional cases and in general, supine imaging with other strategies to reduce motion will yield diagnostic studies and has been shown to have no impact on lesion detection or characterization.[11–13]

The main sequences of the MR enterographic examination include axial and coronal T2-weighted single-shot fast spin echo (SSFSE) sequences with and without fat suppression, axial and coronal balanced steady state free precession (SSFP) sequences, axial T2-weighted FSE with fat suppression, axial diffusion-weighted echoplanar imaging, and coronal three-dimensional (3D) T1-weighted gradient recalled echo (GRE) imaging with fat suppression (**Box 3**). After administration of IV gadolinium-containing contrast material (0.1–0.2 mmol/kg), dynamic coronal 3D T1-weighted GRE sequences with fat suppression are obtained in time intervals of 45 to 55, 70, and 180 seconds. These intervals are not standard but are institutional specific. Delayed axial and coronal postcontrast 2D or 3D T1-weighted sequences with fat suppression are acquired following dynamic imaging. Dynamic postcontrast imaging is considered critical by many as it provides temporal information and has been shown to help differentiate active from fibrotic disease.[2] The postcontrast dynamic acquisition also enables better visualization of progressive transmural bowel wall enhancement and bowel stratification seen with active inflammation in IBD.[13] Regarding motion suppression, there are 2 main strategies in addition to using antiperistaltic agents: (1) breath hold techniques when the patient is cooperative and (2) respiratory triggering or navigator gating technique.[7]

Box 3
Comparison of various imaging sequences

Sequences	Advantages & Pathology Depicted	Artifacts
Single-shot fast spin-echo (SSFSE/HASTE)	• Fast *Good for:* • Edema and fluid in bowel wall and mesentery • Fat suppression increases conspicuity of bowel wall edema, thickening, ulcers; abscesses	• Flow artifacts within bowel lumen
Balanced gradient echo (FIESTA/TRUFISP/BTFE)	• Fast • Good for depicting anatomy, including anastomoses • Depicts mesenteric abnormalities, including lymphadenopathy, engorged vasa recta "comb sign" • Tethering of bowel is easily depicted in fistulizing disease • Global look at vasculature	• Susceptibility artifact from air (increases at 3-T) • Black borders from opposed phase and chemical shift artifact
Diffusion-weighted imaging (DWI)	• Can be performed before or after contrast • Restricted diffusion in bowel wall correlates with areas of active disease at histology	• Distortion at interfaces with air
Dynamic contrast enhanced 3D T1-SPGR (VIBE/LAVA/eTHRIVE)	• High yield sequence • Avid bowel wall hyperenhancement and striated pattern suggest active disease • More bland enhancement suggests chronic/inactive disease or fibrosis (if no coexisting active inflammation)	• Motion artifact from breathing

CINE

Cine sequences are now commonly included in MR enterography protocols. They are acquired as coronal thick slab steady state precession images repeated sequentially from front to back during a period of 2 minutes. The slice thickness can be between 8 and 10 mm, and on average about 18 to 20 images are acquired in each location and can be stacked together to be viewed as 1 acquisition. Cine sequences can be obtained before the first dose of glucagon is given (for single-dose glucagon or split dose protocols), or it can be performed before and after glucagon is given to assess functionality. As this is a fast sequence, there is relative flexibility in its application. The rationale for using cine imaging is to identify abnormal segments of bowel motility. As shown on fluoroscopic barium studies of the small bowel, segments infiltrated by disease, whether infection, inflammation, or tumor, are commonly fixed in place and separated from adjacent bowel loops, and generally do not peristalse normally. Cine can provide added information, especially for equivocal bowel segments, and also aid in the confirmation of true strictures. One study compared cine MR enterographic sequences with conventional sequences in patients with CD and found more abnormal bowel segments with cine than with the standard sequences, but these were not confirmed with histology.[14] The data in this publication are limited, and further studies are needed to validate the utility of this sequence.

DIFFUSION-WEIGHTED IMAGING

DWI also is becoming a standard part of MR enterography protocols in the pediatric population. DWI is an echoplanar sequence obtained in the axial plane with free breathing or respiratory triggering using anywhere between 3 and 5 b-values. There is no consensus on the ideal b-values to use in clinical practice; however, any combination between 0 and 1000 will yield adequate imaging (the authors use b-values of 0, 200, 500, 800, and 1000). The goal of DWI sequences is to help identify actively inflamed segments of bowel. Active disease demonstrates restricted diffusion (mural areas bright on DWI sequence and low or dark signal on the automatically generated apparent diffusion coefficient [ADC] maps). Early investigation into further refinement of diffusion processing techniques is underway, with the incorporation of intravoxel incoherent motion (IVIM) diffusion procession.[15] By using numerous b-values from low (10–50 mm/s^2) to high (800–1000 mm/s^2), this processing aims to separate the "background noise" of Brownian motion from true perfusional changes to better detect inflammation. Further work is needed, however, to refine IVIM and bring it into routine clinical practice. Practically, DWI is most useful when there is a questionable area of bowel abnormality; seeing restricted diffusion can increase reader confidence that the bowel segment is truly abnormal. Anecdotally, the authors have found that in rare cases when IV contrast cannot be given to a patient or if there are areas of suboptimal bowel distention, DWI can be helpful. Some investigators have advocated that there is potential for DWI to replace contrast-enhanced sequences.[16]

DWI is a helpful tool when there is less-than-optimal bowel distention or if IV contrast cannot be given to detect areas of active disease.

3-T VERSUS 1.5-T

Imaging with 3-T scanners is advantageous over imaging with 1.5-T magnets because of the increased signal-to-noise ratio; however, the trade-off for the increased signal-to-noise ratio is a concomitant increase in image artifacts. There are limited published data regarding MR enterographic imaging at 3-T. As described by Dagia and colleagues,[17] single-shot fast spin-echo sequences perform well at 3-T. Although the single-shot sequences still demonstrate flow artifacts within the bowel lumen, intramural and extramural pathology is still clearly depicted (**Fig. 1**A). In the authors' experience, performing single-shot sequences without fat suppression also helps decrease the artifacts encountered. The balanced SSFP sequences are prone to increased susceptibility artifacts, particularly from air in the bowel, especially the colon (see **Fig. 1**B). The pronounced chemical shift artifact at 3-T that occurs at the fat–water interfaces can adversely affect interpretation of bowel-wall pathology either leading to false-negative or false-positive results (see **Fig. 1**C–E).[18] There are a few ways to overcome these challenges at 3-T; one is to remove the sequence that is the most problematic (balanced SSFP) as the other sequences can identify the same abnormalities. The second is to optimize the sequences that withstand 3-T and do better at higher field strengths such as DWI and postcontrast imaging. In the authors' experience, when performing balanced SSFP sequences, increasing the field of view, increasing the number of slices above

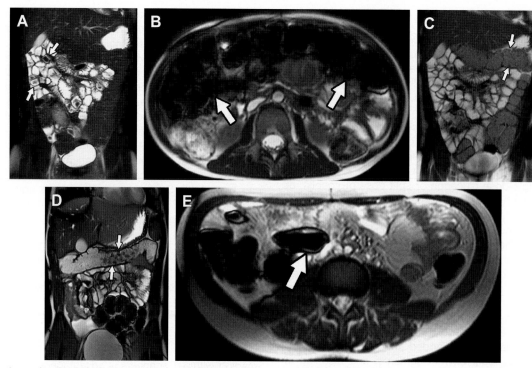

Fig. 1. (*A–E*) Artifacts in the bowel on MR enterography 1.5 and 3 T. (*A*) Coronal T2-weighted (T2W) single-shot fast spin echo (SSFSE) with fat suppression image demonstrating the normal small-bowel loops with the expected flow artifacts in the lumen of the bowel (*arrows*). (*B*) Axial balanced SSFP at 3-T shows the marked susceptibility artifact due to colonic air (*arrows*). (*C*) Coronal balanced SSFP at 1.5-T compared with (*D, E*) coronal and axial balanced SSFP at 3-T in another patient depicts the accentuated opposed phase black border artifact around the bowel (*arrows*) at higher field strength and when repetition time = 5 ms.

and below the area of coverage, and maintaining repetition time less than 4.0 ms improve image quality. High-quality cine sequences are feasible at 3-T.

PERFORMANCE OF MR ENTEROGRAPHY

The conventional gold standard imaging test for small-bowel mucosal involvement in CD is the double-contrast small-bowel barium fluoroscopic enteroclysis with a sensitivity of 93% to 95% and specificity of 92% to 96.5%.[19,20] The invasiveness of this test, lack of extraluminal information, and use of ionizing radiation, however, make this examination impractical, particularly in pediatric patients. In contrast, MR assessment of IBD has been shown to have a sensitivity of 93.0% and specificity of 92.8%, with MR enteroclysis performing slightly better than MR enterography.[21] A review of the literature shows MR enterography (with no contribution from MR enteroclysis studies) having a sensitivity ranging between 81% and 91% and a specificity between 67% and 89% for diagnosis of IBD.[19]

NORMAL FINDINGS ON MR ENTEROGRAPHY

With optimal distention, normal bowel loops should be closely opposed to each other, not separated or fixed, with normal brisk peristalsis on cine images (**Fig. 2**A). Abnormal bowel wall thickening (BWT) is generally considered greater than 3 mm; in children, abnormal measurements of bowel wall are defined as BWT greater than 2.5 mm for small bowel and greater than 2 mm for the colon.[10] The jejunum is an area of potential pitfall because the valvulae conniventes are normally more prominent than in other sections of the small bowel and may simulate BWT (**Fig. 2**B). The enhancement of the normal jejunum is greater than that of the normal ileum (**Fig. 2**C). In addition, when underdistended, the normal jejunum may have an apparent wall thickness of up to 7 mm.[22] Another normal finding is the presence of high signal content within the colon on T1-weighted images related to colonic fecal material (**Fig. 2**D). The cause of this high T1 signal in the colon is unclear.

Prominent mesenteric lymph nodes are commonly seen in normal children on CT and MR

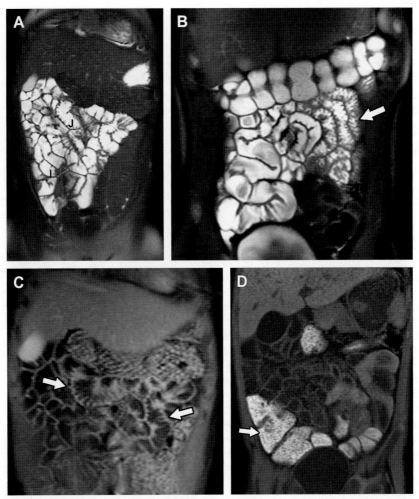

Fig. 2. (*A–D*) Normal findings on MR enterography. (*A*) Coronal T2W SSFSE image demonstrates normal small-bowel loops closely opposed to each other without separation and a normal wall thickness. (*B*) Coronal T2W SSFSE image shows the normal prominent valvulae conniventes of the jejunum (*arrow*). (*C*) Coronal postcontrast 3D T1-weighted (T1W) image depicts increased enhancement of the jejunum and prominent folds (*arrows*). (*D*) Coronal 3D T1W precontrast image shows the normal increased T1W signal of the contents of the colon.

imaging. Normal lymph nodes have a central fatty hilum, tend to be fewer in number, are localized primarily to the right lower quadrant, and only mildly enhance.

INFLAMMATORY BOWEL DISEASE

IBD has been reported to affect approximately 16.6 in 100,000 children and 5.3 in 100,000 children younger than 16 years.[23] Studies have demonstrated an increasing incidence of IBD within the United States, Europe, and Asia.[24–26] UC and CD together encompass most IBD; however, in around 10% of patients, it is categorized as indeterminate.[27]

CD is characterized by asymmetric, granulomatous, and transmural inflammation of the GI tract with periods of remission and relapse. The cause is multifactorial, and evidence suggests that environmental factors may play a significant role. Any portion of the GI tract may be affected, resulting in discontinuous involvement or skip lesions.[28,29] Onset of the disease is typically in late adolescence or early adulthood.[30] A combination of clinical examination, radiological findings, biochemical investigations, and endoscopic and histologic features is utilized to confirm the diagnosis of CD. Different classification systems of CD have been proposed in an attempt to prognosticate, follow disease status, and facilitate implementation of different treatment strategies. Imaging classification systems have been proposed as well. The following is one such classification system proposed by Maglinte and colleagues,[31] in which CD is divided into 4 sub-types (**Box 4**).

Box 4
Classification of Crohn disease based on Maglinte et al

Active inflammatory

Fistulizing/perforating

Fibrostenotic

Regenerative/reparative

Active Inflammatory Subtype

On MR enterography, specific features of active disease include bowel wall thickening, postcontrast hyperenhancement, and increased T2-weighted signal. Some studies have shown a wall thickness of 3 mm or greater to correlate with biologically active disease, whereas others have used a threshold of 4 to 6 mm to differentiate mild or nonactive disease from active inflammation.[32–35] Practically, more than 3 mm in BWT is abnormal. Bowel wall enhancement in active inflammation is transmural and progressive with a layered appearance referred to as mural stratification (**Fig. 3**). This appearance represents edematous submucosa enveloped by an inner layer of enhancing mucosa and an outer layer of enhancing serosa and bowel wall musculature.[31]

Increased mesenteric vascularity is seen in areas with active inflammation resulting in the so-called comb sign (**Fig. 4**). The comb sign is seen when prominence of the vascular arcades, secondary to increased flow, is outlined against a background of fibrofatty proliferation and inflammation. The presence of the comb sign is strongly correlated with active inflammation.[35] The comb sign is well depicted on balanced SSFP or on postcontrast T1 sequences.

Enlarged, enhancing mesenteric lymph nodes are commonly seen adjacent to active inflamed segments of bowel in patients with CD on postcontrast imaging varying in location from the small bowel, along transverse colon, sigmoid, paracolic, and perirectal regions.[36] Lymph nodes with a short axis dimension of 5 mm or greater are shown to positively correlate with active disease.[34] Mesenteric nodes are readily seen as areas of high signal intensity on DWI sequences or low signal structures surrounded by bright fat on SSFP images (**Fig. 5**).

On DWI, increased signal in affected segments combined with decreased ADC values correlates

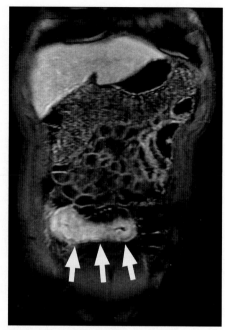

Fig. 3. Active inflammation. A 22-year-old patient with CD. A coronal 3D T1W Spoiled Gradient Echo (SPGR) postcontrast image demonstrating transmural inflammation with mural stratification and hyperenhancement of the distal and terminal ileum (*arrows*).

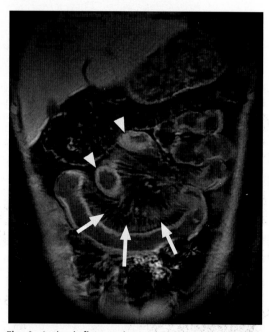

Fig. 4. Active inflammation. A 12-year-old with CD. A coronal 3D T1W SPGR postcontrast image demonstrates diffuse thickening of the distal jejunal and ileal bowel loops (*white arrowheads*) with prominence of the adjacent mesenteric vessels (*white arrows*). The appearance of the prominent mesenteric vasculature represents the comb sign.

Prior investigations have attempted to quantify disease activity using dynamic contrast-enhanced MR enterography and have compared imaging findings with the Crohn's Disease Activity Index, endoscopic scoring, and histology, finding moderate to excellent correlation.[38] Dynamic postcontrast MR enterography therefore may provide accurate differentiation of active from inactive disease to better guide management.[39]

Fistulizing/Perforating Subtype

In the fistulizing or perforating subtype of CD, transmural inflammation extends beyond the bowel wall to involve adjacent mesentery, organs or bowel loops. Inflammatory erosion into adjacent bowel loops or other epithelialized surfaces results in a fistula, whereas a blind ending tract or a connection between bowel and muscle, or mesentery results in a sinus tract (**Figs. 7** and **8**).[36] Sinus tracts and fistulae are well visualized with SSFP, T2-weighted FSE, or postcontrast fat-suppressed GRE sequences.[36,39] Abnormal kinking or tethering of adjacent loops is highly suggestive of fistulae. Enhancement of the fistulous tract can be seen after contrast administration (**Fig. 9**). Fistulous perforation of bowel wall develops initially as deep mucosal ulcers, which may be seen as longitudinal high-intensity lines within the bowel wall on SSFP imaging.[31] These tracts may, on rare occasions, form intramural or subcutaneous abscesses (**Figs. 10** and **11**). A review of IBD including 615 patients with CD found the fistulizing subtype of CD to be an independent risk factor for malignancy

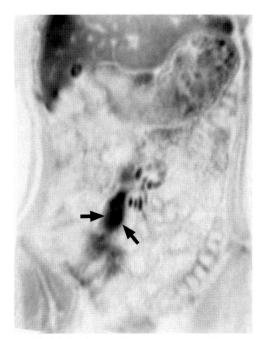

Fig. 5. Nonspecific inflammation. A 17-year-old patient with indeterminate colitis (clinically suspected CD). Coronal DWI (b = 500 s/mm²) image demonstrating lymphadenopathy (*arrows*). Note that the use of an inverted gray-scale image can provide increased conspicuity of lesions.

well with endoscopic and pathologic findings indicating active inflammation.[37] This correlation provides improved diagnostic confidence and can potentially lead to detection of subtle inflammation missed initially on standard sequences (**Fig. 6**).

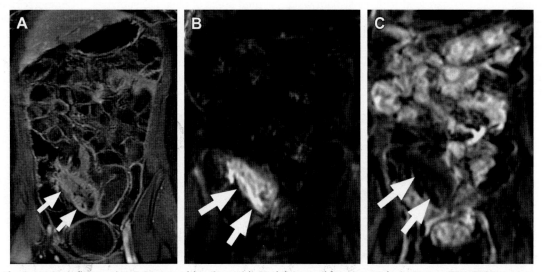

Fig. 6. Active inflammation. A 21-year-old patient with CD. (*A*) Coronal fat-saturated postcontrast T1W SPGR sequence showing extensive inflammation of the terminal ileum (*arrows*). (*B*) Coronal DWI (b = 500 s/mm²) image demonstrates marked DWI signal hyperintensity (*arrows*) corresponding to the area of enhancement. (*C*) Coronal ADC map shows corresponding low signal intensity (*arrows*) in the terminal ileum compatible with true restricted diffusion.

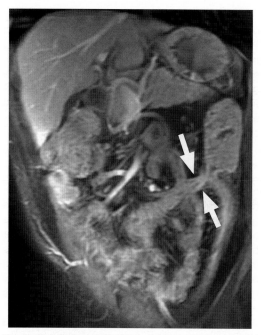

Fig. 7. Fistulizing/perforating subtype. A 22-year-old patient with CD. Coronal postcontrast 3D T1W SPGR image demonstrates a coloenteric fistula (*arrows*) involving the proximal descending colon and a loop of adjacent jejunum.

of the small bowel and colon, and recognition of this subtype should alert the reader to the possibility of a nonbenign lesion, particularly in the older patient.[40]

Fibrostenotic Subtype

Mural thickening can lead to luminal narrowing, but luminal narrowing by itself does not equate to an obstructing stricture/stenosis (both used synonymously in this discussion). True obstructing strictures present as luminal narrowing with associated upstream dilatation. Mural fibrosis leading to irreversible stricture formation is the hallmark of this subtype. Strictures are a cause of obstruction and may be secondary to inflammation, fibrosis, or a combination of both. Differentiation between inflammation and fibrosis is difficult by imaging and prior studies have thus far yielded mixed results. Some studies have demonstrated the inability of MR enterography to distinguish between the fibrotic and inflammatory strictures.[41] On the other hand, Gee and colleagues[2] have described several key features of fibrosis on MR enterography in children and have shown that MR enterography can be accurate in making the distinction between active and fibrotic disease. In their study, bowel wall signal isointense to muscle on T2-weighted sequences, bland enhancement and proximal bowel dilatation with absent early mucosal enhancement were all accurate signs of fibrosis.[2] Marked BWT without enhancement is strongly associated with fibrosis and has a negative correlation with successful medical treatment.[42] MR enterography has been shown to identify fibrostenotic CD at an earlier stage than clinical symptoms alone.[43]

> Hyperenhancement of the bowel wall, postcontrast mural stratification of the bowel wall, mesenteric comb sign, and enhancing lymph nodes are hallmarks of active disease.

Reparative/Regenerative Subtype

No active inflammation is evident in this subtype of CD, although there may be concurrent associated areas of other CD subtypes.[31] Characteristic imaging features include reparative polyps without significant hyperemia or mural edema and luminal narrowing without evidence of obstruction.[31,44] Chronic inflammation tends to involve the bowel wall in an asymmetric manner (**Fig. 12**).

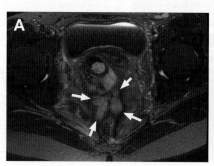
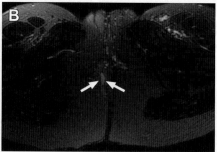

Fig. 8. Fistulizing/perforating subtype. A 15-year-old patient with CD. (*A*) Axial FSE T2W fat-saturated sequence demonstrating 4 separate fistula tracts (*arrows*) originating from the rectum, confirmed on subsequent endoscopy. (*B*) Axial T2W FSE fat-saturated sequence depicts the inferior extent of one of the fistula tracts into the perineal soft tissues (*arrows*).

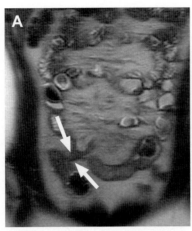
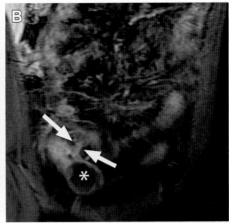

Fig. 9. Fistulizing/perforating subtype. A 18-year-old patient with CD. (*A*) Coronal T2W SSFSE image demonstrating a suspected enteroenteric fistula with a T2W hypointense connection between the terminal ileum and an adjacent small-bowel loop (*arrows*). (*B*) Coronal postcontrast 3D T1W SPGR image also depicts the suspected enteroenteric fistula (*arrows*) between terminal ileum (*asterisk*) and an adjacent loop of ileum. Note the hyperenhancement of the fistula after contrast.

ULCERATIVE COLITIS

UC differs from CD in that it is restricted to the colon and is thus more amenable to diagnosis by endoscopic evaluation. Where colonoscopy is not feasible, MR enterography is a suitable alternative with imaging findings closely correlating with endoscopic findings.[45] In the pediatric population, MR enterography is even more desirable, as it can often be performed without sedation and avoids the risks associated with endoscopy.

MR enterography features of UC are similar to those of CD (**Box 5**). BWT is seen in active UC and is usually of a lesser degree than that seen in CD.[45] Hyperenhancement of involved bowel, which may appear featureless on MR enterography, is common (**Fig. 13**). Surrounding mesenteric changes, including fibrofatty proliferation, are far less prominent than in CD. Inflammation extending contiguously from the rectosigmoid to the more proximal large bowel is the norm, but rarely isolated disease of the right colon may be present.[46] Distal ileum involvement in the form of backwash ileitis can be seen with UC and can complicate the distinction between UC and CD (**Fig. 14**). UC, like CD, demonstrates restricted diffusion in affected segments of bowel (**Fig. 15**). Differentiation of UC from CD is extremely important from a

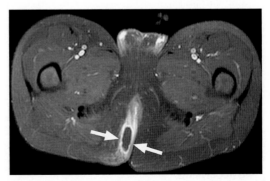

Fig. 10. Fistulizing/perforating subtype. A 16-year-old patient with CD. Axial postcontrast 3D T1W SPGR image demonstrating an intramural abscess in the distal ileum (*arrows*). The fluid collection is separate from the true lumen of the bowel (*asterisk*).

Fig. 11. Fistulizing/perforating subtype. A 14-year-old patient with CD. Axial T1W SPGR postcontrast image showing a rim-enhancing collection in the medial subcutaneous tissues of the right buttock (*arrows*).

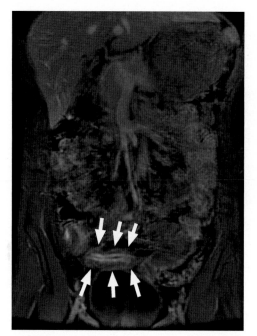

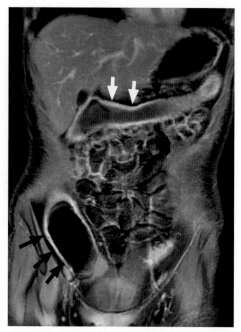

Fig. 12. Chronic inflammation. A 20-year-old patient with CD. Coronal delayed postcontrast 3D T1W SPGR image demonstrating thickening of the terminal ileum with abnormal enhancement limited to the mucosa (*arrows*), suggesting the presence of mural scarring and chronic inflammatory changes.

Fig. 13. Ulcerative colitis. A 11-year-old patient with UC. Coronal postcontrast 3D T1W SPGR image shows hyperenhancing, thickened cecum (*black arrows*), and transverse colon (*white arrows*) with a featureless appearance due to loss of the normal colonic haustra.

Box 5
Extraintestinal pathology of CD and UC

Extraintestinal Pathology	CD	UC
Mesentery		
Vascular engorgement—comb sign	+++	+++
Creeping fat	+++	+
Fluid accumulation	++	+
Fistula/sinus tract formation	++	—
Enlarged lymph nodes	++	+
Pancreaticobiliary system		
Cholelithiasis	++	+
Primary sclerosing cholangitis	+	+++
Autoimmune pancreatitis	+	+
Urogenital tract		
Calculi	+	+
Adhesion/obstruction	++	+
Fistulae	++	—
Cutaneous	+++	+
Skeletal		
Arthropathy	++	+
Osteopenia (secondary to medication/poor nutrition/inflammation)	+	+
Osteomyelitis	++	—
Opthalmic		
Uveitis/iritis	+	++
GI tract malignancy	+	+++

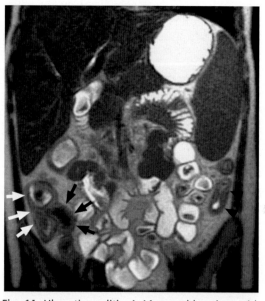

Fig. 14. Ulcerative colitis. A 14-year-old patient with UC. Coronal single-shot FSE T2W image showing wall thickening of the cecum (*white arrows*) and descending colon (*black arrowheads*). Thickening of the terminal ileum (*black arrows*) is also present, consistent with backwash ileitis confirmed on subsequent biopsy.

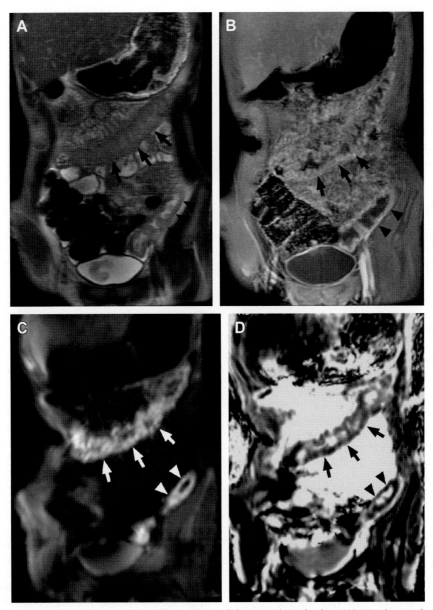

Fig. 15. Ulcerative Colitis. A 14-year-old patient with UC. (*A*) Coronal single-shot FSE T2W image demonstrating diffuse wall thickening of the transverse (*black arrows*) and distal descending colon (*black arrowheads*). (*B*) Coronal postcontrast T1W image also demonstrating diffuse wall thickening and enhancement of the transverse (*black arrows*) and distal descending colon (*black arrowheads*). (*C*) Coronal DWI (b = 500 s/mm²) demonstrating corresponding hyperintense signal in the transverse (*white arrows*) and distal descending colon (*white arrowheads*). (*D*) Coronal ADC map demonstrating diffuse low signal intensity in the transverse (*black arrows*) and distal descending colon (*black arrowheads*), confirming true diffusion restriction.

prognostic and therapeutic viewpoint, and often a combination of pathologic, clinical, and radiological information may be required to arrive at a definitive diagnosis.

COMPLICATIONS OF IBD

Complications of CD may be classified as intestinal or extraintestinal. Examples of common intestinal complications include the development of abscesses; fistulas between the bowel and other pelvic organs such as the bladder, urethra, vagina, prostate, or scrotum; and frank bowel obstruction related to a stricture. Extraintestinal complications include development of perianal manifestations of CD, pancreatobiliary disease and osseous changes (**Fig. 16**A). When perianal disease is the manifesting presentation of CD,

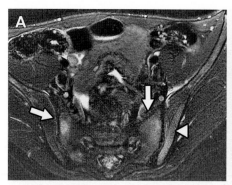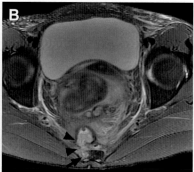

Fig. 16. Complications of IBD: Sacroiliitis and sacral osteomyelitis is 2 different children. (*A*) A 10-year-old with CD. Axial high-resolution T2W FSE fat-saturated image shows abnormal high signal in the sacrum (*arrows*) and in the left ilium (*arrowhead*) representing bilateral sacroiliitis. (*B*) An 11-year-old patient with UC. Axial T2W FSE fat-saturated sequence demonstrating a fistulous tract (*arrowheads*) leading to the distal sacrum. Resulting focal osteomyelitis of the sacrum is present with bone marrow edema and adjacent inflammatory change in the right lateral aspect of the sacrum (*arrow*).

intestinal disease is usually also present. Only a minority of patients have persistent isolated perianal disease.[47] In addition, colonic CD is more likely to have perianal involvement compared with isolated terminal ileum involvement. Due to the prevalence of perianal disease, anatomic coverage to include the pelvis is a crucial part of every MR enterographic study. Perianal abscesses and fistulas are readily seen on T2-weighted and postcontrast T1-weighted images (**Figs. 8B and 11**). In more severe cases, fistula may involve the adjacent bone and lead to osteomyelitis (**Fig. 16B**).

In general, hepatobiliary extraintestinal complications in IBD do not correlate with disease activity, unlike other extraintestinal manifestations affecting the skin, joints, and eyes.[48] Up to 7.5% of patients with IBD develop primary sclerosing cholangitis (PSC), while 70% to 80% of patients with PSC also have underlying IBD.[48,49] Although PSC can occur in CD, it is more prevalent in patients with UC. Magnetic resonance cholangiopancreatography (MRCP) is a noninvasive, sensitive, and radiation-free substitute to the gold standard endoscopic retrograde cholangiopancreatography. Typical features of PSC seen on MRCP include a beaded appearance to the intrahepatic and extrahepatic bile ducts with alternating regions of narrowing and dilation (**Fig. 17**).[49]

- Complications of CD: abscesses, fistulas with other bowel loops or organs, perianal disease, sacroileitis, and chronic osteomyelitis
- PSC is associated with IBD, most commonly UC

INTERPRETATION OF MR ENTEROGRAPHIC STUDIES

The ideal approach to MR enterographic interpretation is a stepwise, systematic approach. Many approaches work; the following is one method of interpretation. In general, as with all MR interpretations, a review of the localizers can reveal pathology outside of the field of view of the examination and is a good habit to develop. Next, assessment of the coronal and axial T2-weighted single-shot FSE and T2-weighted FSE sequences provides an excellent "bird's eye" view of the solid organs, degree of small-bowel distention, presence of fluid collections, and presence of edema and fluid in the bowel wall and mesentery. T2-weighted FSE sequences offer characterization of any incidentally noted liver, biliary, or pancreatic pathology. Coronal SSFP sequences can provide assessment of the overall anatomy. Dynamic postcontrast T1-weighted 3D GRE sequences are critical in assessment of the degree, extent, and distribution of bowel wall enhancement, abdominal vascular structures, and presence of abscesses. These T1-weighted sequences in the coronal plane allow for optimal depiction of the terminal ileum. Finally, cine SSFP sequences can be used to help identify and confirm inflamed segments (which show decreased peristalsis), assess strictures, and verify suspected strictures.[11,14,50,51]

MR ENTEROGRAPHY BEYOND IBD

An additional benefit of MR enterography is the ability to assess the patient with nonspecific chronic abdominal pain when IBD is one part of a broader differential. This ability can limit the number of imaging studies a child needs to under go to arrive at a

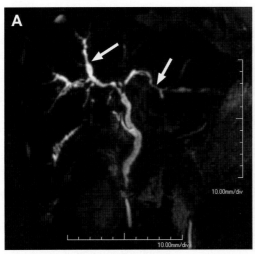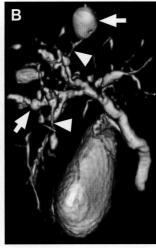

Fig. 17. Complications of IBD. A 17-year-old patient with UC and known primary sclerosing cholangitis. (*A*) Coronal subvolume maximum intensity projection image derived from respiratory gated 3D MRCP demonstrating focal areas of narrowing in the bile ducts (*white arrows*). (*B*) Volume-rendered 3D image derived from respiratory gated 3D MRCP demonstrates focal areas of fusiform dilation of the intrahepatic bile ducts (*arrows*) and long segment strictures (*arrowheads*).

diagnosis as well as minimizes ionizing radiation exposure. Patients presenting with chronic abdominal pain related to appendicitis, infection, polyps, or intestinal masses can be thoroughly assessed with this single examination. The MR enterographic technique for these non-IBD conditions is essentially the same as previously described; however, there are situations in which it may be modified to answer the clinical question at hand.

APPENDICITIS

MR imaging for the appendix is emerging as an alternative to CT in many institutions, especially where US is not available or is equivocal. However, to assess for appendicitis on MR imaging, an enterographic technique is usually not required. In fact, most currently described MR imaging techniques for appendicitis in children do not require oral or IV contrast.[5,52] Fast single-shot FSE sequences with fat suppression are the workhorse for this examination and are usually performed in the coronal and axial planes, with additional sagittal plane if time permits. Two large pediatric studies showed that it is feasible to perform MR imaging of the appendix quickly and without sedation, and that the diagnostic performance is comparable to CT with a sensitivity of 97.6% to 100%, specificity of 97% to 99%, and negative predictive value between 99.4% and 100%.[5,52]

The findings on MR imaging for appendicitis parallel those seen on CT, including

- Enlarged, dilated appendix with T2 hyperintense contents

- Periappendiceal inflammation as high signal on T2-weighted sequences
- Cecal wall thickening
- Free fluid
- Intraluminal appendiceal low-signal structures on T1-weighted and T2-weighted sequences, indicating appendocoliths/fecoliths

> MR imaging for appendicitis can be performed without oral and IV contrasts, using fast T2-weighted single-shot FSE sequences with fat suppression.

SMALL BOWEL OBSTRUCTION

The most common causes of small bowel obstruction in children include adhesions, appendicitis, intussusceptions, inguinal hernias, Meckel diverticula, and volvulus.[53] With adequate bowel distention, the caliber change from dilated to collapsed bowel may be evident on MR imaging, allowing for identification of a transition point. Postoperative adhesions may be visible as fibrous bands that demonstrate low signal on T1- and T2-weighted sequences in the vicinity of the transition point.

> Long imaging times, lack of availability, and the rigorous oral contrast preparation can make MR enterography impractical for evaluation of acute small bowel obstruction in children.

INFECTIONS

Commonly encountered enteritis from viral sources does not warrant imaging with MR enterography. Clinical scenarios in which MR enterography would be helpful include evaluation of atypical enteritis/colitis or suspected typhlitis in immunocompromised patients. Imaging features are nonspecific and tend to overlap with those seen in IBD (**Fig. 18**).[4]

Findings of infection on MR enterography include

- Wall thickening with mural stratification
- Mesenteric inflammation
- Perienteric/pericolic stranding
- Adenopathy with or without necrosis
- Phlegmon, perforation, and abscesses

CELIAC DISEASE

Celiac disease, a gluten-sensitive enteropathy, is traditionally assessed by a combination of serologic markers, clinical symptoms, and direct endoscopic biopsy of the small bowel. Histology is diagnostic with villous atrophy of the jejunum as the hallmark. Celiac disease predominantly

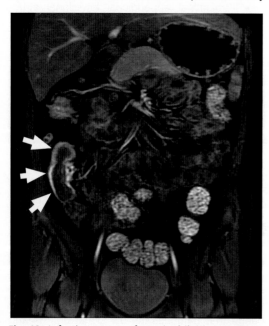

Fig. 18. Infectious cause of terminal ileitis on MR enterography. A 16-year-old girl with systemic lupus with constitutional symptoms and a positive purified protein derivative test. Coronal fat-saturated postcontrast T1W SPGR image demonstrating mucosal hyperenhancement and thickening of the terminal ileum (*arrows*). Subsequent pathology from colonoscopy revealed the presence of acid-fast bacilli in this patient with tuberculosis enteritis.

involves the duodenum and proximal jejunum and can be focal or diffuse. The jejunum will lose its normal feathery folds, whereas the folds in the ileum will become prominent, referred to as reversal of jejunal-ileal folds. MR enterography has been utilized in children and adults to detect rare complications, such as lymphoma, carcinoma, and jejunal strictures.[54]

Findings of celiac disease on MR enterography include

- Reversal of the jejunal-ileal folds, with dilated proximal jejunum
- Nonobstructive small bowel-small bowel intussusceptions,
- Mesenteric vascular engorgement
- Occasional BWT and mesenteric lymphadenopathy

POLYPS

The most common polyposis syndromes encountered in the pediatric population include juvenile polyposis coli, Peutz-Jeghers syndrome (PJS), and familial adenomatous polyposis. A combination of capsule endoscopy (CE), direct upper endoscopy, lower ileocolonoscopy, and double-balloon push enteroscopy has been utilized in the detection, treatment, and surveillance of polyps. There are promising data suggesting that MR enterography can be used as a noninvasive tool to detect large polyps in patients with PJS (**Figs. 19** and **20**). Gupta and colleagues[55] reported that MR enterography was better able to detect polyps greater than 15 mm, was reproducible, and was able to better estimate size and location in comparison to CE. The MR enterographic technique is the same as for IBD.

On reviewing MR enterographic studies for polyps the following are important points:

- SSFP and postcontrast sequences are crucial.
- Luminal flow artifact in single-shot images may mimic polyps.
- Polyps are low signal on balanced SSFP and usually enhance intensely after contrast administration.
- Polyps may adhere to the bowel wall, may have a stalk, and have the potential to cause intussusceptions.

SMALL-BOWEL MASSES

Small-bowel masses are rare in children and comprise benign entities such as lipomas and vascular malformations as well as malignancies such as lymphoma, adenocarcinoma, carcinoid,

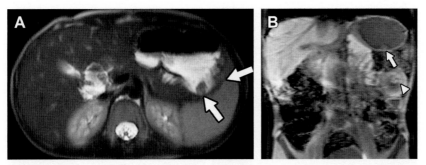

Fig. 19. Gastric and small-bowel polyps in a 12-year-old boy with Peutz-Jegher syndrome. (*A*) Axial single-shot T2W FSE image shows a few focal low-signal polyps in the posterior wall of the stomach (*arrows*). (*B*) Coronal postcontrast T1W 3D SPGR demonstrates moderate enhancement of the gastric polyp (*arrow*), and an additional enhancing polyp is seen protruding into the lumen of the jejunum in the left upper quadrant (*arrowhead*).

and gastrointestinal stromal tumors (**Fig. 21**).[4,54] A full discussion of all these is beyond the scope of this article. It is worthwhile to mention a few important points about the utility of MR enterography for vascular malformations and lymphoma. Usually, children with vascular malformations involving the small or large bowel present with anemia due to occult GI bleeding. These lesions are often visible on CE. On the other hand, lymphoma (usually non-Hodgkin B-cell type, Burkitt subtype) typically presents with intussusceptions, palpable masses, failure to thrive, or early obstructive symptoms.[54]

When performing or reviewing MR enterographic studies for these indications, one should keep in mind the following:

- MR enterography affords better localization and determination of extent of a vascular malformation compared with CT.[56,57]
- Dynamic contrast-enhanced 3D T1-weighted sequences allow for delayed venous phases to capture slow flow vessels within a vascular lesion.
- Lymphoma can involve a single bowel segment or multiple segments.

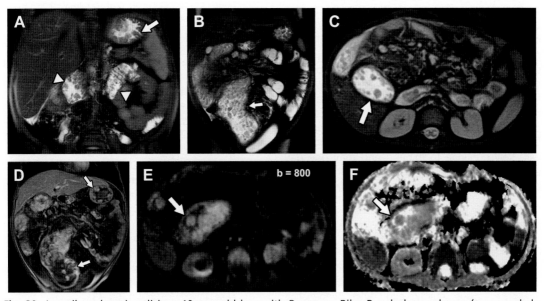

Fig. 20. Juvenile polyposis coli in a 10-year-old boy with Bannayan-Riley-Ruvalcaba syndrome (macrocephaly, developmental delay, and juvenile polyposis). (*A*) Coronal single-shot T2W FSE through the upper abdomen shows numerous low signal intensity polyps in the stomach (*arrow*), duodenum, and jejunum (*arrowheads*). (*B, C*) Coronal single-shot T2W FSE and axial T2W FSE with fat suppression shows a dilated distal ileum filled with numerous low signal polyps (*arrow*). (*D*) Postcontrast coronal T1W 3D SPGR image again show the polyps enhancing intensely compared to the bowel wall (*arrows*). The polyps also demonstrate hyperintense signal on (*E*) axial DWI (b = 800 s/mm^2) and hypointense signal on the (*F*) ADC map indicating restricted diffusion (*arrows*).

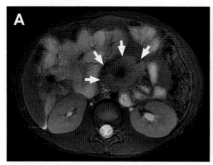 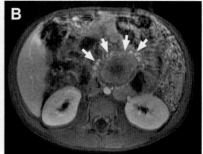

Fig. 21. Mass on MR enterography. A 9-year-old child with chronic iron-deficiency anemia with chronically elevated inflammatory markers and constitutional symptoms. (*A*) Axial T2W radial blade PROPELLER fat-saturated sequence demonstrating a large mesenteric mass (*arrows*) with central T2 hypointensity. (*B*) Axial fat-saturated postcontrast T1W SPGR sequence demonstrates the mass (*arrows*) immediately abutting the short mesenteric arteries. Pathology following resection revealed an enlarged, necrotic mesenteric lymph node with follicular hyperplasia.

- Bowel findings in lymphoma include wall thickening; large intraluminal masses; exophytic, necrotic masses; aneurysmal dilatation of bowel; strictures; or intussusceptions.
- Lymphoma usually demonstrates mild enhancement after IV contrast in contrast to polyps, which enhance more intensely.

SUMMARY

MR enterography has become an important tool for radiologists assessing both pediatric CD and UC. The authors have emphasized how techniques such as DWI and balanced SSFP cine sequences are changing how one interprets these challenging cases because one can now provide both anatomic and functional information. MR enterography can also be utilized in the evaluation of other small-bowel diseases such as infections, polyps, celiac disease, and small-bowel masses. In the future, applications for MR enterography will likely continue to expand and may one day obviate the currently used imaging studies of the bowel that require ionizing radiation.

REFERENCES

1. Absah I, Bruining DH, Matsumoto JM, et al. MR enterography in pediatric inflammatory bowel disease: retrospective assessment of patient tolerance, image quality, and initial performance estimates. AJR Am J Roentgenol 2012;199(3): W367–75.

2. Gee MS, Nimkin K, Hsu M, et al. Prospective evaluation of MR enterography as the primary imaging modality for pediatric Crohn disease assessment. AJR Am J Roentgenol 2011;197(1):224–31.

3. Darge K, Anupindi SA, Jaramillo D. MR imaging of the bowel: pediatric applications. Magn Reson Imaging Clin N Am 2008;16(3):467–78, vi.

4. Fidler JL, Guimaraes L, Einstein DM. MR imaging of the small bowel. Radiographics 2009;29(6): 1811–25.

5. Moore MM, Gustas CN, Choudhary AK, et al. MRI for clinically suspected pediatric appendicitis: an implemented program. Pediatr Radiol 2012;42(9): 1056–63.

6. Young BM, Fletcher JG, Booya F, et al. Head-to-head comparison of oral contrast agents for cross-sectional enterography: small bowel distention, timing, and side effects. J Comput Assist Tomogr 2008;32(1):32–8.

7. Darge K, Anupindi SA, Jaramillo D. MR imaging of the abdomen and pelvis in infants, children, and adolescents. Radiology 2011;261(1):12–29.

8. Grand DJ, Beland MD, Machan JT, et al. Detection of Crohn's disease: comparison of CT and MR enterography without anti-peristaltic agents performed on the same day. Eur J Radiol 2012;81(8):1735–41.

9. Dillman JR, Smith EA, Khalatbari S, et al. IV Glucagon use in Pediatric MR Enterography: Effect on Image Quality, length of examination and patient tolerance. Am J Roentgenol 2013;201(1):185–9.

10. Anupindi SA, Janitz E, Darge K. Bowel imaging in children: a comprehensive look using US and MRI. Semin Roentgenol 2012;47(2):118–26.

11. Griffin N, Grant LA, Anderson S, et al. Small bowel MR enterography: problem solving in Crohn's disease. Insight 2012;3(3):251–63.

12. Cronin CG, Lohan DG, Browne AM, et al. Magnetic resonance enterography in the evaluation of the small bowel. Semin Roentgenol 2009;44(4):237–43.

13. Gee MS, Harisinghani MG. MRI in patients with inflammatory bowel disease. J Magn Reson Imaging 2011;33(3):527–34.

14. Froehlich JM, Waldherr C, Stoupis C, et al. MR motility imaging in Crohn's disease improves lesion detection compared with standard MR imaging. Europe 2010;20(8):1945–51.

15. Freiman M, Perez-Rossello JM, Callahan MJ, et al. Characterization of fast and slow diffusion from diffusion-weighted MRI of pediatric Crohn's disease. J Magn Reson Imaging 2013;37(1): 156–63.

16. Neubauer H, Pabst T, Dick A, et al. Small-bowel MRI in children and young adults with Crohn disease: retrospective head-to-head comparison of contrast-enhanced and diffusion-weighted MRI. Pediatr Radiol 2013;43(1):103–14.

17. Dagia C, Ditchfield M, Kean M, et al. Feasibility of 3-T MRI for the evaluation of Crohn disease in children. Pediatr Radiol 2010;40(10):1615–24.

18. Patak MA, von Weymarn C, Froehlich JM. Small bowel MR imaging: 1.5 T versus 3 T. Magn Reson Imaging Clin N Am 2007;15(3):383–93, vii.

19. Duigenan S, Gee MS. Imaging of pediatric patients with inflammatory bowel disease. AJR Am J Roentgenol 2012;199(4):907–15.

20. Stange E, Travis S, Vermeire S, et al. European evidence based consensus on the diagnosis and management of Crohn's disease: definitions and diagnosis. Gut 2006;55(Suppl 1):i1–15.

21. Horsthuis K, Bipat S, Bennink RJ, et al. Inflammatory bowel disease diagnosed with US, MR, scintigraphy, and CT: meta-analysis of prospective studies. Radiology 2008;247(1):64–79.

22. Baker ME, Walter J, Obuchowski NA, et al. Mural attenuation in normal small bowel and active inflammatory Crohn's disease on CT enterography: location, absolute attenuation, relative attenuation, and the effect of wall thickness. AJR Am J Roentgenol 2009;192(2):417–23.

23. Cosgrove M, Al-Atia RF, Jenkins HR. The epidemiology of paediatric inflammatory bowel disease. Arch Dis Child 1996;74(5):460–1.

24. Jakobsen C, Paerregaard A, Munkholm P, et al. Pediatric inflammatory bowel disease: increasing incidence, decreasing surgery rate, and compromised nutritional status: a prospective population-based cohort study 2007-2009. Inflamm Bowel Dis 2011; 17(12):2541–50.

25. Malaty HM, Fan X, Opekun AR, et al. Rising incidence of inflammatory bowel disease among children: a 12-year study. J Pediatr Gastroenterol Nutr 2010;50(1):27–31.

26. Shen YM, Wu JF, Chen HL, et al. Characteristics and incidences of pediatric Crohn's disease in the decades before and after 2000. Pediatrics 2011;52(6):317–20.

27. Podolsky DK. Inflammatory bowel disease. N Engl J Med 2002;347(6):417–29.

28. Furukawa A, Saotome T, Yamasaki M, et al. Cross-sectional imaging in Crohn disease. Radiographics 2004;24(3):689–702.

29. Lichtenstein GR, Hanauer SB, Sandborn WJ. Management of Crohn's disease in adults. Am J Gastroenterol 2009;104(2):465–83 [quiz: 464, 484].

30. Loftus EV. Clinical epidemiology of inflammatory bowel disease: incidence, prevalence, and environmental influences. Gastroenterology 2004; 126(6):1504–17.

31. Maglinte DD, Gourtsoyiannis N, Rex D, et al. Classification of small bowel Crohn's subtypes based on multimodality imaging. Radiol Clin North Am 2003;41(2):285–303.

32. Chalian M, Ozturk A, Oliva-Hemker M, et al. MR enterography findings of inflammatory bowel disease in pediatric patients. AJR Am J Roentgenol 2011; 196(6):W810–6.

33. Maccioni F, Viscido A, Broglia L, et al. Evaluation of Crohn disease activity with magnetic resonance imaging. Abdom Imaging 2000;25(3): 219–28.

34. Koh DM, Miao Y, Chinn RJ, et al. MR imaging evaluation of the activity of Crohn's disease. AJR Am J Roentgenol 2001;177(6):1325–32.

35. Zappa M, Stefanescu C, Cazals-Hatem D, et al. Which magnetic resonance imaging findings accurately evaluate inflammation in small bowel Crohn's disease? A retrospective comparison with surgical pathologic analysis. Inflamm Bowel Dis 2011;17(4): 984–93.

36. Smith EA, Dillman JR, Adler J, et al. MR enterography of extraluminal manifestations of inflammatory bowel disease in children and adolescents: moving beyond the bowel wall. AJR Am J Roentgenol 2012;198(1):W38–45.

37. Oto A, Zhu F, Kulkarni K, et al. Evaluation of diffusion-weighted MR imaging for detection of bowel inflammation in patients with Crohn's disease. Acad Radiol 2009;16(5):597–603.

38. Del Vescovo R, Sansoni I, Caviglia R, et al. Dynamic contrast enhanced magnetic resonance imaging of the terminal ileum: differentiation of activity of Crohn's disease. Abdom Imaging 2008;33(4):417–24.

39. Grand DJ, Beland M, Harris A. Magnetic resonance enterography. Radiol Clin North Am 2013; 51(1):99–112.

40. Biancone L, Zuzzi S, Ranieri M, et al. Fistulizing pattern in Crohn's disease and pancolitis in ulcerative colitis are independent risk factors for cancer: a single-center cohort study. J Crohns Colitis 2012; 6(5):578–87.

41. Lenze F, Wessling J, Bremer J, et al. Detection and differentiation of inflammatory versus fibromatous Crohn's disease strictures: prospective comparison of (18) F-FDG-PET/CT, MR-enteroclysis,

and transabdominal ultrasound versus endoscopic/histologic evaluation. Inflamm Bowel Dis 2012;18(12):2252–60.

42. Lawrance IC, Welman CJ, Shipman P, et al. Correlation of MRI-determined small bowel Crohn's disease categories with medical response and surgical pathology. World J Gastroenterol 2009; 15(27):3367–75.

43. Rieder F, Lawrance IC, Leite A, et al. Predictors of fibrostenotic Crohn's disease. Inflamm Bowel Dis 2011;17(9):2000–7.

44. Sinha R, Verma R, Verma S, et al. MR enterography of Crohn disease: part 2, imaging and pathologic findings. AJR Am J Roentgenol 2011;197(1): 80–5.

45. Ordas I, Rimola J, Garcia-Bosch O, et al. Diagnostic accuracy of magnetic resonance colonography for the evaluation of disease activity and severity in ulcerative colitis: a prospective study. Gut 2012;1–7.

46. Maccioni F, Colaiacomo MC, Parlanti S. Ulcerative colitis: value of MR imaging. Abdom Imaging 2005;30(5):584–92.

47. Safar B, Sands D. Perianal Crohn's disease. Clin Colon Rectal Surg 2007;20(4):282–93.

48. Navaneethan U, Kochhar G, Venkatesh PG, et al. Duration and severity of primary sclerosing cholangitis is not associated with risk of neoplastic changes in the colon in patients with ulcerative colitis. Gastrointest Endosc 2012;75(5):1045–54.e1.

49. Chavhan GB, Babyn PS, Manson D, et al. Pediatric MR cholangiopancreatography: principles, technique, and clinical applications. Radiographics 2008;28(7):1951–62.

50. Menys A, Atkinson D, Odille F, et al. Quantified terminal ileal motility during MR enterography as a potential biomarker of Crohn's disease activity: a preliminary study. Europe 2012;22(11):2494–501.

51. Wakamiya M, Furukawa A, Kanasaki S, et al. Assessment of small bowel motility function with cine-MRI using balanced steady-state free precession sequence. J Magn Reson Imaging 2011;33(5): 1235–40.

52. Johnson AK, Filippi CG, Andrews T, et al. Ultrafast 3-T MRI in the evaluation of children with acute lower abdominal pain for the detection of appendicitis. AJR Am J Roentgenol 2012;198(6):1424–30.

53. Hryhorczuk AL, Lee EY. Imaging evaluation of bowel obstruction in children: updates in imaging techniques and review of imaging findings. Semin Roentgenol 2012;47(2):159–70.

54. Amzallag-Bellenger E, Oudjit A, Ruiz A, et al. Effectiveness of MR enterography for the assessment of small-bowel diseases beyond Crohn disease. Radiographics 2012;32(5):1423–44.

55. Gupta A, Postgate AJ, Burling D, et al. A prospective study of MR enterography versus capsule endoscopy for the surveillance of adult patients with Peutz-Jeghers syndrome. AJR Am J Roentgenol 2010;195(1):108–16.

56. Jacquier A, Gorincour G, Vidal V, et al. Bowel venous malformation associated with an aneurysm of the portal vein. Pediatr Radiol 2007; 37(7):714–6.

57. Kandpal H, Sharma R, Srivastava DN, et al. Diffuse cavernous haemangioma of colon: magnetic resonance imaging features. Report of two cases. Australas Radiol 2007;51:B147–51.

Magnetic Resonance Imaging of Pediatric Pelvic Masses

Deepa R. Pai, MD, Maria F. Ladino-Torres, MD*

KEYWORDS

- Pelvic masses • Rhabdomyosarcoma • Surgical planning

KEY POINTS

- Magnetic resonance (MR) evaluation of pediatric pelvic masses is advantageous, given its excellent soft-tissue contrast resolution and lack of ionizing radiation.
- Rhabdomyosarcoma is the most common primary malignant neoplasm of the lower genitourinary tract. There is a peak incidence between 2 and 4 years of life, with a second peak in adolescence.
- Most pediatric ovarian masses are benign and functional. Functional ovarian cysts are the most commonly encountered entity and the most common abdominal mass in a newborn female. Malignant ovarian neoplasms are uncommon.
- Germ-cell tumors are the most common type of ovarian neoplasm encountered in the pediatric population. The most common type of pediatric ovarian germ-cell tumor is a mature teratoma.
- Uterine tumors are uncommon in pediatric patients, but when encountered in this population they are more likely to be malignant.
- Other miscellaneous tumors found in the pelvis in the pediatric population include those in the presacral space; these can be classified as congenital, developmental, neurogenic, inflammatory, mesenchymal, and osseous (extension of sacral neoplasms).

INTRODUCTION

Both benign and malignant pelvic masses are encountered in the pediatric population. Although ultrasonography remains the modality of choice for initial evaluation of a pediatric pelvic mass, magnetic resonance (MR) imaging is often used for further evaluation and lesion characterization. MR evaluation of pediatric pelvic masses is advantageous, given its multiplanar capabilities, excellent soft-tissue contrast resolution, and ability to specifically characterize certain types of tissues (ie, fat and blood). Contrast-enhanced MR imaging assists in mass characterization, presurgical planning, and staging when a malignancy is suspected. The lack of ionizing radiation is another advantage of MR imaging, particularly given the radiosensitivity of the gonads, and when multiple consecutive studies are needed to monitor therapy response in malignant conditions.

Pediatric pelvis masses can arise from a variety of pelvic structures, including the ovaries, lower genitourinary tract, musculature, neurovascular structures, lymph nodes, and adjacent osseous structures. Although the MR appearance of many pelvic masses is nonspecific, some masses demonstrate characteristic imaging features. For example, ovarian teratomas typically demonstrate areas of hyperintense signal on T1-weighted and T2-weighted sequences compatible with fat. Dysgerminomas contain internal fibrovascular septations that enhance on postcontrast sequences. Given its excellent soft-tissue contrast resolution, MR is useful in evaluating the full extent of a mass, including the relationship of the mass with adjacent critical pelvic structures, which may be

Section of Pediatric Radiology, Department of Radiology, C.S. Mott Children's Hospital, University of Michigan Health System, 1540 E. Hospital Drive, Ann Arbor, MI 48109–4252, USA
* Corresponding author.
E-mail address: marialad@med.umich.edu

Magn Reson Imaging Clin N Am 21 (2013) 751–772
http://dx.doi.org/10.1016/j.mric.2013.07.002
1064-9689/13/$ – see front matter © 2013 Elsevier Inc. All rights reserved.

important for presurgical planning and staging especially when a pelvic malignancy is suspected.

PROTOCOL
Pelvic Mass MR Imaging Protocol

The authors perform MR imaging for pelvic masses at both 1.5 and 3 T, but prefer 3 T imaging because of its improved signal to noise ratio (SNR), allowing for shorter image acquisition times and improved spatial resolution. During imaging, a multichannel torso surface coil is placed over the patient's pelvis and lower abdomen anteriorly. Parallel imaging can be used to reduce scan times. A routine pelvic mass protocol includes coronal T1-weighted fast spin-echo, coronal short-tau inversion recovery (STIR), axial T2-weighted fat-suppressed fast spin-echo, axial T1-weighted dual-gradient echo in-phase and opposed-phase, axial diffusion-weighted, axial 3D T1-weighted fat-suppressed spoiled gradient recalled echo before intravenous contrast, and axial, sagittal, and coronal postcontrast 3D T1-weighted fat-suppressed spoiled gradient recalled echo acquisitions. In female patients, if a detailed evaluation of the uterus is indicated, the authors include T2-weighted fast

spin-echo sequences in short and long axis relative to the uterus, and sagittal T2-weighted fast spin-echo sequence. Details of their institutional pelvic mass protocol are included in **Table 1**. Standard intravenous gadolinium-based contrast material dosing is calculated based on the patient's weight. The authors do not routinely administer glucagon or other antiperistaltic agents before pelvic MR imaging.

When evaluating bladder masses, dynamic T1-weighted 3D-SPGR postcontrast sequences are performed to evaluate bladder-wall enhancement and tumor extension before excreted contrast reaches the bladder. Dynamic T1-weighted post-contrast sequences in the arterial, venous, and delayed phases are also used to evaluate patients with suspected vascular malformations involving the pelvis.

OVARY

The majority of pediatric ovarian masses are functional and benign. The functional ovarian cyst is the most commonly encountered entity and the most common abdominal mass in a newborn female.[1] Malignant ovarian neoplasms are uncommon,

---

Table 1
Sample pediatric pelvic mass protocol pulse sequences and key parameters at 3 T

Sequence	Plane	Fat Saturation (Yes/No)	Flip Angle (°)	TE (ms)	TR (ms)	Slice Thickness/ Gap (mm)	NSA
T1-weighted fast spin-echo	Coronal	No	90	8	Shortest	5/1	2
Short-tau inversion recovery (STIR)	Coronal		None	60	Shortest	5/1	1
T2-weighted fast spin-echo	Axial	Yes	90	75	Shortest	5/1	1
T1-weighted dual gradient echo in-phase and opposed-phase	Axial	No	55	In-phase = 2.3 Opposed-phase = 1.15	180	5/0.5	1
T2-weighted fast spin-echo[a]	Sagittal	No	90	75	Shortest	5/1	1
T2-weighted fast spin-echo[a]	Short and long axis relative to the uterus	No	90	90	Shortest	4/0	1
Diffusion-weighted	Axial	Yes	90	Shortest	Shortest	5/0	4
Precontrast 3D-SPGR	Axial	Yes	10	Shortest	Shortest	1.5–3	1
Postcontrast 3D-SPGR	Coronal, axial, sagittal	Yes	10	Shortest	Shortest	1.5–3	1

Shortest = TE and/or TR set to be the shortest allowed by scanner.
Abbreviations: 3D-SPGR, 3-dimensional spoiled gradient recalled acquisition; NSA, number of signal averages; TE, echo time; TR, repetition time.
[a] Female patients for detailed evaluation of the uterus.

accounting for approximately 1% to 2% of malignant pediatric neoplasms and 10% of all ovarian neoplasms.[2,3] Ovarian malignancies rarely develop in infants younger than 1 year.[4] Ovarian malignancy is more frequently encountered in older children (age 9–19 years). Suspicion of an ovarian malignancy must be maintained if a girl presents with an abdominopelvic mass, especially in prepubertal girls (between infancy and the onset of puberty), who uncommonly have functional ovarian lesions.[4]

Classification of ovarian tumors is based on their cell of origin and includes germ-cell, epithelial, and sex-cord stromal tumors. Germ-cell tumors are the most common and comprise 60% to 90% of pediatric ovarian neoplasms, followed by sex-cord stromal (10%–13%) and epithelial tumors (5%–11%).[5] Ovarian neoplasms can be either benign or malignant, and often contain cystic and solid components; in general, the solid component is a predictor of malignancy.[6] The most common benign tumors are teratomas, followed by cystadenomas.

A suspected pelvic mass in a female child should be initially investigated with ultrasonography. Depending on the sonographic findings, cross-sectional imaging may be indicated. MR imaging has proved useful in further characterization of ovarian masses, provides staging information, and assists in preoperative planning. Clinical presentations of pelvic masses vary and include

nonspecific abdominal pain, increasing abdominal circumference, ovarian torsion, and, occasionally, symptoms related to excess hormone production by the tumor. Treatment is variable depending on the tumor; general treatment options include surgery and chemotherapy. Some malignant tumors such as dysgerminomas and granulosa cell tumors are also radiosensitive.[5] **Table 2** summarizes the imaging characteristics of the most common ovarian lesions.

Functional Ovarian Lesions

Functional ovarian lesions such as follicular cysts and corpus luteal cysts are the most common adnexal masses seen in children, accounting for approximately 45% of all adnexal abnormalities.[7] Functional ovarian lesions are occasionally encountered in the neonatal period when there is exposure to maternal hormones, but are most common in the postmenarchal period.[8] The functional ovarian cyst is also the most commonly encountered intra-abdominal mass in females in utero. Most cysts encountered are simple, but complex cysts also occur. Any cystic lesion identified between infancy and the onset of puberty should be viewed with a higher degree of suspicion, as functional ovarian cysts are only rarely encountered in this age group.[7]

Although ultrasonography is typically adequate for detection and characterization of ovarian

---

Table 2
Common ovarian lesions and MR imaging characteristics

Ovarian Lesion	Imaging Characteristics
Simple cyst	Low signal on T1-weighted and high on T2-weighted sequences with a thin rim of peripheral enhancement
Hemorrhagic cyst	Commonly high signal on T1-weighted sequences given presence of blood products, although variable depending on evolution of blood products. Peripheral enhancement common, but no nodular/central enhancement should be present
Torsion	Intermediate to high signal on T2-weighted sequences because of edema. Variable degrees of nonenhancement depending on degree of infarction
Teratoma	High signal on T1-weighted and T2-weighted sequences given presence of fat. Most present as unilocular cystic masses
Dysgerminoma	Solid mass with calcifications and enhancement of fibrous septa
Sertoli-Leydig neoplasm	Can have multiple cystic areas and demonstrate areas of low signal on T1-weighted and T2-weighted sequences, owing to fibrosis
Serous epithelial	Unilocular or multilocular components with thin septations; usually large at presentation. Papillary and solid components more predictive of malignancy
Mucinous epithelial	Typically multilocular with the multiple cysts containing fluid demonstrating variable signal; usually large at presentation. Papillary and solid components more predictive of malignancy

cysts, MR imaging can be useful in certain cases.[9] MR imaging can confirm the presence of a cyst when the ultrasound imaging characteristics are atypical or when an underlying mass is suspected. A simple ovarian cyst should demonstrate homogeneous T1-weighted hypointense and T2-weighted hyperintense signal characteristics with uniform peripheral or rim enhancement after the administration of gadolinium-containing contrast material (**Fig. 1**). Functional hemorrhagic cysts classically have been described to demonstrate hyperintense signal on T1-weighted images[10]; however, the MR appearance of hemorrhagic cysts can vary somewhat depending on the evolutionary stage of blood products.[11] Kanso and colleagues[11] described only 36% of hemorrhagic cysts demonstrating intermediate or hyperintense signal on T1-weighted sequences (**Fig. 2**). A corpus luteum cyst that has involuted can have wavy and irregular borders and may also demonstrate heterogeneous signal, depending on the presence of blood products (see **Fig. 2**). There should be no central or nodular enhancement in any of these benign, functional ovarian cysts.

Treatment is usually conservative unless there is associated ovarian torsion or the cyst reaches a particular size that would significantly increase the risk of torsion.

Ovarian Torsion

Ovarian torsion is a surgical emergency that results from twisting of the ovary on its vascular pedicle with resultant vascular compromise. Fifteen percent of ovarian torsion occurs in the pediatric population.[12] Ovarian torsion is commonly associated with other ovarian abnormalities in the adult population; however, in children ovarian torsion is more commonly associated with benign lesions or normal ovaries.[13] Ovarian torsion can occur from inherent hypermobility of the ovary, or

secondary to a mass acting as a lead point. Clinical presentations include abdominal pain, nausea and vomiting, and palpable mass (detected in 40%–70% of patients).[12]

Ultrasonography is the initial modality of choice in suspected ovarian torsion, and is usually the only imaging test obtained before surgical intervention. In rare cases, MR imaging with contrast may assist in the diagnosis when sonographic findings are confounding or when there is suspicion for an underlying mass acting as a lead point. With torsion, ovarian follicles may migrate to the periphery of the ovary, which has been described as resembling a "string of pearls."[14] Postcontrast imaging will assist with detection of solid/nodular components if an underlying mass is present. Nonenhancement of ovarian parenchyma is compatible with infarction (**Fig. 3**). The torsed ovary can have variable degrees of T2-weighted signal intensity from intermediate to high, depending on the amount of edema present. Torsion can occur in utero. After birth, the nonviable ovary can appear as a complex cystic lesion and may eventually involute into a calcified mass.[2]

The treatment for ovarian torsion is emergent surgery. Early diagnosis is critical for preserving fertility and maximizing chances of ovarian salvage. Unfortunately, one large series reported that approximately 58% of patients are treated with oophorectomy because of delays in diagnosis.[13]

Germ-Cell Neoplasms

Germ-cell tumors are the most common type of ovarian neoplasm encountered in the pediatric population, in contrast to the adult population in which the majority of ovarian malignancies are epithelial in origin. Germ-cell tumors comprise between 60% and 90% of pediatric ovarian malignancies, depending on the cited study.[4,6] Children with gonadal dysgenesis are at increased risk for developing germ-cell tumors.[15]

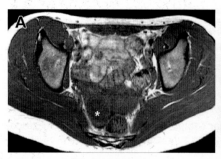
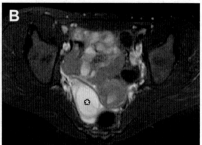

Fig. 1. A 16-year-old girl with a simple right ovarian cyst. Axial T1-weighted (*A*) and axial T2-weighted fat-suppressed (*B*) images of the right ovary demonstrate the characteristic homogeneous T1-weighted hypointense and T2-weighted hyperintense signal of a simple cyst (*asterisks*). No central enhancement should be present on postcontrast imaging.

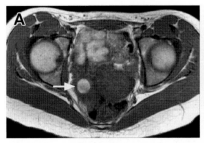 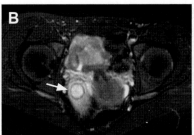 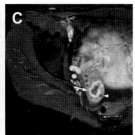

Fig. 2. An 18-year-old girl with functional ovarian cyst. Axial T1-weighted image (*A*) of the right ovary (*arrow*) demonstrates the commonly seen T1-weighted hyperintense signal changes with functional hemorrhagic cysts. Axial T2-weighted fat-suppressed image (*B*) of the right ovary demonstrates hyperintense signal changes of the cyst with a low signal border (*arrow*) compatible with blood products. (*C*) Axial T1-weighted postcontrast fat-suppressed sequence of the same patient demonstrates the characteristic wavy borders of an involuting corpus luteum cyst (*arrow*). Note the lack of central enhancement. Arrowhead denotes a normal ovarian follicle, which also demonstrates thin, peripheral enhancement.

Germ-cell tumors include mature teratomas, immature teratomas, dysgerminomas, endodermal sinus tumors, embryonal carcinomas, and choriocarcinomas. The most common type of pediatric ovarian germ-cell tumor is a mature teratoma, which is benign. All of the other types are malignant and have the potential to metastasize to the liver, lungs, and peritoneum.[16]

Mature teratomas account for 67% of pediatric ovarian tumors and are bilateral 25% of the time.[17,18] They comprise at least 2 of the 3 embryonic germ-cell layers: ectoderm, mesoderm, and

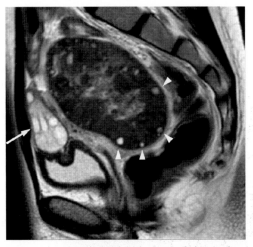

Fig. 3. An 11-year-old girl with acute abdominal pain and ovarian torsion. Sagittal T2-weighted sequence through the pelvis demonstrates a hypointense "mass" with peripherally located hyperintense follicles (*arrowheads*), described as a "string of pearls." These findings are consistent with ovarian torsion. No underlying mass was detected at the time of surgery. Arrow denotes the patient's other ovary, which was normal.

endoderm. Imaging features of mature teratomas range from completely cystic lesions to solid, predominantly fat-containing masses. Most teratomas present as a unilocular cystic mass (**Fig. 4**)[2] and commonly contain a Rokitansky nodule (a soft-tissue plug containing hair, fat, and calcific and/or sebaceous components), which extends into the lumen of the cyst (**Fig. 4**).[19] The imaging appearance of a mature teratoma varies, particularly on ultrasonography, depending on the size of the Rokitansky nodule and the distribution of calcifications and fat.[2] However, their appearance on MR imaging is more characteristic. The presence of macroscopic fat in an ovarian tumor is diagnostic of a mature teratoma, and can be exquisitely demonstrated with the use of in-phase/opposed-phase imaging and fat-suppressed MR sequences (**Fig. 5**). The fatty component of the tumor will demonstrate hyperintense signal on T1-weighted and T2-weighted non–fat-suppressed sequences, and will subsequently lose signal with fat suppression. Lesions that contain hemorrhage or proteinaceous material will demonstrate hyperintense signal on T1-weighted sequences both with and without fat suppression.

The remaining tumors in this category, including dysgerminomas, yolk sac tumors, and choriocarcinomas, generally demonstrate a nonspecific imaging appearance. However, MR imaging is useful for preoperative planning and staging. Dysgerminoma is the most common malignant ovarian neoplasm (**Fig. 6**). Imaging may demonstrate a solid mass with small calcifications. Dysgerminomas demonstrate low signal intensity on T1-weighted sequences and intermediate to high signal on T2-weighted sequences, depending on the amount of necrosis present. Intralesional fibrous septa demonstrate low signal intensity on T2-weighted sequences and enhance on postcontrast

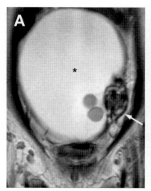
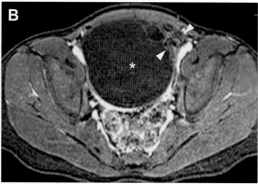

Fig. 4. An 8-year-old girl with an ovarian mature teratoma. Coronal T2-weighted image through the pelvis (*A*) demonstrates a large unilocular cystic lesion (*asterisk*) with a peripheral nodular component. This solid component is likely the Rokitansky nodule protruding into the cyst lumen (*arrow*). Axial T1-weighted fat-suppressed postcontrast image (*B*) demonstrates mild enhancement of the nodule (*arrowheads*) and nonenhancement of the central cystic component (*asterisk*).

sequences.[5] Other types of germ-cell tumors may be distinguished by their hormonal markers. For example, endodermal sinus tumors may have elevated levels of α-fetoprotein (AFP), whereas embryonal carcinomas may have elevated levels of both AFP and β–human chorionic gonadotropin.

Stromal Cell Tumors

Tumors of stromal cell origin constitute the second most common category of pediatric ovarian neoplasms. Although there are several types, the most commonly encountered are granulosa cell tumors (75%) followed by Sertoli-Leydig tumors (25%).[5] Because of their functional nature, patients with granulosa tumors can present with precocious puberty arising from the estrogen exposure. On the other hand, oligomenorrhea and virilization can be presenting features in patients with Sertoli-Leydig tumors, as a result of excess androgen production.[5] Granulosa tumors

have a variable MR appearance, and can present as cystic or solid masses containing areas of hemorrhage and infarction.[20] Sertoli-Leydig tumors are well defined, can contain multiple cystic areas, and can demonstrate hypointense signal on T1-weighted and T2-weighted sequences owing to fibrosis.[2,20]

Epithelial Tumors

Epithelial ovarian neoplasms are the least common group of pediatric ovarian malignancies.[21] The majority of epithelial tumors are benign (approximately 58%) followed by those categorized as having borderline to low malignant potential. High-grade malignant epithelial tumors are rare.[21] Serous and mucinous cystadenomas, the most common types of epithelial neoplasms, are typically large at presentation and can present with ovarian torsion.[2,22] Serous cystadenomas usually have a significant unilocular or multilocular

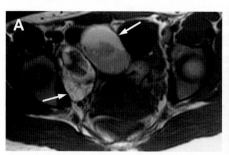
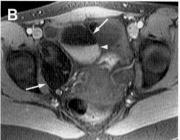

Fig. 5. An 18-year-old girl with bilateral mature teratomas. Axial T1-weighted image without fat-suppression (*A*) demonstrates 2 complex pelvic masses. Arrows denote the fatty components of the masses, which are hyperintense on this non–fat-suppressed T1-weighted sequence. Axial T1-weighted image with fat suppression (*B*) through the same level demonstrates loss of signal of the fatty components of the masses (*arrows*). Arrowhead denotes a fluid-fluid level within the mass, possibly from hemorrhage.

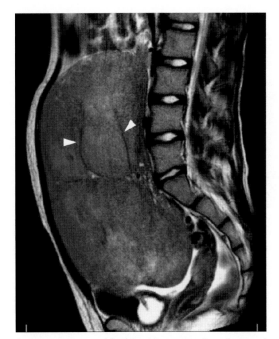

Fig. 6. A 16-year-old girl with an ovarian dysgerminoma. Sagittal T2-weighted image demonstrates a large space-occupying solid mass within the pelvis with predominantly low signal and displacement of bowel. Imaging features are nonspecific. Arrowheads denote fibrous septations within the mass.

cystic component and thin septations. Mucinous cystadenomas are typically multilocular, septated masses, with the multiple cysts containing fluid demonstrating varying signal intensities (**Fig. 7**).[2] Papillary projections and solid, enhancing components may be present and are more predictive of malignancy (**Fig. 8**).[6]

Metastatic Disease to the Ovary

Although uncommon, metastases to the ovaries have been reported in the pediatric population. Reported pediatric malignancies metastasizing to the ovaries include alveolar rhabdomyosarcoma, Burkitt lymphoma, colonic adenocarcinoma, Wilms tumor, retinoblastoma, and neuroblastoma (**Fig. 9**).[1,23] The MR imaging appearance of ovarian metastases can be variable, but may be similar to that of the primary tumor.

UTERUS

Uterine tumors are uncommon in pediatric patients, but when encountered in this age group they are likely to be malignant.[24] Uterine sarcomas, such as leiomyosarcomas, mixed mesodermal tumors, and endometrial carcinomas have been reported but are extremely rare.[24] In general, uterine leiomyosarcomas tend to occur in a younger population, in contrast to mixed mesodermal tumors.

The most commonly encountered benign tumors in the uterus overall are leiomyomas; however, these are also uncommon in the pediatric population. Although most leiomyomas present as well-circumscribed masses, unusual patterns of growth have been described. The appearance on MR imaging can vary depending on the size of tumors, particularly larger lesions that may outgrow their blood supply and infarct centrally. Nondegenerated leiomyomas typically are hypointense on T2-weighted sequences relative to myometrium, and demonstrate relatively little enhancement (**Fig. 10**). Occasionally these tumors may demonstrate more pronounced enhancement and increased signal on T2-weighted sequences.

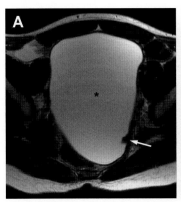
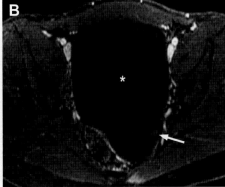

Fig. 7. An 18-year-old girl with serous ovarian neoplasm. Axial T2-weighted image through the pelvis (A) demonstrates a mass with large cystic component (*asterisk*) with peripherally located papillary projection (*arrow*). Axial T1-weighted fat-suppressed image through the same level (B) demonstrates mild enhancement of the papillary projection. Although pathology revealed a serous cystadenoma, the enhancing papillary projection would raise the possibility of a cystadenocarcinoma.

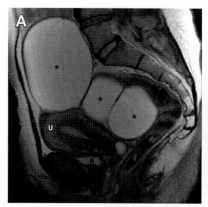
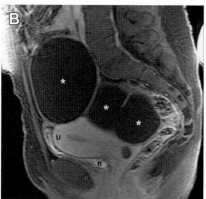

Fig. 8. A 17-year-old with a mucinous cystadenoma. Sagittal T2-weighted image (*A*) demonstrates a multilocular, septated cystic mass (*asterisks*) just above the uterus. These are typical MR imaging characteristics of a mucinous tumor. Sagittal T1-weighted fat-suppressed postcontrast image (*B*) shows peripheral enhancement of the cysts and septations. B, bladder; U, uterus.

Areas of degeneration manifest as lack of enhancement on postcontrast sequences.[25] Unusual presentations such as leiomyomatosis are uncommon, but have been described (**Fig. 11**).[26]

Although uncommon, a mass-like nonneoplastic condition described in the adolescent population is uterine adenomyosis.[27] In adolescents presenting with severe refractory dysmenorrhea, MR imaging may help establish this diagnosis. MR imaging classically demonstrates focal or diffuse thickening of the junctional zone with discrete foci of T2-hyperintense signal corresponding to islands of ectopic endometrial tissue.[28] A junctional-zone thickness of greater than 12 mm is predictive of adenomyosis.[28] Adenomyoma is a localized mass-like form of adenomyosis. Adenomyotic cysts have been described but are generally uncommon.[28] MR

findings can occasionally mimic those of uterine malignancy (**Fig. 12**).[28]

VAGINA AND CERVIX

The most commonly encountered pediatric vaginal and cervical neoplasm is rhabdomyosarcoma. This tumor is usually found in the vagina of infants and children younger than 2 years. Clinically these tumors may present with vaginal bleeding or as a polypoid mass protruding from the vaginal introitus (sarcoma botryoides). Uterine rhabdomyosarcoma is rare, with peak incidence in the second decade of life. On MR imaging these tumors demonstrate intermediate to high signal intensity on T2-weighted sequences and low to intermediate signal intensity on T1-weighted sequences. Contrast enhancement is variable, depending on

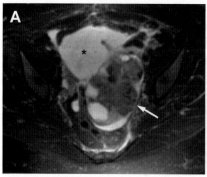
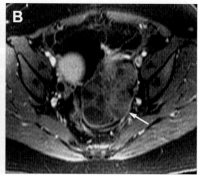

Fig. 9. A 26-year-old woman with history of colonic adenocarcinoma presenting with an adnexal mass later proven to be metastatic disease. Axial T2-weighted fat-suppressed (*A*) and axial T1-weighted fat-suppressed postcontrast (*B*) images through the pelvis demonstrate a mixed cystic and solid enhancing left adnexal mass (*arrow*) compatible with metastatic colonic adenocarcinoma. A large amount of adjacent free fluid is present (*asterisk*).

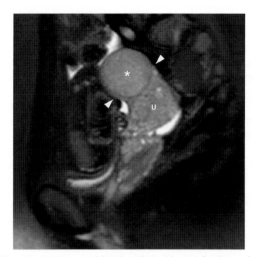

Fig. 10. A 17-year-old girl with incidental finding of a uterine fibroid while undergoing magnetic resonance urography. Sagittal T2-weighted fat-suppressed image through the pelvis demonstrates an exophytic, homogeneous, well-circumscribed, isointense (relative to the uterus) mass (*asterisk*) arising from the anterior aspect of the uterus (U) compatible with a subserosal fibroid. Note the rim of uterine tissue extending along the anterior and posterior margins of the mass (*arrowheads*), indicating that the mass is arising from the uterus. A small amount of free fluid is seen anterior and posterior to the uterus.

the degree of tumor necrosis (with necrotic portions of the tumor not enhancing). Degree and change in tumor enhancement after chemotherapy are also useful in assessing response to treatment.

Other less common malignancies encountered in the lower genital tract include endodermal sinus tumors and clear-cell adenocarcinomas.[29] Endodermal sinus tumors more commonly occur in children younger than 3 years.[29] Tumor markers such

as AFP are helpful in clinically following these tumors. Clear-cell adenocarcinoma has been associated with exposure to diethylstilbestrol. Cervical carcinomas are rare in children, but have been reported (**Fig. 13**). Cervical carcinomas typically demonstrate intermediate signal intensity on T2-weighted sequences, and are seen distorting the normal T2-weighted hypointense stroma of the cervix. The tumor can be exophytic, infiltrative, or endocervical. Although these tumors are detectable with T2-weighted imaging, smaller tumors may be more apparent owing to early enhancement on dynamic postcontrast sequences.[30]

Gartner duct cysts are uncommon in the pediatric population[31] and are located posteriorly within the vaginal wall, arising from embryologic remnants of the Wolffian duct. Gartner duct cysts are typically located above the inferiormost margin of the pubic symphysis (**Fig. 14**).[32] On MR imaging, this lesion typically demonstrates features of a cyst; it is homogeneously hyperintense on T2-weighted sequences and hypointense on T1-weighted sequences, with only peripheral enhancement on postcontrast sequences.

Cysts and abscesses of the Bartholin glands are exceedingly uncommon before puberty; however, there have been several case reports of Bartholin-gland abscesses in neonates.[33] Bartholin glands are outgrowths of the urogenital sinus. Blockage of a Bartholin duct leads to cystic enlargement of the gland, which can then become infected. In contrast to cysts of the Gartner duct, Bartholin cysts are located within the posterolateral inferior vagina, below the level of the pubic symphysis, and are associated with the labia majora.[32] An uncomplicated Bartholin-duct cyst should demonstrate uniform T2-weighted signal hyperintensity and thin peripheral enhancement; however, the cyst may have heterogeneous internal signal and

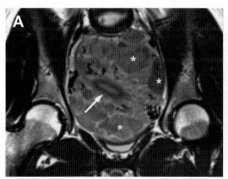
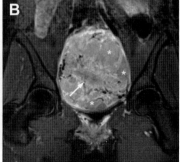

Fig. 11. A 16-year-old girl with diffuse uterine leiomyomatosis. Coronal T2-weighted (*A*) and coronal T1-weighted fat-suppressed postcontrast (*B*) images through the pelvis demonstrate a markedly enlarged uterus replaced by numerous enhancing, heterogeneously T2-hypointense masses (*asterisks*). Arrow denotes the endometrial canal.

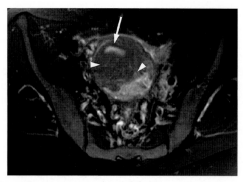

Fig. 12. An 18-year-old girl with pelvic mass with history of Wilms tumor at age 5 years treated with radiation. Initial imaging was concerning for a radiation-induced leiomyosarcoma; however, pathology was consistent with uterine adenomyosis. Axial T2-weighted image with fat suppression through the pelvis demonstrates an enlarged uterus with distortion of the endometrial canal (*arrow*). Arrowheads denote focal areas of T2-weighted hyperintense signal within the myometrium, compatible with islands of ectopic endometrium.

irregular or thick peripheral enhancement when infected (**Fig. 15**).[32]

VULVA

Vulvar masses in children are rare, and when encountered they are typically benign. Entities include retention cysts, vascular lesions, lipomas, benign perineal granulomas, and condylomata acuminata (**Figs. 16** and **17**). Presentation is variable, and treatment is reserved for lesions that are symptomatic.[24] MR imaging features depend on the histology of the lesion. Rarely, malignant tumors such as rhabdomyosarcoma and endodermal sinus tumors have been reported.

BLADDER AND PROSTATE

Bladder masses are relatively uncommon in children; however, benign, primary, and secondary malignant bladder masses do occur in the pediatric population. Tumors arising from the epithelial surface can be benign or malignant, and include papillomas and urothelial carcinomas. Nonepithelial tumors originate from the other layers of the bladder wall and may be benign, such as hemangiomas, paragangliomas, and neurofibromas, or malignant, such as rhabdomyosarcoma. Uncommonly, mass-like inflammatory changes of the bladder wall, known as pseudotumoral cystitis or bladder pseudotumor, may mimic a polypoid bladder neoplasm.[34,35]

Although rare in children, a variety of benign lesions have been described including hemangioma, fibroma, fibroepithelial polyp, and inverted papilloma.[5,34,36] Neurofibromas of the bladder are rarely found in isolation, but may occur in patients with neurofibromatosis type 1.[37,38]

Rhabdomyosarcoma is the most common primary malignant neoplasm of the lower urinary tract. Lower urinary tract sites account for 15% to 20% of all rhabdomyosarcomas in infants and children.[39] Other malignant neoplasms are rarely found in the first decades of life. Urothelial (transitional cell) carcinoma[40] and rhabdoid tumors have been reported.[41] Secondary involvement of the bladder has been reported in patients with lymphoma and leukemia.

Rhabdomyosarcoma

Rhabdomyosarcoma is a tumor derived from primitive mesenchyme. There is a peak of incidence between 2 and 4 years of life with a second peak in adolescence. Although this tumor occurs in both boys and girls, bladder rhabdomyosarcoma has a male predominance of 2.5 to 1.[42] While rhabdomyosarcomas usually present in patients without underlying disorders, an association with familial cancer syndromes including Li-Fraumeni, Beckwith-Wiedeman, and Gorlin syndrome has been reported.[43]

Histologic subtypes include embryonal, which is by far the most common subtype of genitourinary rhabdomyosarcoma; sarcoma botryoides, a polypoid subtype of embryonal rhabdomyosarcoma that arises from the submucosa; and rarely the alveolar subtype, which has the worst prognosis.[44] Rhabdomyosarcoma commonly arises in the bladder trigone or neck (**Fig. 18**). Cases of primary prostatic rhabdomyosarcoma may occur in boys (**Fig. 19**). The botryoid rhabdomyosarcoma does not infiltrate the overlying epithelium but rather protrudes to the lumen of the bladder or the vagina (**Fig. 20**).[34] Most lower urinary tract rhabdomyosarcomas are of the embryonal subtype.[45,46] Clinical presentation is related to the location of the mass and includes urinary obstruction, urinary frequency, urinary retention, and hematuria.

Rhabdomyosarcoma of the female genital tract usually arises from the vagina during infancy and early childhood (**Fig. 21**).[34] Symptoms include vaginal bleeding or vaginal masses that may protrude from the introitus.[34,44]

Paratesticular rhabdomyosarcoma accounts for 7% of the genitourinary tumors. This tumor usually presents as a painless scrotal mass occurring in young infants or teenagers. Microscopic

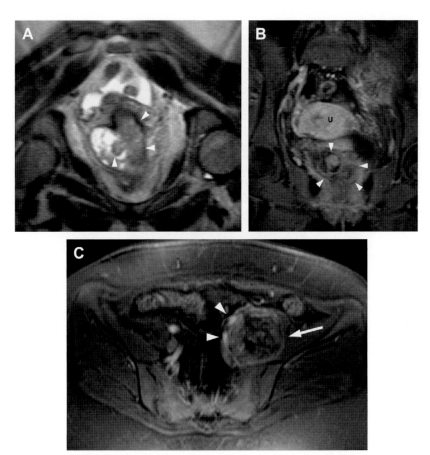

Fig. 13. A 17-year-old girl with aggressive cervical carcinoma. Axial T2-weighted (*A*) and coronal T1-weighted postcontrast fat-suppressed images (*B*) through the pelvis demonstrate a heterogeneously enhancing solid mass within the cervix (*arrowheads*). U, uterus. Axial T1-weighted postcontrast fat-suppressed image (*C*) through the lower abdomen demonstrates a heterogeneously enhancing conglomerate of lymph nodes (*arrow*) compatible with metastatic disease. Arrowheads denote vessels that appear to be partially encased by these lymph nodes.

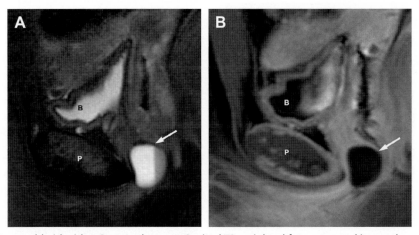

Fig. 14. A 13-year-old girl with a Gartner duct cyst. Sagittal T2-weighted fat-suppressed image through the pelvis (*A*) demonstrates a cystic lesion within the posterior vaginal wall with fluid-fluid levels (*arrow*). Sagittal T1-weighted fat-suppressed postcontrast image (*B*) demonstrates lack of internal enhancement. Note the relationship of the cyst with the pubic symphysis (P); the cyst does not extend beyond the inferior margin of the pubic symphysis. B, bladder.

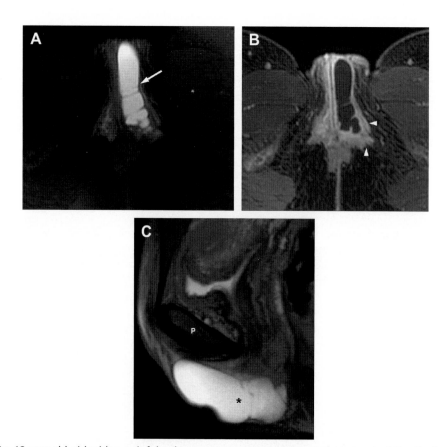

Fig. 15. An 18-year-old girl with a painful vulvar mass consistent with an infected cyst of the Bartholin gland. Axial T2-weighted fat-suppressed image (*A*) demonstrates a septated T2-hyperintense mass within the inferior vagina involving the left labia majora (*arrow*). Axial T1-weighted postcontrast fat-suppressed image (*B*) demonstrates enhancement of the septations and exuberant enhancement of the surrounding soft tissues (*arrowheads*), which would raise the possibility of infection. Sagittal T2-weighted fat-suppressed image through the pelvis (*C*) demonstrates the location of this cyst (*asterisk*) within the inferior vagina, inferior to the pubic symphysis (P). Compare this with the location of the Gartner-duct cyst described in **Fig. 14.**

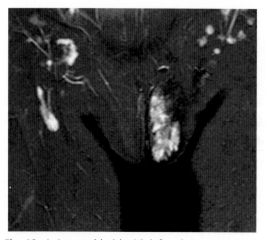

Fig. 16. A 4-year-old girl with left vulvar malformation. Coronal T2-weighted fat-suppressed image demonstrate a lobulated T1-hypointense and heterogeneously T2-weighted hyperintense mass within the left vulva.

metastases to the retroperitoneum are present in 30% to 40% of the patients.[42]

On MR imaging, rhabdomyosarcomas typically demonstrate low to intermediate signal intensity on T1-weighted images and intermediate to high signal intensity on T2-weighted images. For tumors arising from the bladder, T2-weighted images provide excellent contrast between the fluid-filled bladder lumen, hypointense bladder wall, prostate, and surrounding soft tissues. Postcontrast dynamic images, acquired before excreted contrast reaches the bladder, are very useful in assessment of heterogeneous tumor enhancement. Given the exquisite soft-tissue contrast resolution, MR is the imaging modality of choice to evaluate for local invasion as well as regional lymph node enlargement. Diffusion-weighted imaging may also assist in the detection of metastatic lymph nodes.

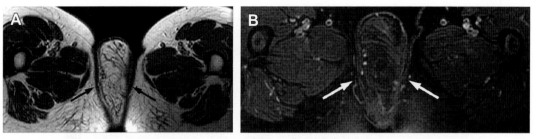

Fig. 17. A 17-year-old girl with a vulvar lipoma. Axial T1-weighted (*A*) and axial T2-weighted fat-suppressed (*B*) images through the vulva demonstrate a septated mass that follows the signal intensity of fat on both sequences (*arrows*). While the lesions contains numerous thin septations, there are no solid/nodular components were present to suggest malignancy.

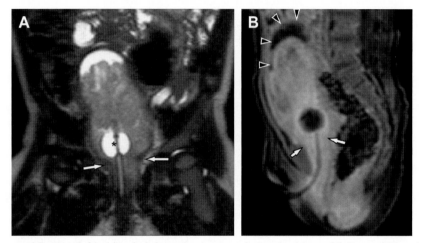

Fig. 18. A 2-year-old girl with bladder rhabdomyosarcoma, embryonal subtype. (*A*) Coronal T2-weighted image reveals a large, heterogeneous soft-tissue mass at the bladder base, extending into the bladder neck and proximal urethra (*arrows*). Foley catheter is present (*asterisk*). (*B*) Sagittal postcontrast fat-saturated T1-weighted image demonstrates diffuse enhancement (*arrows*). The bladder wall is seen superiorly (*arrowheads*).

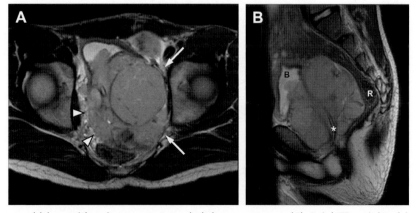

Fig. 19. A 6-year-old boy with primary prostate rhabdomyosarcoma. (*A*) Axial T2-weighted image demonstrates a large multinodular, mildly hyperintense mass (*arrows*) arising from the prostate with extension into the bladder wall (*arrowheads*). (*B*) Sagittal T2-weighted image. Note elevation and anterior displacement of the bladder (B) and mass effect on the rectum (R). A catheter is present along the posterior urethra (*asterisk*). (*Courtesy of* D. Jaramillo, MD, Children's Hospital of Philadelphia, Philadelphia, PA.)

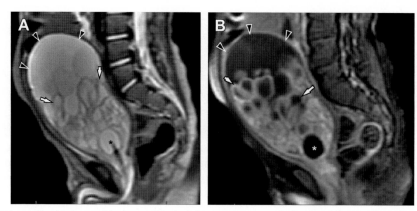

Fig. 20. A 27-month-old boy with botryoid rhabdomyosarcoma of the bladder. (*A*) Sagittal fat-saturated T2-weighted image shows multiple hyperintense cystic intraluminal masses (*arrows*) extending from the bladder base. The bladder wall is displaced superiorly (*arrowheads*). A Foley catheter is present (*asterisk*). (*B*) Sagittal postcontrast fat-saturated T1-weighted image. Peripheral enhancement of the mass is clearly depicted. Images were obtained early, before contrast was excreted into the bladder.

Rhabdomyosarcoma staging is based on primary tumor extension, involvement of lymph nodes, and metastatic disease. Treatment includes neoadjuvant chemotherapy and surgical excision, with the goal of preservation of the bladder function.[42,43] Multidisciplinary treatment protocols, including initial chemotherapy and delayed definitive surgery, are preferred to preserve the vagina and uterus if possible (**Fig. 22**).[44]

PRESACRAL SPACE

The presacral space lies between the rectum and the sacrum above the presacral fascia. This space contains structures derived from the embryologic hindgut, neuroectoderm, and notochord.[47,48]

Masses in the presacral space may be congenital, developmental, neurogenic, inflammatory, mesenchymal, and osseous (extension of sacral neoplasms).[48,49] The clinical presentation is determined by etiology, size and location of the lesion, and the age of the patient at diagnosis. Possible symptoms include constipation, palpable mass, urinary symptoms, and lower back pain. Some presacral masses may remain asymptomatic.

Ultrasonography and computed tomography (CT) evaluation of presacral masses is often limited by a poor sonographic window resulting from the adjacent osseous structures and bowel gas, and

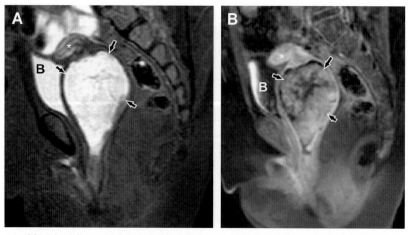

Fig. 21. A 2-year-old girl with vaginal botryoid rhabdomyosarcoma. (*A*) Sagittal short-tau inversion recovery (STIR) image shows a hyperintense, slightly heterogeneous intravaginal mass (*arrows*). The cervix and uterus (*asterisk*) are superiorly displaced. Mass effect is noted on the fluid-filled bladder (B). (*B*) Sagittal postcontrast fat-saturated T1-weighted image. Intense, heterogeneous enhancement of the mass (*arrows*) is noted. The cervix and uterus (*asterisk*) are separate from the mass.

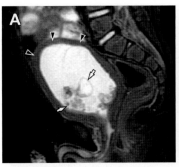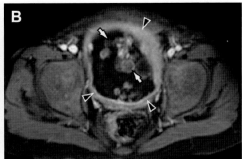

Fig. 22. A 27-month-old boy with botyroid rhabdomyosarcoma (same patient as in **Fig. 20**, after initial chemotherapy). (*A*) Sagittal STIR reveals decreased size of cystic masses (*arrows*). Thickening of the bladder wall is likely related to post-therapeutic changes (*arrowheads*). (*B*) Axial postcontrast fat-saturated T1-weighted image demonstrates enhancement of the masses (*arrows*), as well as enhancement of the thickened bladder wall (*arrowheads*), more prominent at site of prior involvement.

the limited soft-tissue contrast resolution available with CT. The excellent soft-tissue contrast resolution and multiplanar capability of MR make it optimal for presacral mass detection, characterization, and assessment of infiltration into surrounding structures.

Sacrococcygeal Germ-Cell Tumors

Sacrococcygeal teratoma (SCT) is the most common presacral tumor in neonates and infants.[49,50] This tumor arises from totipotent somatic cells that originate from the Hensen node.[51]

Most SCT are benign, although malignant or immature elements may be present. The median age at diagnosis in cases with malignant elements is significantly greater.[50,52]

SCT is classified into 4 different types based on the extrapelvic component and the degree of extension into the pelvic cavity:

- Type I: tumors are predominantly external with minimal presacral component
- Type II: both internal and external components, predominantly external
- Type III: both internal and external components, predominantly internal
- Type IV: entirely internal presacral mass with no external component[53]

Benign SCT are predominantly cystic and may contain mature tissues including fat, soft tissue, and areas of calcification. Areas of macroscopic fat are readily identified on MR as foci of high T1-weighted and T2-weighted signal, which lose signal on fat-saturated images. Calcifications may be hyperintense on T1-weighted images or may demonstrate hypointense signal on gradient-echo sequences. Postcontrast imaging demonstrates enhancement of any soft-tissue components, as

well as enhancement of the cyst walls or internal septa in multicystic masses (**Fig. 23**). Tumors with immature tissues or malignant elements usually have large solid components that are highly vascular and demonstrate heterogeneous enhancement. Areas of internal hemorrhage or necrosis may be present.[49] Although intraspinal extension is uncommon, with only a few cases reported in the literature,[54–56] MR imaging is the ideal modality for evaluating the spinal canal and its contents.

SCT is the most common congenital pelvic neoplasm. When diagnosed in utero, SCT has high morbidity and mortality rates, with a high risk of preterm delivery. Poor prognosis is associated with solid highly vascularized masses, hemorrhage, or development of fetal hydrops. Prenatal MR imaging provides precise information regarding tumor extension, solid components, foci of hemorrhage, and compression of adjacent organs (**Fig. 24**).[51,57]

Treatment includes surgical resection with coccygectomy. Malignant tumors are also treated with chemotherapy either before or after surgical resection.[58] Recurrence can be seen in cases of incomplete excision. Immature and malignant histology of the primary tumor are also predictors of recurrence.[59]

Anterior Sacral Meningocele

Anterior sacral meningocele is an uncommon form of spinal dysraphism that consists of herniation of dura mater–lined spinal canal contents through a sacral defect or a sacral foramen.[60] An anterior meningocele may also include neural elements, and can be asymptomatic or may present with mass effect, neurologic deficit, meningitis, or rupture.[49] Sacral hypoplasia, vertebral scalloping, and scimitar sacrum may be present.

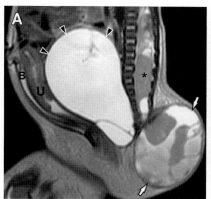
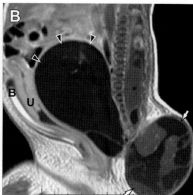

Fig. 23. A newborn baby girl with a large sacrococcygeal teratoma. (*A*) Sagittal fat-saturated T2-weighted image demonstrates large external mass (*arrows*), with both cystic solid components and large predominantly cystic intrapelvic mass extending to the lower abdomen (*arrowheads*). Mass effect on the uterus (U) and bladder (B) is noted. (*B*) Sagittal postcontrast fat-saturated T1-weighted image shows only minimal enhancement of solid components. Note intraspinal extension of the mass to the level of the conus medullaris (*asterisk*) which can be seen on both T2-weighted and postcontrast images.

An interesting association with anterior sacral meningocele is the so-called Currarino triad. This association consists of sacral dysplasia, anterior sacral mass, and different forms of anorectal malformation.[61] The syndrome is often familial, with autosomal dominant inheritance.[62,63]

MR imaging is excellent for evaluation of the anterior meningocele neck, sac, and contents. MR is also optimal in determining the presence of nerve roots within the sac, which is of critical importance for surgical planning (**Fig. 25**).

Tumors of the Sacrum

Although primary tumors of the sacrum are uncommon, when encountered they may extend into the presacral space. Benign tumors such as giant-cell tumors and aneurysmal bone cysts can arise from the sacrum. Ewing sarcoma is a primary malignant tumor that can originate from the sacrum. Other malignant bone tumors, including osteosarcoma and chordoma, have also been described.[49,60]

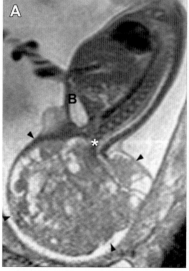
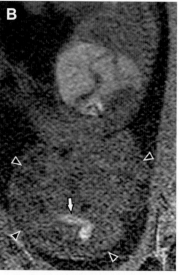

Fig. 24. Fetal MR image of a fetus of 24 weeks gestational age with a large sacrococcygeal teratoma. (*A*) Sagittal T2-weighted image demonstrates a large external mass (*arrowheads*) with solid and cystic components and only minimal intrapelvic extension. Note the posterior displacement of distal sacrum and coccyx (*asterisk*). (*B*) Sagittal T1-weighted image reveals focal areas of increased T1-weighted signal (*white arrow*), consistent with fat or blood products within the mass.

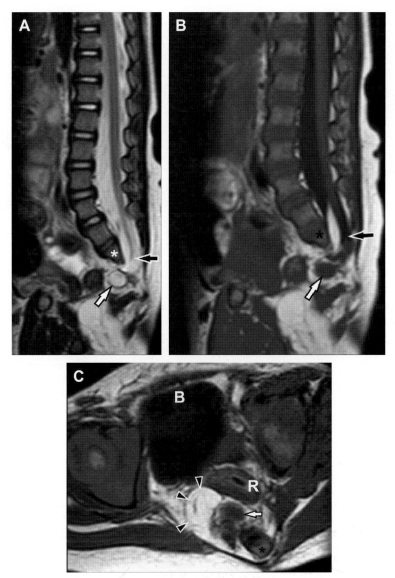

Fig. 25. A 13-month-old girl with tethered spinal cord to a fat-containing lesion extending into the presacral space. Sagittal T2-weighted image (*A*), sagittal T1-weighted image (*B*), and axial T1-weighted image (*C*) show a low-lying tethered cord (*black arrow*) and a fat-containing presacral mass (*arrowheads*). A small anterior sacral meningocele is also present (*white arrow*). Note dysplastic sacrum displaced to the left (*asterisk*) as well as displacement of the rectum (R) and bladder (B).

NEUROBLASTOMA

Neuroblastoma is the most common pediatric extracranial tumor, with incidence peaking in children younger than 4 years. This tumor arises from primordial neural crest cells, precursors of the sympathetic nervous system. Approximately 1% to 2% occur in the pelvis, most commonly in the presacral region, or arising from the organ of Zuckerkandl.[64]

On MR imaging, neuroblastoma is predominantly solid with heterogeneous signal intensity and variable degrees of enhancement. These tumors may contain areas of necrosis or small foci of calcification, which may be difficult to detect on MR. MR imaging is especially helpful for assessment of local extension, evaluation of spinal involvement, and detection of bone marrow metastasis. MR imaging also allows for staging and presurgical planning, including details regarding tumor size, vessel encasement, and the relationship between the tumor and the sacral plexus and pelvic floor.[64]

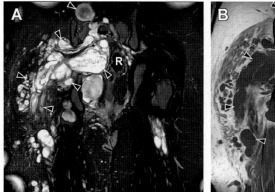
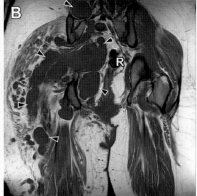

Fig. 26. A 15-year-old girl with history of neurofibromatosis type 1. Coronal STIR (*A*) and coronal T1-weighted (*B*) images demonstrate multiple plexiform neurofibromas (*arrowheads*) in the right hemipelvis extending from the right L5-S1 neural foramen as well as the right sacral foramina, and into the sciatic notch along the sciatic nerve. Note leftward displacement of the rectum (R).

MISCELLANEOUS
Cysts

Enteric duplication cysts are an uncommon congenital abnormality that may arise anywhere along the gastrointestinal tract. The ileum is the most commonly involved segment of the bowel. Rectal duplication cysts are rare, representing approximately 5% of overall intestinal duplication cysts. Duplication cysts may be asymptomatic or may present with abdominal distention, vomiting, palpable abdominal mass, and bleeding, especially in cysts containing gastric mucosa. MR imaging typically demonstrates a well-circumscribed T2-weighted hyperintense lesion that may be associated with the bowel wall. T1-weighted signal characteristics are variable depending on cyst contents, which sometimes include blood products or infection. Peripheral enhancement may be irregular in the setting of secondary infection.

Peritoneal inclusion cysts are predominantly diagnosed in reproductive-age females and have been reported in adolescent females. These cysts are most commonly seen in patients with a history of abdominal surgery, and may present with pelvic pain.[65,66] MR imaging features are typical of simple cysts, including homogeneous low T1-weighted signal, high T2-weighted signal, and thin rim enhancement.

Systemic Disorders

Diffuse involvement of the pelvis can be seen in patients with systemic disorders such as neurofibromatosis type 1. In the abdomen and pelvis,

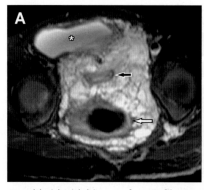
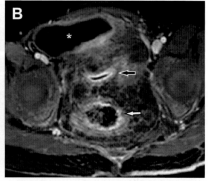

Fig. 27. A 10-year-old girl with history of neurofibromatosis type 1. Axial STIR (*A*) and axial T1-weighted postcontrast (*B*) images show widespread involvement of the pelvis by multiple plexiform neurofibromas surrounding the rectum (*white arrow*), vagina/uterus (*black arrow*), and the majority of the bladder (*asterisk*). Postcontrast image demonstrates very mild, predominantly peripheral enhancement of the masses. Note diffuse enhancement of the posterior wall of the bladder, owing to focal involvement.

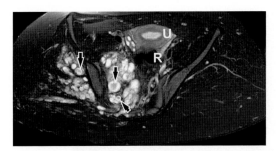

Fig. 28. A 15-year-old girl with history of neuro-fibromatosis type 1. Axial STIR image showing several plexiform neurofibromas with the typical target sign (*arrows*), with central low T2-weighted signal intensity and peripheral high signal intensity. R, rectum; U, uterus.

plexiform neurofibromas most commonly affect the retroperitoneum.[38] In the pelvis, plexiform neu-rofibromas can arise from the sacral nerve roots or from the pelvic plexus of nerves (**Fig. 26**). Bladder and rectal involvement due to mass effect can be seen, or may present as circumferential or focal infiltration (**Fig. 27**).

On MR imaging, plexiform neurofibromas demonstrate low signal intensity on T1-weighted images and increased signal on T2-weighted im-ages. On T2-weighted images some neurofi-bromas may exhibit a target-like appearance, with a central area of low signal intensity (**Fig. 28**). Relatively homogeneous enhancement is noted on postcontrast sequences, although pe-ripheral enhancement may be seen.

Malignant peripheral nerve sheath tumor occurs in 2% to 29% of patients with neurofibromatosis type 1.[67] Rapid growth of an existing tumor may indicate malignant transformation. Other imaging findings suggestive of malignant degeneration include loss of typical target sign,[67] development of hemorrhage, and a heterogeneous enhance-ment pattern indicating necrosis.[38]

Vascular Malformations

Slow-flow vascular malformations, including venous malformations and lymphatic malforma-tions, may primarily arise in the pelvis or extend into the pelvis from the abdomen or lower ex-tremities. Complex combined malformations, such as those seen in Klippel-Trenaunay syn-drome, commonly affect the lower limbs, with occasional extension into the perineum or pelvis.[68]

Fast spin-echo sequences are used to delin-eate the anatomy. STIR images provide homoge-neous fat suppression to determine the extent of the malformation. T1-weighted images are useful for evaluation of internal hemorrhage and throm-bosis. Gradient-echo sequences are especially helpful for evaluation of hemosiderin and calcifi-cation or phleboliths within the lesion. Phleboliths are exclusively present in venous malforma-tions.[68] Dynamic postcontrast imaging not only reveals the pattern and comparative timing of arterial and venous enhancement but also provides anatomic information about extent and

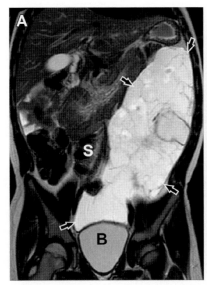
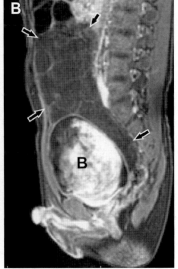

Fig. 29. A 3-year-old boy with large abdominopelvic lymphatic malformation. (*A*) Coronal T2-weighted image demonstrates homogeneous fluid signal intensity with multiple thin septations and significant mass effect on the bowel (*arrows*), including the sigmoid colon (S). (*B*) Sagittal postcontrast fat-saturated T1-weighted image reveals minimal enhancement of the internal septations. Contrast material is seen in the bladder (B).

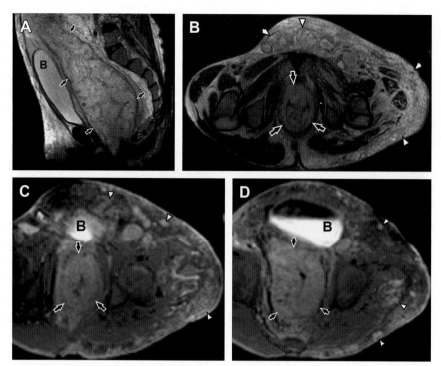

Fig. 30. A 16-year-old boy with history of Klippel-Trenaunay-Weber syndrome involving the abdomen, pelvis, rectum, left thigh, and left lower extremity. Sagittal T2-weighted image (*A*), axial T2-weighted image (*B*), and axial delayed postcontrast fat-saturated T1-weighted images (*C, D*) reveal marked wall thickening, increased signal, and enhancement involving the sigmoid colon and rectum (*black arrows*), consistent with extensive venous malformation. Note asymmetry of the soft tissues of the left pelvis, inguinal and gluteal regions with relative enlargement and abnormal hyperintense tubular structures, with delayed enhancement (*white arrowheads*) representing multiple dilated venous structures. B, bladder.

venous drainage. Pelvic lymphatic malformations do not internally enhance (peripheral and septal enhancement is common), whereas venous malformations fill with contrast material on delayed imaging (**Figs. 29** and **30**).

SUMMARY

The role of MR imaging in the assessment of pediatric pelvic masses goes beyond lesion detection to include detailed characterization, assessment of disease staging, and assistance in presurgical planning. MR imaging also provides a measure whereby we can assess response to therapy. Pelvic MRI has numerous advantages over CT in the pediatric population, including superior contrast resolution, ability to acquire multiple postcontrast imaging phases, and lack of ionizing radiation.

REFERENCES

1. Anthony EY, Caserta MP, Singh J, et al. Adnexal masses in female pediatric patients. AJR Am J Roentgenol 2012;198(5):W426–31.

2. Epelman M, Chikwava KR, Chauvin N, et al. Imaging of pediatric ovarian neoplasms. Pediatr Radiol 2011;41(9):1085–99.

3. von Allmen D. Malignant lesions of the ovary in childhood. Semin Pediatr Surg 2005;14(2):100–5.

4. Brookfield KF, Cheung MC, Koniaris LG, et al. A population-based analysis of 1037 malignant ovarian tumors in the pediatric population. J Surg Res 2009;156(1):45–9.

5. Shah RU, Lawrence C, Fickenscher KA, et al. Imaging of pediatric pelvic neoplasms. Radiol Clin North Am 2011;49(4):729–48, vi.

6. Oltmann SC, Garcia N, Barber R, et al. Can we preoperatively risk stratify ovarian masses for malignancy? J Pediatr Surg 2010;45(1):130–4.

7. Spinelli C, Di Giacomo M, Cei M, et al. Functional ovarian lesions in children and adolescents: when to remove them. Gynecol Endocrinol 2009;25(5):294–8.

8. Strickland JL. Ovarian cysts in neonates, children and adolescents. Curr Opin Obstet Gynecol 2002;14(5):459–65.

9. Nemec U, Nemec SF, Bettelheim D, et al. Ovarian cysts on prenatal MRI. Eur J Radiol 2012;81(8):1937–44.

10. Outwater EK, Dunton CJ. Imaging of the ovary and adnexa: clinical issues and applications of MR imaging. Radiology 1995;194(1):1–18.

11. Kanso HN, Hachem K, Aoun NJ, et al. Variable MR findings in ovarian functional hemorrhagic cysts. J Magn Reson Imaging 2006;24(2):356–61.

12. McCloskey K, Grover S, Vuillermin P, et al. Ovarian torsion among girls presenting with abdominal pain: a retrospective cohort study. Emerg Med J 2013;30(1):e11.

13. Guthrie BD, Adler MD, Powell EC. Incidence and trends of pediatric ovarian torsion hospitalizations in the United States, 2000-2006. Pediatrics 2010; 125(3):532–8.

14. Servaes S, Zurakowski D, Laufer MR, et al. Sonographic findings of ovarian torsion in children. Pediatr Radiol 2007;37(5):446–51.

15. Cools M, Looijenga LH, Wolffenbuttel KP, et al. Disorders of sex development: update on the genetic background, terminology and risk for the development of germ cell tumors. World J Pediatr 2009; 5(2):93–102.

16. Stranzinger E, Strouse PJ. Ultrasound of the pediatric female pelvis. Semin Ultrasound CT MR 2008;29(2):98–113.

17. Garel L, Dubois J, Grignon A, et al. US of the pediatric female pelvis: a clinical perspective. Radiographics 2001;21(6):1393–407.

18. Outwater EK, Siegelman ES, Hunt JL. Ovarian teratomas: tumor types and imaging characteristics. Radiographics 2001;21(2):475–90.

19. Jung SE, Lee JM, Rha SE, et al. CT and MR imaging of ovarian tumors with emphasis on differential diagnosis. Radiographics 2002;22(6): 1305–25.

20. Jung SE, Rha SE, Lee JM, et al. CT and MRI findings of sex cord-stromal tumor of the ovary. AJR Am J Roentgenol 2005;185(1):207–15.

21. Hazard FK, Longacre TA. Ovarian surface epithelial neoplasms in the pediatric population: incidence, histologic subtype, and natural history. Am J Surg Pathol 2013;37(4):548–53.

22. Morowitz M, Huff D, von Allmen D. Epithelial ovarian tumors in children: a retrospective analysis. J Pediatr Surg 2003;38(3):331–5 [discussion: 331–5].

23. McCarville MB, Hill DA, Miller BE, et al. Secondary ovarian neoplasms in children: imaging features with histopathologic correlation. Pediatr Radiol 2001;31(5):358–64.

24. Hanprasertpong J, Chandeying V. Gynecologic tumors during childhood and adolescence. J Med Assoc Thai 2006;89(Suppl 4):S192–8.

25. Murase E, Siegelman ES, Outwater EK, et al. Uterine leiomyomas: histopathologic features, MR imaging findings, differential diagnosis, and treatment. Radiographics 1999;19(5):1179–97.

26. Pai D, Coletti MC, Elkins M, et al. Diffuse uterine leiomyomatosis in a child. Pediatr Radiol 2012; 42(1):124–8.

27. Dietrich JE. An update on adenomyosis in the adolescent. Curr Opin Obstet Gynecol 2010; 22(5):388–92.

28. Tamai K, Togashi K, Ito T, et al. MR imaging findings of adenomyosis: correlation with histopathologic features and diagnostic pitfalls. Radiographics 2005;25(1):21–40.

29. Choi CM, Majmudar B, Horowitz IR. Malignant neoplasms of the vagina and cervix in the neonate, child, and adolescent. In: Carpenter SE, Rock JA, editors. Pediatric and adolescent gynecology. 2nd edition. Philadelphia: Lippincott Williams & Wilkens; 2000.

30. Nicolet V, Carignan L, Bourdon F, et al. MR imaging of cervical carcinoma: a practical staging approach. Radiographics 2000;20(6):1539–49.

31. Paradies G, Zullino F, Caroppo F, et al. Gartner's duct cyst: report of three cases. Pediatr Med Chir 2011;33(5–6):247–52 [in Italian].

32. Hahn WY, Israel GM, Lee VS. MRI of female urethral and periurethral disorders. AJR Am J Roentgenol 2004;182(3):677–82.

33. El Kady S, Al Zahrani A, Jednak R, et al. Bartholin's gland abscess in a neonate: a case report. Can Urol Assoc J 2007;1(2):117–9.

34. Agrons GA, Wagner BJ, Lonergan GJ, et al. From the archives of the AFIP. Genitourinary rhabdomyosarcoma in children: radiologic-pathologic correlation. Radiographics 1997;17(4):919–37.

35. Rosenberg HK, Eggli KD, Zerin JM, et al. Benign cystitis in children mimicking rhabdomyosarcoma. J Ultrasound Med 1994;13(12):921–32.

36. Huppmann AR, Pawel BR. Polyps and masses of the pediatric urinary bladder: a 21-year pathology review. Pediatr Dev Pathol 2011;14(6):438–44.

37. Wong-You-Cheong JJ, Woodward PJ, Manning MA, et al. From the Archives of the AFIP: neoplasms of the urinary bladder: radiologic-pathologic correlation. Radiographics 2006;26(2):553–80.

38. Zacharia TT, Jaramillo D, Poussaint TY, et al. MR imaging of abdominopelvic involvement in neurofibromatosis type 1: a review of 43 patients. Pediatr Radiol 2005;35(3):317–22.

39. Crist WM, Anderson JR, Meza JL, et al. Intergroup rhabdomyosarcoma study—IV: results for patients with nonmetastatic disease. J Clin Oncol 2001; 19(12):3091–102.

40. Lerena J, Krauel L, Garcia-Aparicio L, et al. Transitional cell carcinoma of the bladder in children and adolescents: six-case series and review of the literature. J Pediatr Urol 2010;6(5):481–5.

41. Savage N, Linn D, McDonough C, et al. Molecularly confirmed primary malignant rhabdoid tumor of the urinary bladder: implications of accurate diagnosis. Ann Diagn Pathol 2012;16(6):504–7.

42. Wu HY, Snyder HM 3rd. Pediatric urologic oncology: bladder, prostate, testis. Urol Clin North Am 2004;31(3):619–27, xi.

43. Castellino SM, Martinez-Borges AR, McLean TW. Pediatric genitourinary tumors. Curr Opin Oncol 2009;21(3):278–83.

44. Grimsby GM, Ritchey ML. Pediatric urologic oncology. Pediatr Clin North Am 2012;59(4):947–59.

45. Treetipsatit J, Kittikowit W, Zielenska M, et al. Mixed embryonal/alveolar rhabdomyosarcoma of the prostate: report of a case with molecular genetic studies and literature review. Pediatr Dev Pathol 2009;12(5):383–9.

46. Freling NJ, Merks JH, Saeed P, et al. Imaging findings in craniofacial childhood rhabdomyosarcoma. Pediatr Radiol 2010;40(11):1723–38 [quiz: 1855].

47. Bullard Dunn K. Retrorectal tumors. Surg Clin North Am 2010;90(1):163–71 [table of contents].

48. Glasgow SC, Dietz DW. Retrorectal tumors. Clin Colon Rectal Surg 2006;19(2):61–8.

49. Kocaoglu M, Frush DP. Pediatric presacral masses. Radiographics 2006;26(3):833–57.

50. Sebire NJ, Fowler D, Ramsay AD. Sacrococcygeal tumors in infancy and childhood; a retrospective histopathological review of 85 cases. Fetal Pediatr Pathol 2004;23(5–6):295–303.

51. Danzer E, Hubbard AM, Hedrick HL, et al. Diagnosis and characterization of fetal sacrococcygeal teratoma with prenatal MRI. AJR Am J Roentgenol 2006;187(4):W350–6.

52. Davenport KP, Blanco FC, Sandler AD. Pediatric malignancies: neuroblastoma, Wilm's tumor, hepatoblastoma, rhabdomyosarcoma, and sacrococcygeal teratoma. Surg Clin North Am 2012;92(3):745–67, x.

53. Altman RP, Randolph JG, Lilly JR. Sacrococcygeal teratoma: American Academy of Pediatrics Surgical Section Survey—1973. J Pediatr Surg 1974;9(3):389–98.

54. Kunisaki SM, Maher CO, Powelson I, et al. Benign sacrococcygeal teratoma with spinal canal invasion and paraplegia. J Pediatr Surg 2011;46(9):e1–4.

55. Powell RW, Weber ED, Manci EA. Intradural extension of a sacrococcygeal teratoma. J Pediatr Surg 1993;28(6):770–2.

56. Teal LN, Angtuaco TL, Jimenez JF, et al. Fetal teratomas: antenatal diagnosis and clinical management. J Clin Ultrasound 1988;16(5):329–36.

57. Avni FE, Guibaud L, Robert Y, et al. MR imaging of fetal sacrococcygeal teratoma: diagnosis and assessment. AJR Am J Roentgenol 2002;178(1):179–83.

58. De Corti F, Sarnacki S, Patte C, et al. Prognosis of malignant sacrococcygeal germ cell tumours according to their natural history and surgical management. Surg Oncol 2012;21(2):e31–7.

59. Derikx JP, De Backer A, van de Schoot L, et al. Factors associated with recurrence and metastasis in sacrococcygeal teratoma. Br J Surg 2006;93(12):1543–8.

60. Diel J, Ortiz O, Losada RA, et al. The sacrum: pathologic spectrum, multimodality imaging, and subspecialty approach. Radiographics 2001;21(1):83–104.

61. Currarino G, Coln D, Votteler T. Triad of anorectal, sacral, and presacral anomalies. AJR Am J Roentgenol 1981;137(2):395–8.

62. Isik N, Elmaci I, Gokben B, et al. Currarino triad: surgical management and follow-up results of four [correction of three] cases. Pediatr Neurosurg 2010;46(2):110–9.

63. Pfluger T, Czekalla R, Koletzko S, et al. MRI and radiographic findings in Currarino's triad. Pediatr Radiol 1996;26(8):524–7.

64. Nour-Eldin NE, Abdelmonem O, Tawfik AM, et al. Pediatric primary and metastatic neuroblastoma: MRI findings: pictorial review. Magn Reson Imaging 2012;30(7):893–906.

65. Amesse LS, Gibbs P, Hardy J, et al. Peritoneal inclusion cysts in adolescent females: a clinicopathological characterization of four cases. J Pediatr Adolesc Gynecol 2009;22(1):41–8.

66. Dillman JR, DiPietro MA. Hemorrhagic 'spider-in-web': atypical appearance of a peritoneal inclusion cyst. Pediatr Radiol 2009;39(11):1252.

67. Laor T. MR imaging of soft tissue tumors and tumor-like lesions. Pediatr Radiol 2004;34(1):24–37.

68. Dubois J, Alison M. Vascular anomalies: what a radiologist needs to know. Pediatr Radiol 2010;40(6):895–905.

Müllerian Duct and Related Anomalies in Children and Adolescents

Monica Epelman, MD[a],*, David Dinan, MD[a],
Michael S. Gee, MD, PhD[b,c], Sabah Servaes, MD[d],
Edward Y. Lee, MD, MPH[e], Kassa Darge, MD, PhD[f]

KEYWORDS

• Müllerian anomalies • Children • Uterine anomalies • Vaginal anomalies

KEY POINTS

- Müllerian duct anomalies represent a more frequent entity than previously believed.
- Various magnetic resonance imaging sequences allow detection of specific tissue and fluid elements that may have diagnostic implications, such as blood products, fibrous tissue, or calcifications.
- Best results for correction of genital tract outflow obstruction are achieved at the first attempt; therefore, accurate initial diagnosis is of utmost importance.
- Strong consideration should be given to evaluating potential genital tract anomalies in females with antenatal or postnatal diagnoses of renal agenesis, ureteral ectopia, or a multicystic dysplastic kidney with or without associated hydrocolpos.
- In clinical practice, it is important to distinguish between septate and bicornuate uteri, because the management and therapeutic interventions for these entities are different. However, this task is challenging and not always possible in pediatric patients.

INTRODUCTION

Developmental abnormalities of the Müllerian duct system encompass a wide spectrum of anomalies resulting from nondevelopment, defective fusion, or incomplete septal regression during fetal life.[1–3] The prevalence of Müllerian duct anomalies (MDAs) is unclear, because many are asymptomatic and may go unnoticed.[4] In women with a previous history of infertility and miscarriage, the prevalence may be as high as 25%.[5] Previously reported prevalence in unselected populations ranged from 0.4% to 1%.[6,7] In 2 more recent meta-analyses, Chan and colleagues[5] and Saravelos and colleagues[7] reported a prevalence of 5.5% and 6.7%, respectively, for MDAs in the general population. Therefore, MDAs represent a more frequent entity than previously believed. This fact might be at least partly related to the availability of noninvasive and accurate diagnostic imaging methods.[4] MDAs are also commonly inaccurately reported and ineffectively managed.[4,8] An accurate

[a] Department of Medical Imaging, Nemours Children's Hospital, 13535 Nemours Parkway, Orlando, FL 32827, USA; [b] Section of Pediatric Imaging, Department of Radiology, Massachusetts General Hospital, Harvard Medical School, 55 Fruit Street, Ellison 237, Boston, MA 02114, USA; [c] Section of Abdominal Imaging & Intervention, Department of Radiology, Massachusetts General Hospital, Harvard Medical School, 55 Fruit Street, Ellison 237, Boston, MA 02114, USA; [d] Computed Tomography, Department of Radiology, The Children's Hospital of Philadelphia, Perelman School of Medicine, University of Pennsylvania, 34th Street and Civic Center Boulevard, Philadelphia, PA 19104, USA; [e] Division of Thoracic Imaging, Magnetic Resonance Imaging, Department of Radiology, Boston Children's Hospital and Harvard Medical School, 300 Longwood Avenue, Boston, MA 02115, USA; [f] Division of Body Imaging, Department of Radiology, The Children's Hospital of Philadelphia, Perelman School of Medicine, University of Pennsylvania, 34th Street and Civic Center Boulevard, Philadelphia, PA 19104, USA
* Corresponding author.
E-mail address: Monica.Epelman@nemours.org

Magn Reson Imaging Clin N Am 21 (2013) 773–789
http://dx.doi.org/10.1016/j.mric.2013.04.011
1064-9689/13/$ – see front matter © 2013 Elsevier Inc. All rights reserved.

initial diagnosis is of utmost importance, because the best surgical results for correction of outflow tract obstruction are achieved at the first attempt.[8]

The most common types of MDA in the general population are, in order of frequency, the arcuate uterus, septate and subseptate defects, and the bicornuate uterus.[5] Environmental factors, chromosomal abnormalities, and hormonal factors are considered to be possible mechanisms in the development of MDAs, although most of the cases are idiopathic.[9,10]

MDAs are frequently associated with renal or axial skeletal anomalies. Consequently, strong consideration should be given to evaluating potential genital tract anomalies in women with antenatal or postnatal diagnoses of renal agenesis, ureteral ectopia, or a multicystic dysplastic kidney with or without a sonographically visible pelvic mass (**Fig. 1**).[11–14] Prenatal imaging may often detect a renal abnormality before identification of an associated uterine anomaly. Anorectal malformations may also be associated with this condition. It is important to be aware of this association, because it may have management implications. In such patients, the concomitant performance of a sigmoid colovaginoplasty or vaginal pull-through at the time of the anorectoplasty may potentially improve their outcome.[15]

An increased incidence of ovarian maldescent, which is defined as ovaries that are positioned at or above the level of the iliac artery bifurcation on magnetic resonance (MR) imaging, has been reported in association with MDAs.[16,17] Inguinal ovaries have also been reported in association with uterine malformations (**Fig. 2**).[18]

This article reviews the embryology, classification, and MR imaging findings of Müllerian duct and related anomalies in children and adolescents. Understanding the proper imaging techniques as well as the characteristic MR imaging appearance of various MDAs aids in accurate diagnosis and thus contributes to optimal patient care.

EMBRYOLOGY

The Müllerian (or paramesonephric) ducts are the primal components of the female genital tract, giving rise to the fallopian tubes, uterus, cervix, and the upper two-thirds of the vagina. Given the dual origin of the vagina, the upper two-thirds originate independently from the Müllerian ducts, whereas the lower one-third originates from the urogenital sinus[19]; vaginal anomalies, such as septa, duplication, and aplasia/hypoplasia, may or may not coexist with uterine anomalies.[8]

The normal development of the uterus is completed in 3 stages: organogenesis, fusion, and septal resorption.[3] Uterine anomalies may be caused by failed organogenesis of 1 or both ducts, resulting in uterine hypoplasia/agenesis or a unicornuate uterus. Abnormal or absent fusion of the ducts may cause the formation of a didelphys or bicornuate uterus. Failure of septal resorption, once the Müllerian ducts have fused, may result in a septate or arcuate uterus. In addition, a T-shaped uterus, which is an unusual anomaly in uterine morphology, was reported in the past in association with diethylstilbestrol (DES) exposure.[1,3,4,20–22]

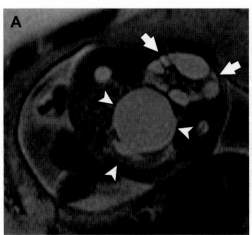
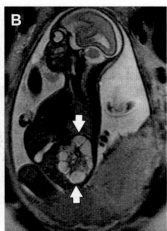

Fig. 1. Axial (*A*) and sagittal (*B*) fetal single-shot fast spin-echo MR images show a multicystic dysplastic kidney (*arrows*) and contralateral ureteropelvic junction obstruction (*arrowheads*) in a fetus, in whom later postnatal US revealed a uterine anomaly.

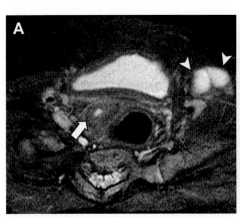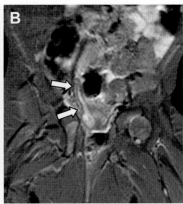

Fig. 2. Infant with multiple congenital anomalies and a left inguinal mass. (*A*) Axial fat-suppressed T2-weighted MR image through the pelvis shows an ectopic ovary (*arrowheads*) in the left inguinal canal. Note the multifollicular appearance of the ovary. There is a single uterine horn seen in the right pelvis (*arrow*). The lumbosacral spine is dysmorphic. (*B*) Coronal fat-suppressed T2-weighted MR image through the pelvis shows a banana-shaped unicornuate uterus (*arrows*) deviated to the right in this patient with MURCS (Müllerian duct aplasia, unilateral renal aplasia, and cervicothoracic somite dysplasia) association.

IMAGING

During the neonatal period, evaluation of the uterus by transabdominal ultrasonography (US) is facilitated by the effects of maternal hormones, avoiding the need for MR imaging (and possible sedation). As the influence of maternal hormones on the uterus diminishes, the uterus becomes small and tubular, precluding optimal evaluation. Thus, some advocate follow-up evaluation be delayed until the pubertal period in suspicious cases.[12,13] Transvaginal three-dimensional (3D) US, which seems to be highly accurate for the diagnosis and classification of Müllerian anomalies, is a recommended method for the initial evaluation of adult women[23–25]; however, this procedure is not safely performed in pediatric or sexually nonactive adolescent patients.[26] Transabdominal US may often provide enough information for making management decisions and prognostication. However, the findings may not always be conclusive, especially when the ovaries are not definitively identified or when the presence or absence of Müllerian remnants cannot be determined with high confidence. In these instances, MR imaging is usually recommended for a complete assessment.

MR imaging is widely considered to be the standard for MDA evaluation, especially in patients who are not sexually active, with reported diagnostic accuracies of almost 100%.[26–29] Recent advances in pediatric pelvic MR imaging, including more rapid sequences, isotropic volumetric image acquisition, and higher field strengths (with an increase in the MR signal-to-noise ratio on newer 3-T scanners compared with the classic 1.5-T systems), have allowed not only faster examinations but also improvements in the overall image quality. Various pulse sequences allow evaluation and characterization of a range of tissues and fluids and accurately detect specific components that may have diagnostic implications, such as blood products, fibrous (vs muscular) tissue, or calcifications.[30]

MR imaging protocols for the evaluation of MDAs vary across institutions. However, as a rule of thumb, water-sensitive sequences, such as T2-weighted sequences with or without fat suppression, are considered to be the pillars of female pelvic imaging. They allow for optimal visualization of the uterine zonal anatomy and clearly distinguish among the hyperintense endometrium, the hypointense junctional zone/inner myometrium, and the intermediate signal intensity of the outer myometrium (**Fig. 3**).[27,30,31] Initial T2-weighted sequences are usually performed in the sagittal plane to identify the position and orientation of the uterus. These sequences are followed by images that are parallel to the long axis and short axis of the uterus.[32] Images oriented along the long axis of the uterus in the coronal-oblique plane are crucial for depicting the external fundal contour.[27,29,31] Alternatively, high-resolution, volumetric, 3D T2-weighted fast spin-echo or balanced steady-state free precession images may be obtained, and multiplanar reformatting in any desired plane can be performed retrospectively at a work station, thereby potentially decreasing the total scan times (**Fig. 4**).[1,30] Axial fat-suppressed T1-weighted images are also obtained to evaluate for the presence of blood products in cases of obstruction and hemato(metro)colpos.[27,30,31] The uterus has a uniform signal intensity on T1-weighted images, which are therefore of limited value for the assessment of the uterine zonal anatomy.

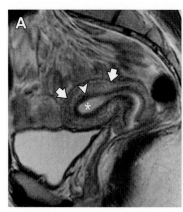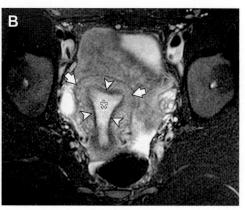

Fig. 3. Sagittal (*A*) and coronal (*B*) T2-weighted MR images without (*A*) and with (*B*) fat suppression, showing the normal uterine zonal anatomy. Note the hyperintense endometrium (*asterisk*), the hypointense junctional zone/inner myometrium (*arrowheads*), and the intermediate signal of the outer myometrium (*arrows*).

Evaluation of the kidneys and renal collecting systems is recommended in patients with MDAs,[2,33,34] because as many as 40% of the patients have concomitant renal anomalies.[35] The common associated anomalies are unilateral agenesis, ectopia, renal hypoplasia, multicystic dyspalstic kidney, and hydronephrosis.[35] Such evaluation can be accomplished by a single-shot fast spin-echo sequence providing a large field of view in the coronal plane, which can capture the renal fossae, expected course of ureters, and urinary bladder (**Fig. 5**).[32,36]

CLASSIFICATION

There is considerable controversy regarding the classification and nomenclature of MDAs. The most widely accepted classification system is the one developed in 1988 by the American Fertility Society (AFS), now known as the American Society of Reproductive Medicine (**Fig. 6**).[20] The anomalies are grouped based on similar uterine anatomy and the impact on pregnancy outcome/fetal survival.[4,7,20,21,37] This system classifies anomalies into 7 major anatomic uterine types, with additional subdivisions (**Box 1**).

Despite its widespread use, the AFS classification is by no means accepted by all. There are several drawbacks, especially the absence of a system for classifying a uterus that shows 2 or more anomalies from different classes.[14,27,37,38] This classification system is best suited to postpubescent females, because the neonatal or prepubescent uterus may be too small to allow definitive characterization. For example, by definition, the external fundal cleft in a bicornuate uterus

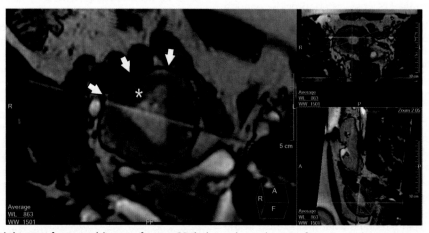

Fig. 4. Multiplanar reformatted images from a 3D balanced steady-state free precession sequence, showing a mild indentation (*asterisk*) at the inner fundus caused by incomplete resorption of the uterovaginal septum, representing an arcuate uterus. Note the chemical shift artifact seen at the fat-water interface between the uterus and surrounding peritoneal fat, which delineates the normal convex external uterine fundal contour (*arrows*).

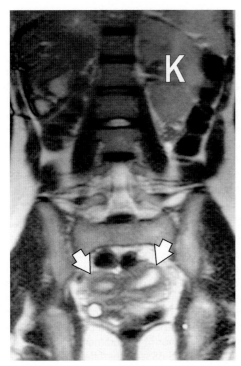

Fig. 5. Coronal single-shot fast spin-echo image through the abdomen and pelvis shows a uterine anomaly (*arrows*) and a normal-appearing single left kidney (K). The right kidney is congenitally absent and bowel loops are seen filling the right renal fossa.

must measure at least 10 mm.[1] In prepubescent girls, the entire normal uterus may measure only 20 mm,[39] and the typical findings sought for the differentiation between bicornuate and septate uteri in premenopausal women, such as the criteria for fundal contours and measurements, may not be applicable to fetuses, neonates, infants, or prepubescent females. There is also debate regarding whether an arcuate uterus should be included in the same class with a septate uterus, should be placed in a separate class within the classification system,[21] or should be considered a normal variant and thus excluded from the classification system.[3]

The classification system refers only to the uterus and lacks a systematic approach to obstructive anomalies, which are usually caused by cervical or vaginal anomalies and are responsible for many of the symptoms, especially in the pediatric population.[21,22]

Because of the difficulty in classifying MDAs using this system, perhaps the best approach may be to thoroughly describe the anatomy, including the number of cervices and uterine horns, (or lack of communication) of any atrophic horn, and the MR signal characteristics, if present, of any uterine or vaginal septa and any evidence of obstruction. Although many anomalies do not require treatment, in certain MDA cases, surgery may be necessary to enable sexual activity or to preserve fertility.[40] In these cases, a thorough but concise description may best guide the surgical treatment or clinical management.[36,38] Given the lack of standardized terminology, communication and joint reviews of cases between surgeons and radiologists are essential to ensure that appropriate clinical decisions are made and that inconsistencies in

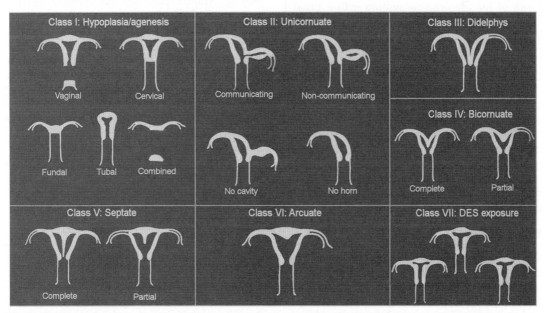

Fig. 6. Classification system developed by the AFS, now the American Society for Reproductive Medicine. (*Reproduced from* Copyright © 2005 by the American Society for Reproductive Medicine; with permission.)

Box 1
Classification of MDAs

Class I: Müllerian hypoplasia or agenesis

a. Vaginal

b. Cervical

c. Fundal

d. Tubal

e. Combined

Class II: unicornuate uterus (agenesis or hypoplasia of 1 of the Müllerian ducts)

a. Rudimentary horn with a communicating cavity

b. Rudimentary horn with a noncommunicating cavity

c. Rudimentary horn without a cavity

d. Complete absence of 1 horn

Class III: uterus didelphys (failure of lateral fusion of the Mullerian ducts)

Class IV: bicornuate uterus (incomplete Mullerian ductal fusion at the level of the body and fundus)

a. Complete

b. Partial

Class V: septate uterus (incomplete resorption or nonresorption of the uterovaginal septum)

a. Complete

b. Partial

Class VI: arcuate uterus (near-complete resorption of the uterovaginal septum with a trivial inner notch in the fundus and without external cleft)

Class VII: DES-related uterine hypoplasia and luminal changes

---

terminology do not lead to the incorrect decisions or to differences in management.[40] A multidisciplinary team of health care workers (including psychological counselors) is typically necessary to optimally manage these patients and to prepare them to adapt to their congenital anomalies, both at the time of diagnosis and later in life, especially in adolescents with class I anomalies.[41]

Class I Anomalies

Uterine agenesis or hypoplasia accounts for approximately 5% to 10% of uterine anomalies and is caused by failure of the Müllerian ducts to develop at approximately 5 weeks of gestation, resulting in various degrees of agenesis or hypoplasia of the upper two-thirds of the vagina, cervix, or uterus.[3,27]

Type I Mayer-Rokitansky-Küster-Hauser (MRKH) syndrome is the extreme form of this anomaly and consists of complete agenesis of the uterus, cervix, and proximal two-thirds of the vagina. Because normal ovaries are usually present, this disorder is characterized by a normal female phenotype, but primary amenorrhea during adolescence (**Fig. 7**).[35] If Müllerian duct agenesis or hypoplasia occurs with renal, ear, or skeletal anomalies, then the terms MURCS (Müllerian duct aplasia, unilateral renal aplasia, and cervicothoracic somite dysplasia) association or type II MRKH syndrome are sometimes used.[35]

Class II Anomalies

Unicornuate uterus accounts for close to 20% of all uterine anomalies and is the result of incomplete or absent development of 1 of the paired Müllerian ducts.[27,42] This type of anomaly is commonly associated with renal anomalies, which may be observed in as many as 40% of patients,[1] particularly with renal agenesis ipsilateral to the rudimentary or absent horn.[42] A rudimentary horn may be present in up to 65% of the affected patients and may contain endometrium in nearly 50% of cases; moreover, in nearly 70% of cases, the rudimentary horn does not communicate with the primary horn and may contain T1-weighted hyperintense blood products (**Fig. 8**).[27,42] The AFS recognizes 4 subtypes: (a) rudimentary horn with a communicating cavity; (b) rudimentary horn with a noncommunicating cavity; (c) rudimentary horn without a cavity (nonfunctional); and (d) complete absence of 1 horn (**Fig. 9**). Type b in particular may obstruct and present at menarche with dysmenorrhea, hematometra, and hematosalpinx.[2,3,42] In these patients, endometriosis may be a source of chronic pelvic pain. Endometriosis, defined as the presence of endometrial glands and stroma outside the uterus, is believed to occur secondary to obstruction, with retrograde menstruation and implantation of functional endometrium within the peritoneal cavity.[1,2,42] MR imaging may reveal the banana-shaped or cigar-shaped unicornuate uterus, determine the presence or absence of a rudimentary horn and whether it communicates with the contralateral horn, and evaluate for the presence of associated renal anomalies.[1,31]

Class III Anomalies

Uterus didelphys is the result of nonfusion of the Müllerian ducts and accounts for nearly 5% of cases.[27] This anomaly is characterized by the presence of 2 noncommunicating uterine cavities with 2 cervices, and a very deep fundal cleft is typically shown on MR imaging (**Fig. 10**). It is not uncommon

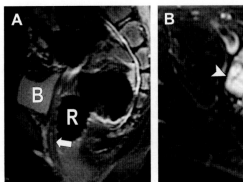
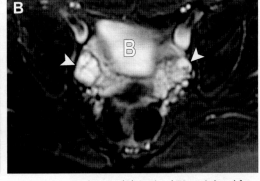

Fig. 7. A 17-year-old with Meyer-Rokitansky-Kuster-Hauser syndrome. (*A*) Sagittal T2-weighted fat-suppressed MR image shows a hypoplastic, blind-ending vagina (*arrow*) between the bladder (B) and rectum (R). No normal uterine tissue is identified. (*B*) Axial T2-weighted MR image showing absence of expected normal uterine tissue posterior to the bladder (B). Normal ovaries (*arrowheads*) are present and are responsible for the normal female phenotype.

for some of these patients to present with an associated obstructed hemivagina and ipsilateral renal agenesis, which is a syndrome referred to as OH-VIRA (obstructed hemivagina and ipsilateral renal agenesis) or Herlyn-Werner-Wunderlich syndrome **(Fig. 11)**.[43] Associated complications, such as hematosalpinx and endometriosis, may occur secondary to retrograde menstruation.[2,12,44] These complications are best evaluated on T1-weighted images with fat suppression, in which blood products appear hyperintense. These patients typically present during postpubescence with normal pubertal development, worsening dysmenorrhea, and a palpable pelvic mass. Many of these cases are often initially misdiagnosed or correct diagnosis is delayed, because regular menses occur from the nonobstructed hemiuterus.[2,43]

Class IV Anomalies

Bicornuate uterus accounts for approximately 10% of uterine anomalies and is caused by

incomplete fusion of the Müllerian ducts.[1,27] On MR imaging, the anomaly is characterized by the presence of 2 widely divergent uterine cornua, with a normal zonal anatomy that is fused caudally at the lower uterine segment or uterine isthmus, a concave outward external uterine contour, and a fundal cleft greater than 10 mm in depth.[1,2,31] Bicornuate uteri may present with or without cervix duplication, constituting a bicornuate bicollis uterus or a bicornuate unicollis uterus, respectively **(Fig. 12)**.[2]

Class V Anomalies

Septate uteri are the most common type of uterine anomalies, accounting for more than 50% of cases.[1,27] The fibrous or fibromuscular septum may be partial or complete and is caused by a failure to be resorbed. This anomaly is typically diagnosed during adulthood because of its poor reproductive outcome, because the live birth rate may be as low as 5%.[31] The fibrous septum of a

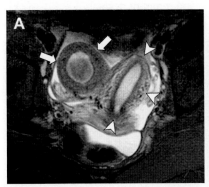
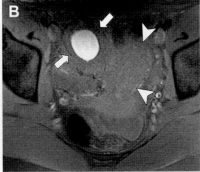

Fig. 8. Right lower quadrant pain in a 15-year-old girl. Axial T2-weighted fat-saturated (*A*) and axial T1-weighted fat-saturated (*B*) MR images show a class IIb uterine anomaly consistent with a unicornuate uterus with a noncommunicating right uterine horn. The obstructed, amorphous right uterine horn (*arrows*) shows intermediate T2-weighted (shading) and increased T1-weighted signal within the endometrial cavity, consistent with retained blood products. The left uterine horn (*arrowheads*) is nonobstructed and functional.

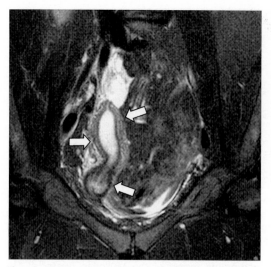

Fig. 9. Unicornuate uterus consisting of a single normal uterine horn (class type IId). Coronal fat-saturated T2-weighted MR image shows the characteristic banana-shaped appearance of a single, nonobstructed unicornuate uterus (*arrows*) with no rudimentary horn.

septate uterus is characterized by signal hypo-intensity on T1-weighted and T2-weighted images, as would be expected with fibrous tissue (**Fig. 13**).[29] The external fundal contour may be convex, flat, or mildly concave (with the fundal cleft measuring <10 mm).[2] In clinical practice and in cases of infertility, it is important to distinguish between septate and bicornuate uteri, because the management and therapeutic interventions for these entities are different. Although the fibrous septum is surgically resected by a transvaginal approach in septate uteri, a transabdominal approach is required for bicornuate uteri to ensure appropriate hemostasis. However, in some patients, no intervention may be necessary for bicornuate uteri.[29,31] As previously mentioned,

in pediatric patients, the differentiation between the 2 entities may be challenging, particularly in prepubertal patients with a small uterus.[22] In such cases, it may be best to describe the findings, and to counsel the patient and her parents or guardians regarding the imaging results and informing that additional imaging may be necessary in the future.

Class VI Anomalies

Considered a normal variant by many investigators, arcuate uterus is the result of near complete resorption of the uterovaginal septum, except for a small portion causing a mild, smooth, and saddle-shaped indentation at the endometrial fundus, with a T2-weighted signal that is isointense to the myometrium and without evidence of hypointense fibrous tissue. The external fundal contour is preserved and typically shows convex outward margins (**Fig. 14**).[1,2,27]

Class VII Anomalies

Class VII anomalies are related to exposure to DES, which is a synthetic estrogen that was prescribed to prevent miscarriages until 1971, when Herbst and colleagues[45] reported the association of this drug with adenocarcinoma of the vagina. Therefore, this anomaly is unexpected nowadays in pediatric patients. DES exposure causes a so-called T-shaped uterus (uterine cavity), which consists of a hypoplastic uterus with a shortened upper uterine segment.[1]

VAGINAL DISORDERS

Congenital disorders of the vagina fall into 1 of the following 3 major groupings: obstructive outflow tract disorders, congenital absence of the vagina, and remnant cysts.[8]

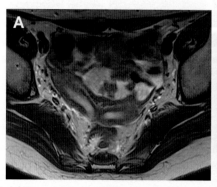
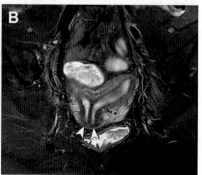

Fig. 10. (*A*) Axial T2-weighted and (*B*) coronal-oblique T2-weighted fat-suppressed MR images show widely divergent uterine horns separated by a very deep fundal cleft caused by failure of Mullerian duct fusion. Two cervices (*arrowheads*) are present, consistent with uterus didelphys (vs bicornuate bicollis uterus).

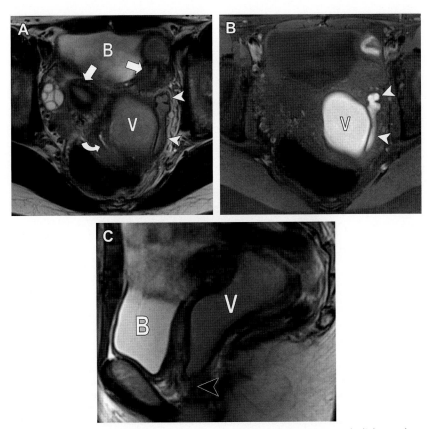

Fig. 11. Didelphys uterus with obstructed hemivagina in Herlyn-Werner-Wunderlich syndrome. Axial T2-weighted (*A*) and axial T1-weighted fat-suppressed (*B*) MR images show widely divergent uterine horns (*arrows*) superior to an obstructed left hemivagina (V). There is high signal within the obstructed hemivagina, consistent with blood products and hematocolpos. The ipsilateral left fallopian tube is also distended with blood products, representing hematosalpynx (*white arrowheads*). The right hemivagina is unobstructed (*curved arrow*). (*C*) Sagittal T2-weighted MR image shows the distended upper left hemivagina (V), with intermediate signal blood products as a result of obstruction by a transverse vaginal septum. The lower portion of this hemivagina (*black arrowhead*) is collapsed. B, bladder.

Obstructive Outflow Tract Disorders

Vaginal obstructive outflow tract disorders typically manifest either at birth or at puberty.[34,46] In neonates, fluid accumulation in the vagina, termed hydrocolpos, may result from cervical secretions or from urine in cases that are associated with a persistent urogenital sinus or cloacal dysgenesis.[34] A transient fluid accumulation in the vagina, known as a vaginal reflux, is infrequently seen during voiding and usually disappears when the patient stands up. Vaginal reflux can be seen during US examinations of the bladder or at voiding cystourethrography and should not be confused with hydrocolpos. Hydrometrocolpos is the term used to describe the concomitant dilatation of the vagina and uterus. During the newborn period, most cases of hydrometrocolpos result from a persistent urogenital sinus or cloacal dysgenesis.[34] Both anomalies (urogenital sinus and

cloacal dysgenesis) occur only in female phenotypes and are believed to be caused by failure of the urorectal septum to join the cloacal membrane during the fourth to sixth weeks of gestation.[10,47] The resulting spectrum of congenital urogenital malformations is highly variable, with a multitude of differing combinations and degrees of fusion of parts of the urinary, genital, and intestinal tracts.[33] In persistent urogenital sinus, there is a single external exit for the bladder and vagina, with a separate opening for the gastrointestinal tract; therefore, affected girls clinically present with 2 external openings in the introitus. In cloacal dysgenesis, there is a single, common perineal opening for the urinary, genital, and gastrointestinal tracts.[10,22,47,48]

On US and MR imaging, neonates with a persistent urogenital sinus usually show hydrometrocolpos, which displaces the bladder anteriorly. The typical US finding of a fluid-debris level is believed

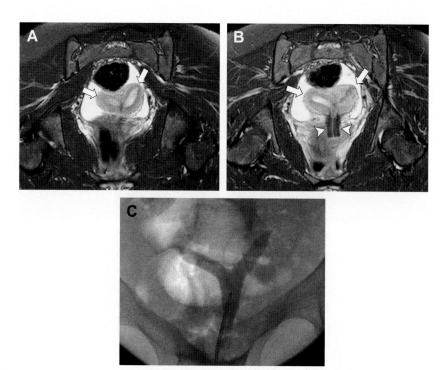

Fig. 12. Bicornuate uterus in a 16-year-old with multiple congenital anomalies. (*A*, *B*) Coronal-oblique fat-saturated T2-weighted MR images in the plane of the uterus show an apparent bicornuate unicollis uterus with 2 divergent uterine horns (*arrows*) and a single cervix (*arrowheads*). This uterus technically does not fulfill the criteria for a bicornuate uterus, because the external fundal cleft is not deep enough. This is an example of why accurate, descriptive terminology should be used rather than rigid classification in the pediatric population. (*C*) Fluoroscopic spot image favors the presence of a bicornuate uterus as well.

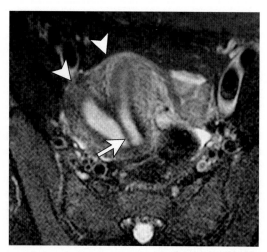

Fig. 13. Septate uterus. T2-weighted fat-suppressed MR image shows a septate uterus, with the arrow denoting the hypointense fibrous septum. The arrowheads show a flattened outer external contour without a fundal cleft.

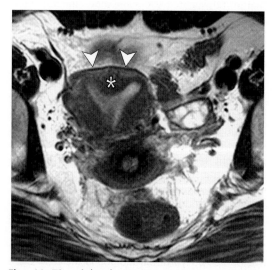

Fig. 14. T2-weighted MR image shows an arcuate uterus, considered by many a normal variant. It is the result of incomplete resorption of the uterovaginal septum. Note the smooth, mild indentation (*asterisk*) at the inner fundus and the normal convex external uterine fundal contour (*arrowheads*), without a cleft.

to reflect the admixture of urine with uterovaginal secretions.[34] Similarly, in cloacal dysgenesis, the fluid-debris level most likely reflects a mixture of urine with uterovaginal secretions and meconium.[34]

Although abdominal radiography is of limited value as a definitive diagnostic tool, it may occasionally aid in diagnosis, for example, by revealing a midline pelvic mass that displaces the bowel loops cranially. Rarely, gas may be observed within a midline pelvic mass, suggesting a rectovaginal communication.[33] US is the examination of choice for suspected hydrometrocolpos or for characterizing a pelvic mass in a child. However, CT and MR imaging may also show these findings, aid in the diagnosis, and serve as a baseline. Several investigators advocate the use of an inert gel during MR imaging to distend the vagina and to better evaluate for any anomalies[49,50]; such technique is possible in older and sexually active adolescents, but may be inappropriate and poorly tolerated in young girls and pediatric patients. Fluoroscopic imaging in combination with US and MR imaging may more clearly delineate the anatomy, particularly the levels of abnormal fistulous communications, in complex cases, although in certain instances, volumetric MR imaging sequences may suffice (**Fig. 15**).[51] Because postsurgical changes can make follow-up imaging studies difficult to interpret, several investigators advocate preoperative MR imaging as a baseline for follow-up studies.[22,44]

Correlations with preexisting fetal images may also be useful and may provide additional information regarding the presence or absence of a cloacal anomaly and the associated hydrometrocolpos, which may be observed as a dilated cystic structure in the pelvis on fetal US or fetal MR imaging. The diagnosis of hydrometrocolpos in fetal images is usually made by the location, morphology, and fluid signal intensity of the lesion. Fetal MR imaging may be especially helpful in determining if the rectum is separate from the lesion, because this finding has prognostic implications.[22,52,53] The absence of a fistulous communication between the lesion and the rectum may be inferred by showing a compressed rectum with an expected, normal hyperintense signal of meconium on the T1-weighted images.[52,53] This finding may increase the level of confidence of the radiologist who is performing the postnatal fluoroscopic examination to assess whether a fistulous communication is present, targeting the fluoroscopic examination, decreasing its duration, and consequently reducing radiation exposure (**Fig. 16**).[52]

Infrequently, ambiguous genitalia with enlargement of the clitoris and signs of virilization is observed in some neonates with urogenital sinus

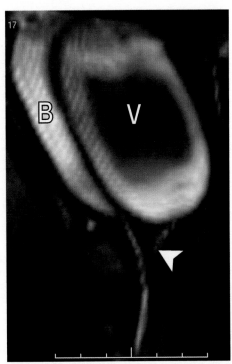

Fig. 15. A 9-month-old female with multiple congenital anomalies including clinical and US findings consistent with urogenital sinus and hydrometrocolpos. A catheter was placed into her vagina percutaneously to drain the fluid. Multiple fluoroscopic studies failed to show the level of communication (*images not shown*). Before surgical correction and to further delineate the anatomy, MR imaging was performed. Sagittal-oblique reformatted MR image from a 3D balanced steady-state free precession sequence shows a catheterized bladder (B) and the dilated vagina, which was distended with saline via the indwelling suprapubic catheter. A small vaginourethral communication (*arrowhead*) is shown, which was subsequently confirmed on cystoscopy.

or cloacal defects. The cause and incidence of the ambiguous genitalia in these patients is uncertain. McMullin and Hutson[54] suggested that the associated genitalia ambiguity in these patients may result from the early derangement of urogenital development, which prevents the normal, androgen-dependent growth-control mechanisms. This phenomenon also allows for autonomous phallic growth and fusion of the genital folds. In addition, abnormal cloacal and urogenital sinus formation may interfere with normal development of the ureteric bud, leading to ureteric agenesis and secondary renal agenesis.[33,54]

For patients who have begun menstruating, the terms hematometra, hematocolpos, and hematometrocolpos are used, thus implying that blood products are also present in the uterus or the

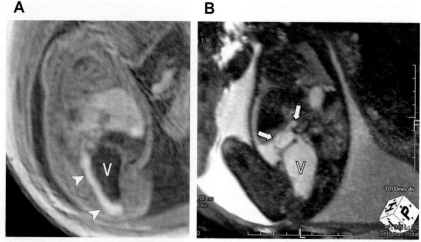

Fig. 16. Fetal hydrometrocolpos. (*A*) Midline sagittal T1-weighted fetal MR image shows the expected hyperintense signal within the rectum caused by meconium (*arrowheads*). The distended vagina (V) shows fluid signal. (*B*) Frontal 3D maximum intensity projection image from a fluid-sensitive pulse sequence shows an apparent bicornuate uterus (*arrows*). The vagina (V) is dilated related to the presence of a urogenital sinus proved on postnatal imaging.

vagina or both.[10,22] During adolescence, a common and benign cause of vaginal obstruction is an imperforate hymen, which usually manifests at the onset of menses and has a characteristic appearance on clinical examination. This condition is not a Müllerian anomaly and should be differentiated from vaginal atresia or from longitudinal or transverse vaginal septa,[34,37,46] which are Müllerian anomalies. These more complex anomalies may result in vaginal obstruction and may be associated with other predominantly renal or skeletal anomalies.[8,34,46]

Congenital Absence of the Vagina

Complete vaginal agenesis may be isolated or associated with agenesis or hypoplasia of the uterus. The most common cause is MRKH syndrome, with a prevalence of 1:4000 to 5000 live births.[8,55,56] Affected patients usually have a normal female karyotype and normal external female genitalia. Gonadal dysgenesis or Turner syndrome (45XO), Klippel-Feil syndrome, Holt-Oram syndrome, and velocardiofacial syndrome have also been reported in association with agenesis or hypoplasia of the uterus and vagina.[10,22,56]

Congenital Vaginal Septa

Congenital vaginal septa, may be transverse or longitudinal (**Fig. 17**), occurring either in isolation or in conjunction with other MDAs. Transverse vaginal septa are variable in thickness and believed to result from incomplete vertical fusion between the Müllerian ductal system and the urogenital sinus,

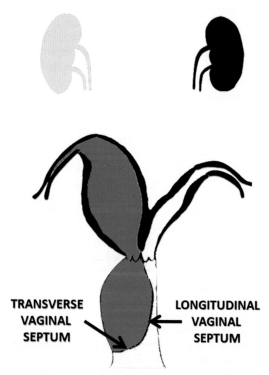

Fig. 17. Congenital vaginal septa. The transverse vaginal septum is the result of failed vertical fusion between the Müllerian duct and the urogenital sinus and is characteristically ipsilateral to the side of renal agenesis and vaginal obstruction (*red*). Failed lateral fusion of the Müllerian ducts results in a longitudinal vaginal septum.

leaving a transverse septum, which may occur at variable levels in the vagina. However, longitudinal vaginal septa reflect disordered lateral fusion between the lower aspects of the 2 Müllerian ducts. This anomaly is usually associated with didelphys uteri (**Fig. 18**).[2,8,22,55,57] Symptoms in affected patients typically arise with the onset of menses, because these patients may present with difficulty inserting tampons into the abnormal vagina or the inserted tampon may occlude only 1 hemivagina.[8] Dyspareunia has been also associated with this anomaly. Longitudinal vaginal septa may be present in as many as 75% of patients with uterine didelphys[37] and are sometimes further complicated by a transverse septum obstructing 1 hemivagina, usually the right more than the left.[8,12] As noted earlier, OHVIRA or Herlyn-Werner-Wunderlich syndrome are the terms used when the congenital obstruction of 1 hemivagina, in cases of didelphys uteri, and ipsilateral renal agenesis are concomitantly present (see **Fig. 18**).[12,58] Recurrent, cyclic episodes of pelvic pain and a palpable pelvic mass caused by hemihematometrocolpos is a common clinical presentation with the onset of menses in OHVIRA.[12,58]

Vaginal Cysts

Congenital cysts of the vagina include Müllerian and Gartner duct cysts, which may be found incidentally on MR imaging examinations performed for other reasons. MR imaging is not routinely used in the diagnosis of congenital or acquired vaginal cysts, most of which are Müllerian remnant cysts or epidermal inclusion cysts.[8] Gartner duct cysts are less common, result from remnants of Wolffian (mesonephric) ducts, and are typically located in the anterolateral wall of the vagina and are usually located above the level of the inferiormost aspect of the pubic symphysis (**Fig. 19**)[59]; by contrast, Müllerian duct cysts may be found in several locations. The clinical relevance of differentiating between these types of cysts is of limited clinical significance.[60] Gartner duct cysts should also be differentiated from urethral diverticula, a distinction that should not be challenging, because diverticula typically are centered around the urethra, whereas Gartner duct cysts are located more posteriorly in the anterolateral vaginal wall.[59] Gartner and Müllerian duct cysts usually display low signal intensities on T1-weighted images when the cysts contain simple fluids and intermediate signal intensities when internal protein, mucin, or blood products are present. High signal intensity on T2-weighted images is generally observed.[55] Several investigators have reported on the association between Gartner duct cysts; ipsilateral renal hypoplasia, dysplasia, or agenesis; and ectopic ureters. This association may prompt imaging of the kidneys and urinary tract when evaluating patients who present with Gartner duct cysts.[61]

Bartholin glands are homologous to Cowper glands in males, are of urogenital sinus origin, and are located more caudally, inferiorly and posteriorly

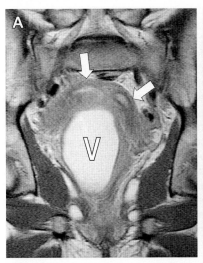 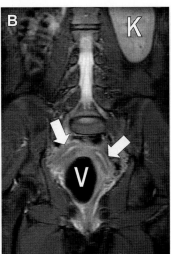 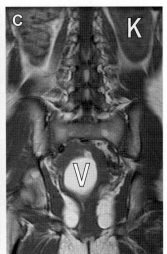

Fig. 18. OHVIRA or Herlyn-Werner-Wunderlich syndrome. (*A*) Coronal T2-weighted and (*B*) coronal inversion recovery MR images show a uterus didelphys with widely divergent uterine horns (*arrows*) superior to an obstructed right hemivagina (V). Hypointense vaginal fluid signal on the inversion recovery imaging confirms the presence of complex fluid, likely blood products (simple fluid should appear hyperintense). (*C*) Coronal T1-weighted MR image shows high signal within the obstructed hemivagina, again consistent with blood products and hematocolpos. Note the absence of the right kidney and the presence of a single left orthotopic kidney (K).

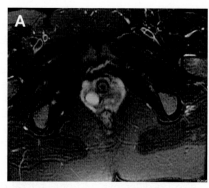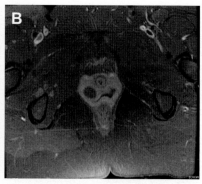

Fig. 19. A 17-year-old girl with a history of ulcerative colitis. (*A*) Axial T2-weighted and (*B*) axial T1-weighted postcontrast MR images obtained as part of an MR enterography examination show a rounded cystic lesion located anterolaterally in the vaginal wall, consistent with a Gartner duct cyst. (*Courtesy of* Ethan A. Smith, MD, Section of Pediatric Radiology, Department of Radiology, C. S. Mott Children's Hospital, University of Michigan Health System.)

in the vaginal wall compared with Gartner duct cysts.[55,61] Obstruction secondary to infection or inspissated mucus results in cyst formation. Uncomplicated Bartholin gland cysts may normally show restricted diffusion on diffusion-weighted images (**Fig. 20**).[62] Wall thickening on either US or MR imaging or wall hyperenhancement on postcontrast T1-weighted MR imaging suggests infection in both Gartner duct cysts and Bartholin gland cysts.[55]

METANEPHRIC BLASTEMA AND URETERAL BUD

Renal abnormalities often accompany uterine anomalies.[14,33,44,54] Therefore, a renal evaluation

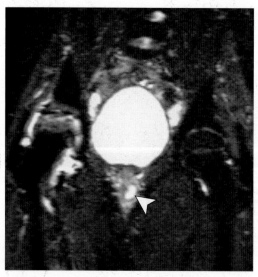

Fig. 20. Coronal diffusion-weighted MR image (with b value of 1000 s/mm²) shows restricted diffusion in an incidentally noted Bartholin gland cyst (*arrowhead*) in a patient being evaluated for right hip osteonecrosis.

should always be performed in patients with congenital uterine abnormalities. Renal evaluation can be easily performed concurrently with the patient's pelvic US[36] or pelvic MR imaging. Merrot and colleagues[11] found that 15% of patients with a multicystic dysplastic kidney had ipsilateral genitourinary tract anomalies. In a recent review of 113 patients with MDAs, Hall-Craggs and colleagues[14] found renal agenesis in close to 32% of the patients showing lower ureteric remnants, with ectopic insertions in the gynecologic tract present in as many as 25% of cases. These remnants may fill with urine or menstrual blood and become the source of chronic pain, incontinence, or infection. This finding is clinically relevant, because precise knowledge of orthotopic or ectopic ureteric course is important before the surgeon embarks on the complex laparoscopic and vaginal surgery needed for the successful correction of obstructed MDAs as well as for the surgeon to anticipate the need for urologic input.[14] A horseshoe kidney, which is the result of fusion of the metanephrogenic blastema before ascent, and an ectopic kidney, which is caused by failed migration of the metanephric blastema and ureteral bud to the renal fossa, may also be encountered in association with Müllerian anomalies. As noted earlier, prenatal US screening may reveal a renal abnormality before detection of a uterovaginal abnormality, with the uterine or vaginal anomalies being detected later (eg, in the third trimester, during the neonatal period, or even after menarche).[22,63]

CANAL OF NUCK

The processus vaginalis in females, known as the canal of Nuck, is a rudimentary peritoneal sac that travels with the round ligament through the inguinal canal, thereby terminating in the labia

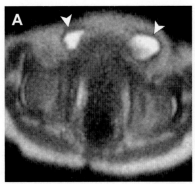 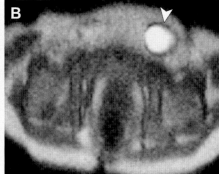

Fig. 21. Bilateral hydroceles of the canal of Nuck in an infant. (*A, B*) Axial T2-weighted MR image of the pelvis shows bilateral, left larger than right, well-delineated inguinal lesions (*arrowheads*), showing fluid signal.

majora. The canal of Nuck forms at approximately 6 months of gestation and obliterates during the first year of life.[64] Persistent patency may cause an indirect inguinal hernia or the formation of a cyst, which is equivalent to an encysted hydrocele of the spermatic cord in males (**Fig. 21**). Affected patients typically present with painless, fluctuating inguinolabial swelling.[50,61,64]

SUMMARY

Despite transabdominal US being the initial imaging modality for evaluating the reproductive system in the pediatric population, MR imaging is being increasingly used and is considered the standard modality for imaging MDAs by many investigators. Correct management of these anomalies is imperative, and their detailed anatomic depiction, as can be achieved only with MR imaging, may be of utmost importance for definitive diagnosis and possibly surgical planning, particularly in the evaluation of the most complex anomalies.

REFERENCES

1. Behr SC, Courtier JL, Qayyum A. Imaging of Müllerian duct anomalies. Radiographics 2012;32(6): E233–50.
2. Junqueira BL, Allen LM, Spitzer RF, et al. Müllerian duct anomalies and mimics in children and adolescents: correlative intraoperative assessment with clinical imaging1. Radiographics 2009;29(4): 1085–103.
3. Chandler TM, Machan LS, Cooperberg PL, et al. Müllerian duct anomalies: from diagnosis to intervention. Br J Radiol 2009;82(984):1034–42.
4. Acién P, Acién MI. The history of female genital tract malformation classifications and proposal of an updated system. Hum Reprod Update 2011; 17(5):693–705.
5. Chan YY, Jayaprakasan K, Zamora J, et al. The prevalence of congenital uterine anomalies in unselected and high-risk populations: a systematic review. Hum Reprod Update 2011;17(6):761–71.
6. Stampe Sorensen S. Estimated prevalence of Mullerian anomalies. Acta Obstet Gynecol Scand 1988;67(5):441–5.
7. Saravelos SH, Cocksedge KA, Li T- C. Prevalence and diagnosis of congenital uterine anomalies in women with reproductive failure: a critical appraisal. Hum Reprod Update 2008;14(5):415–29.
8. Edmonds DK. Congenital malformations of the genital tract and their management. Best Pract Res Clin Obstet Gynaecol 2003;17(1):19–40.
9. Dang Y, Qin Y, Tang R, et al. Variants of the WNT7A gene in Chinese patients with Müllerian duct abnormalities. Fertil Steril 2012;97(2):391–394.e391.
10. Servaes S, Epelman M. The current state of imaging pediatric genitourinary anomalies and abnormalities. Curr Probl Diagn Radiol 2013; 42(1):1–12.
11. Merrot T, Lumenta DB, Tercier S, et al. Multicystic dysplastic kidney with ipsilateral abnormalities of genitourinary tract: experience in children. Urology 2006;67(3):603–7.
12. Orazi C, Lucchetti MC, Schingo PM, et al. Herlyn-Werner-Wunderlich syndrome: uterus didelphys, blind hemivagina and ipsilateral renal agenesis. Sonographic and MR findings in 11 cases. Pediatr Radiol 2007;37(7):657–65.
13. Capito C, Echaieb A, Lortat-Jacob S, et al. Pitfalls in the diagnosis and management of obstructive uterovaginal duplication: a series of 32 cases. Pediatrics 2008;122(4):e891–7.
14. Hall-Craggs MA, Kirkham A, Creighton SM. Renal and urological abnormalities occurring with Müllerian anomalies. J Pediatr Urol 2013;9(1):27–32.
15. Wester T, Tovar JA, Rintala RJ. Vaginal agenesis or distal vaginal atresia associated with anorectal malformations. J Pediatr Surg 2012;47(3):571–6.
16. Allen JW, Cardall S, Kittijarukhajorn M, et al. Incidence of ovarian maldescent in women with Müllerian duct anomalies: evaluation by MRI. Am J Roentgenol 2012;198(4):W381–5.

17. Dabirashrafi H, Mohammad K, Moghadami-Tabrizi N. Ovarian malposition in women with uterine anomalies. Obstet Gynecol 1994;83(2):293–4.

18. Demirel F, Kara O, Esen I. Inguinal ovary as a rare diagnostic sign of Mayer-Rokitansky-Kuster-Hauser syndrome. J Pediatr Endocrinol Metab 2012;25(3–4):383–6.

19. Sadler TW, Langman J. Langman's medical embryology. 8th edition. Philadelphia: Lippincott Williams & Wilkins; 2000.

20. The American Fertility Society classifications of adnexal adhesions, distal tubal occlusion, tubal occlusion secondary to tubal ligation, tubal pregnancies, Mullerian anomalies and intrauterine adhesions. Fertil Steril 1988;49(6):944–55.

21. Grimbizis GF, Campo R. Congenital malformations of the female genital tract: the need for a new classification system. Fertil Steril 2010;94(2):401–7.

22. Servaes S, Victoria T, Lovrenski J, et al. Contemporary pediatric gynecologic imaging. Semin Ultrasound CT MR 2010;31(2):116–40.

23. Faivre E, Fernandez H, Deffieux X, et al. Accuracy of three-dimensional ultrasonography in differential diagnosis of septate and bicornuate uterus compared with office hysteroscopy and pelvic magnetic resonance imaging. J Minim Invasive Gynecol 2012;19(1):101–6.

24. Ghi T, Casadio P, Kuleva M, et al. Accuracy of three-dimensional ultrasound in diagnosis and classification of congenital uterine anomalies. Fertil Steril 2009;92(2):808–13.

25. Bermejo C, Martínez Ten P, Cantarero R, et al. Three-dimensional ultrasound in the diagnosis of Müllerian duct anomalies and concordance with magnetic resonance imaging. Ultrasound Obstet Gynecol 2010;35(5):593–601.

26. Santos XM, Krishnamurthy R, Bercaw-Pratt JL, et al. The utility of ultrasound and magnetic resonance imaging versus surgery for the characterization of Müllerian anomalies in the pediatric and adolescent population. J Pediatr Adolesc Gynecol 2012;25(3):181–4.

27. Olpin JD, Heilbrun M. Imaging of Mullerian duct anomalies. Top Magn Reson Imaging 2010;21(4):225–35.

28. Pellerito JS, McCarthy SM, Doyle MB, et al. Diagnosis of uterine anomalies: relative accuracy of MR imaging, endovaginal sonography, and hysterosalpingography. Radiology 1992;183(3):795–800.

29. Carrington B, Hricak H, Nuruddin R, et al. Mullerian duct anomalies: MR imaging evaluation. Radiology 1990;176:715–20.

30. Church DG, Vancil JM, Vasanawala SS. Magnetic resonance imaging for uterine and vaginal anomalies. Curr Opin Obstet Gynecol 2009;21(5):379–89.

31. Marcal L, Nothaft M, Coelho F, et al. Mullerian duct anomalies: MR imaging. Abdom Imaging 2011;36(6):756–64.

32. Dykes TM, Siegel C, Dodson W. Imaging of congenital uterine anomalies: review and self-assessment module. AJR Am J Roentgenol 2007;189(Suppl 3):S1–10.

33. Jaramillo D, Lebowitz RL, Hendren WH. The cloacal malformation: radiologic findings and imaging recommendations. Radiology 1990;177(2):441–8.

34. Blask AR, Sanders RC, Gearhart JP. Obstructed uterovaginal anomalies: demonstration with sonography. Part I. Neonates and infants. Radiology 1991;179(1):79–83.

35. Morcel K, Camborieux L, Guerrier D. Mayer-Rokitansky-Kuster-Hauser (MRKH) syndrome. Orphanet J Rare Dis 2007;2:13.

36. Coley BD. Pediatric gynecologic ultrasound. Ultrasound Clin 2012;7(1):107–21.

37. Troiano RN, McCarthy SM. Mullerian duct anomalies: imaging and clinical issues. Radiology 2004;233(1):19–34.

38. Levine D. Solving the problem pelvic ultrasound with magnetic resonance imaging. Ultrasound Q 2006;22(3):159–68.

39. Ivarsson SA, Nilsson KO, Persson PH. Ultrasonography of the pelvic organs in prepubertal and postpubertal girls. Arch Dis Child 1983;58(5):352–4.

40. Creighton SM, Hall-Craggs MA. Correlation or confusion: the need for accurate terminology when comparing magnetic resonance imaging and clinical assessment of congenital vaginal anomalies. J Pediatr Urol 2012;8(2):177–80.

41. Edwards JE. Anomalies of the derivatives of the aortic arch system. Med Clin North Am 1948;32:925–49.

42. Khati NJ, Frazier AA, Brindle KA. The unicornuate uterus and its variants: clinical presentation, imaging findings, and associated complications. J Ultrasound Med 2012;31(2):319–31.

43. Vallerie AM, Breech LL. Update in Mullerian anomalies: diagnosis, management, and outcomes. Curr Opin Obstet Gynecol 2010;22(5):381–7.

44. Lang IM, Babyn P, Oliver GD. MR imaging of paediatric uterovaginal anomalies. Pediatr Radiol 1999;29(3):163–70.

45. Herbst AL, Ulfelder H, Poskanzer DC. Adenocarcinoma of the vagina. Association of maternal stilbestrol therapy with tumor appearance in young women. N Engl J Med 1971;284(15):878–81.

46. Blask AR, Sanders RC, Rock JA. Obstructed uterovaginal anomalies: demonstration with sonography. Part II. Teenagers. Radiology 1991;179(1):84–8.

47. Chauvin NA, Epelman M, Victoria T, et al. Complex genitourinary abnormalities on fetal MRI: imaging findings and approach to diagnosis. AJR Am J Roentgenol 2012;199(2):W222–31.

48. Berrocal T, López-Pereira P, Arjonilla A, et al. Anomalies of the distal ureter, bladder, and urethra in children: embryologic, radiologic, and pathologic features. Radiographics 2002;22(5):1139–64.

49. Papaioannou G, Koussidis G, Michala L. Magnetic resonance imaging visualization of a vaginal septum. Fertil Steril 2011;96(5):1193–4.

50. Hosseinzadeh K, Heller MT, Houshmand G. Imaging of the female perineum in adults. Radiographics 2012;32(4):E129–68.

51. Jarboe MD, Teitelbaum DH, Dillman JR. Combined 3D rotational fluoroscopic-MRI cloacagram procedure defines luminal and extraluminal pelvic anatomy prior to surgical reconstruction of cloacal and other complex pelvic malformations. Pediatr Surg Int 2012;28(8):757–63.

52. Epelman M, Victoria T, Meyers KE, et al. Postnatal imaging of neonates with prenatally diagnosed genitourinary abnormalities: a practical approach. Pediatr Radiol 2012;42(Suppl 1):S124–41.

53. Huisman T, van der Hoef M, Willi U, et al. Pre- and postnatal imaging of a girl with a cloacal variant. Pediatr Radiol 2006;36(9):991–6.

54. McMullin ND, Hutson JM. Female pseudohermaphroditism in children with cloacal anomalies. Pediatr Surg Int 1991;6(1):56–9.

55. Siegelman ES, Outwater EK, Banner MP, et al. High-resolution MR imaging of the vagina. Radiographics 1997;17(5):1183–203.

56. Kimberley N, Hutson JM, Southwell BR, et al. Vaginal agenesis, the hymen, and associated anomalies. J Pediatr Adolesc Gynecol 2012;25(1):54–8.

57. Saleem SN. MR imaging diagnosis of uterovaginal anomalies: current state of the art. Radiographics 2003;23(5):e13.

58. Gholoum S, Puligandla PS, Hui T, et al. Management and outcome of patients with combined vaginal septum, bifid uterus, and ipsilateral renal agenesis (Herlyn-Werner-Wunderlich syndrome). J Pediatr Surg 2006;41(5):987–92.

59. Hahn WY, Israel GM, Lee VS. MRI of female urethral and periurethral disorders. Am J Roentgenol 2004; 182(3):677–82.

60. Kondi-Pafiti A, Filippidou-Giannopoulou A, Papakonstantinou E, et al. Epidermoid or dermoid cysts of the ovary? Clinicopathological characteristics of 28 cases and a new pathologic classification of an old entity. Eur J Gynaecol Oncol 2012;33(6): 617–9.

61. Eilber KS, Raz S. Benign cystic lesions of the vagina: a literature review. J Urol 2003;170(3): 717–22.

62. Feuerlein S, Pauls S, Juchems MS, et al. Pitfalls in abdominal diffusion-weighted imaging: how predictive is restricted water diffusion for malignancy. AJR Am J Roentgenol 2009;193(4):1070–6.

63. Odibo AO, Turner GW, Borgida AF, et al. Late prenatal ultrasound features of hydrometrocolpos secondary to cloacal anomaly: case reports and review of the literature. Ultrasound Obstet Gynecol 1997;9(6):419–21.

64. Khanna PC, Ponsky T, Zagol B, et al. Sonographic appearance of canal of Nuck hydrocele. Pediatr Radiol 2007;37(6):603–6.

Magnetic Resonance Imaging of Anorectal Malformations

Daniel J. Podberesky, MD[a],*, Alexander J. Towbin, MD[a],
Mohamed A. Eltomey, MD[b], Marc A. Levitt, MD[c]

KEYWORDS

- Anorectal malformation • Cloaca • Cloacal malformation • MR imaging • Children

KEY POINTS

- Anorectal malformation (ARM) comprises a diverse spectrum of congenital malformations of the anus and rectum with an incidence of approximately 1 in 5000 newborns.
- Fetal MR imaging plays an increasingly important role for ARM patients; it helps in providing appropriate parental counseling and enables proper antenatal and postnatal management.
- With the advent of faster imaging sequences and more advanced imaging techniques, MR imaging is increasingly being relied on to aid definitive surgical correction planning.
- MR imaging is increasingly being called on to aid in the evaluation of postoperative complications following the original corrective surgery in ARM patients.
- MR imaging has the potential to serve as an ionizing radiation-free, one-stop shop for the imaging evaluation of ARM patients

INTRODUCTION

Anorectal malformation (ARM) comprises a diverse spectrum of congenital malformations of the anus and rectum. These malformations can range in severity from minor and easily treated with excellent prognosis, such as rectoperineal or rectovestibular fistulae, to those that are complex and difficult to manage with relatively poor prognosis, such as cloacal malformation and caudal regression syndrome. Overall, congenital ARM affects approximately 1 in 5000 newborns, with a slight male predominance.[1] The incidence of cloacal malformations has frequently been reported in the literature as approximately 1 in 40,000 to 50,000 newborns,[2] although the incidence is likely more frequent (approximately 1 in 20,000) because many of these patients were previously erroneously diagnosed with a rectovaginal fistula.[3]

> Anomalies of the gastrointestinal, genitourinary, skeletal, nervous, and cardiovascular systems are frequently associated with ARM.

Associated anomalies are frequently found in patients with congenital ARM. Although all organ systems can be affected, abnormalities of the gastrointestinal, genitourinary, skeletal, nervous, and cardiovascular systems are most common.[4] Anomalies of the gastrointestinal tract outside of

Funding Sources: None.

Conflicts of Interest. Dr D.J. Podberesky: Toshiba of America Medical Systems, Professional Speaker Bureau member; General Electric Healthcare, travel reimbursement; Philips Healthcare, travel reimbursement; Amirsys, royalties. Dr A.J. Towbin: Amirsys, royalties. Dr M.A. Eltomey and Dr M.A. Levitt: None.

[a] Department of Radiology, Cincinnati Children's Hospital Medical Center, University of Cincinnati College of Medicine, 3333 Burnet Avenue, MLC 5031, Cincinnati, OH 45229, USA; [b] Department of Radiology and Medical Imaging, Tanta University, Elbahr Street, Medical Compound, Tanta 31111, Egypt; [c] Department of Surgery, Colorectal Center, Cincinnati Children's Hospital Medical Center, University of Cincinnati College of Medicine, 3333 Burnet Avenue, MLC 2023, Cincinnati, OH 45229, USA

* Corresponding author.

E-mail address: daniel.podberesky@cchmc.org

the primary ARM include esophageal atresia and duodenal atresia. Anomalies of the genitourinary tract include but are not limited to absent, dysplastic, or horseshoe kidney; hypospadias; bifid scrotum; vesicoureteral reflux and hydroureteronephrosis; undescended testes; vaginal abnormalities; and Müllerian structure anomalies. Common skeletal abnormalities include sacral agenesis or dysgenesis, spinal dysraphism, vertebral segmentation and fusion anomalies, and scoliosis. Specific spine abnormalities encountered in ARM patients include tethered spinal cord, meningoceles and myelomeningoceles, intradural lipomas, and diastematomyelia. Cardiovascular anomalies are present in 12% to 22% of ARM patients, with tetralogy of Fallot and ventricular septal defect most commonly encountered.[4]

Three specific associations typically encountered with congenital ARM are the Currarino triad; caudal regression syndrome; and the syndrome of vertebral defects, anorectal anomalies or atresia, cardiac defects, tracheoesophageal fistula, renal anomalies, and limb defects (VACTERL). In 1971, Currarino and colleagues[5] first described the triad of ARM, partial agenesis of the sacrum (typically a sickle-shaped sacrum), and presacral mass (typically a teratoma or anterior meningocele). The triad is inherited in an autosomal dominant pattern secondary to a mutation in the HLXB9 homeobox gene.[6]

Caudal regression syndrome is a rare disorder that affects the lower half of the body to varying degrees, including the lower extremities, low back or spine, genitourinary tract, and gastrointestinal tract, including ARM (typically imperforate anus). Approximately 15% to 25% of cases of caudal regression syndrome occur in children of a diabetic mother.[7]

VACTERL is a nonrandom cluster of a group of congenital anomalies. Typically, at least three malformations are required to be diagnosed with the association. The VACTERL association occurs in approximately 1 in 10,000 to 1 in 40,000 newborns, with approximately 55% to 90% of these patients having an ARM.[8]

Currarino triad = ARM, partial agenesis of the sacrum, and presacral mass.

VACTERL = vertebral defects, anorectal anomalies, cardiac defects, tracheoesophageal fistula, renal anomalies, and limb defects.

As with most complex congenital malformations, imaging has long played a critical role in the evaluation and management of patients with ARM. From the first invertogram radiograph described by Wangensteen and Rice[9] in 1930, to contrast fluoroscopic examinations such as contrast enemas, distal high-pressure colostograms, and voiding cystourethrograms, to cross-sectional modalities of today such as ultrasound, CT, and (most recently) MR imaging, diagnostic imaging helps provide the surgeon with the information needed to correct the malformation. To accomplish a successful postoperative outcome, an accurate preoperative imaging assessment is required. This includes assessment of the level and type of malformation, the presence of a fistula, the developmental state of the sphincter muscle complex, and the presence of associated anomalies. In the postoperative patient, accurate imaging is required for identification of postoperative complications, potential reoperative planning, other associated anomalies that may have initially been inconspicuous, and predicting morbidity and quality of life. MR imaging is ideally suited to fulfill these requirements because of its lack of ionizing radiation, excellent intrinsic contrast resolution, and multiplanar imaging capabilities. Disadvantages of MR imaging in ARM patients include the frequent need for sedation, relative high cost, and relative lack of expertise and access to the technique. Despite these disadvantages, MR imaging is increasingly being used by radiologists in the diagnostic work-up of ARM patients, including in the prenatal state, before definitive surgical repair, and postoperatively.

EMBRYOLOGY, CLASSIFICATION, AND ANATOMY

A basic understanding of the normal and pathologic embryology and anatomy of the anorectum, particularly the sphincter mechanism, is helpful when interpreting MR imaging studies in the ARM patient (**Fig. 1**). The process of normal and abnormal development of the hindgut is not fully understood, although various theories have been offered over the years.[10–15] Cranially, the hindgut is in continuity with the midgut; caudally, it is in direct contact with the ectoderm, thus forming the cloacal membrane. When development progresses, the caudal part of the hindgut, the cloaca, differentiates into two separate organ systems, the urogenital tract and the anorectal tract.[16] Normal anorectal and genitourinary development depends on the normal development of the dorsal cloaca and the cloacal membrane, the latter having a crucial role in the pathogenesis of ARM.[17,18] Cloacal membrane defects are thought to also affect development of the genitourinary system and mesenchymal tissue leading to genital malformation and abnormal pelvic floor and sphincter muscle development.[16]

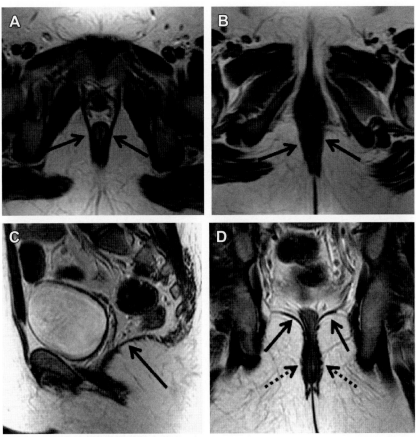

Fig. 1. Fourteen-year-old girl with normal pelvic-sphincter muscle anatomy. (*A*) Axial T2-weighted image at the level of the pubic symphysis showing the innermost fibers of the levator ani muscles surrounding the rectum (*arrows*). (*B*) Axial T1-weighted image at the level of the inferior pubic rami showing the external anal sphincter around the anal canal (*arrows*). (*C*) Paramidline sagittal T2-weighted image shows the normal gently curved levator sling (*arrow*). (*D*) Coronal T2-weighted image shows the levator sling (*solid arrows*) forming the shape of a funnel continuing caudally and seamlessly transitioning into the external sphincter (*dashed arrows*).

The rectum is the terminal end of the colon, beginning anterior to the level of the third sacral vertebra and extending to the anal canal. The anal canal extends from the anorectal junction to the anal verge.[19] In normal individuals, the muscle groups of the anal sphincter mechanism include the voluntary, striated muscles of the external sphincter and the levator musculature, and the involuntary, smooth muscle internal sphincter. The levator ani muscle is a series of striated muscle groups composed of ischiococcygeus, iliococcygeus, pubococcygeus, and puborectalis. These muscles are continuous with each other. The levator ani muscles extend from the pubic bone, the lowest portion of the sacrum, and the middle of the pelvis downward and medial to join with the external sphincter. The confluence of muscles forms a funneled appearance on coronal imaging planes (see **Fig. 1D**). For all practical purposes, no anatomic distinction between the individual

muscles of the levator ani or the external anal sphincter can be routinely discerned by MR imaging and their distinction is of no clinical value in the setting of ARM correction. During perineal reconstruction, the surgeon places the mobilized rectum within this muscular funnel, ensuring its correct trajectory through the levator ani, and tacks it to the posterior edge of the muscle complex to end at the neoanus.[1]

> No anatomic distinction between the individual muscles of the levator ani or the external anal sphincter can be routinely discerned by MR imaging, and their distinction is of no clinical value in the setting of ARM correction.

Traditionally, ARM patients were classified into high, intermediate, and low malformations.[20] However, this classification system has been found to be arbitrary and somewhat inaccurate.[1] A more practical classification scheme is one that groups ARMs that share common diagnostic, therapeutic, and prognostic features as proposed by Levitt and Peña[1] (**Table 1**).

MR IMAGING IN THE PRENATAL PERIOD

The ability to identify and characterize ARM on prenatal imaging is important because it allows for appropriate parental counseling, helps to determine the delivery site and plan, and helps the surgeon to plan antenatal and postnatal management.[21,22] Diagnosing ARM via prenatal ultrasound is challenging. It can be suggested when a fluid-filled, distended rectum is seen in conjunction with a cystic pelvic structure in a female fetus.[22] Even when this combination is seen, typically a wide differential diagnosis must be offered including cystic sacrococcygeal teratoma, anterior meningocele or myelomeningocele, and megacystis-microcolon.

Fetal MR imaging has the potential to diagnose ARM more accurately and with increased confidence relative to ultrasound.[21–23] As fetal MR imaging availability and expertise becomes more widespread, it will assuredly continue to play an increasing role in the evaluation of suspected ARMs detected during screening prenatal ultrasound.

What the Referring Physician Needs to Know

The referring physician needs to know

- Presence of a cystic pelvis mass in a female fetus suggesting a cloacal malformation
- Presence of signs indicating mixture of urine and meconium

Table 1
Classification of ARM

Male	Female
Rectovesical (bladder neck) fistula	Rectoperineal fistula
Rectourethral (prostatic) fistula	Rectovestibular fistula
Rectourethral (bulbar) fistula	Cloaca with short common channel (<3 cm)
Rectoperineal fistula	Cloaca with long common channel (>3 cm)
Imperforate anus without fistula	Imperforate anus without fistula
Rectal atresia	Rectal atresia

Adapted from Levitt MA, Peña A. Anorectal malformations. Orphanet J Rare Dis 2007;2:33.

- Presence of associated anomalies of the spine, gastrointestinal, genitourinary, and skeletal systems

Imaging Protocol

Fetal MR imaging for ARM is typically performed in the third trimester of pregnancy. It is important that it not be performed before 20 weeks gestational age because, before this time, the distribution of meconium cannot be accurately defined within the colon and rectum.[21] Fetal MR imaging studies most commonly are performed in a 1.5-T scanner using a phased-array body coil. Neither fetal nor maternal sedation are required. The following sequences are typically obtained in all three planes (relative to the fetus) without fat saturation: (1) T2-weighted single-shot fast spin-echo, (2) two-dimensional (2D) balanced steady-state free precession (bSSFP), and (3) T1-weighted fast gradient recalled echo.

Fetal MR imaging in ARM patients should be performed after approximately 20 weeks gestation. Before this time, abnormal meconium distribution cannot be accurately defined.

Imaging Findings

The normal appearance of the distal colon and rectal cul-de-sac on fetal MR imaging (**Fig. 2**) has been well described.[24,25] The rectum should always be identifiable; it should be closely apposed to the bladder regardless of gender, and it should extend at least 10 mm below the bladder neck (increases from 10 to 23 mm with increasing gestation age after 20 weeks).[21,24] The intraluminal contents of the distal colon and rectum should be hypointense on T2-weighted images, intermediate signal intensity on bSSFP images, and hyperintense on T1-weighted images.[21,24] The normal maximum distal colon diameter increases with gestational age from approximately 8 mm at 24 weeks to approximately 16 to 18 mm by 35 to 38 weeks.[24]

Normal fetal MR imaging features of the rectum include close apposition to the bladder, extension at least 10 mm below the bladder neck, and meconium signal intensity characteristics.

Prenatal gastrointestinal MR imaging findings that have been described with ARM include dilation of the distal colon and rectum (**Fig. 3**A), abnormal

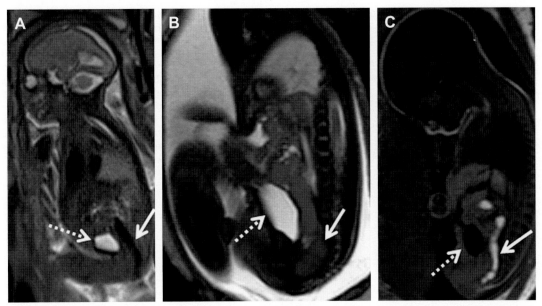

Fig. 2. Prenatal MR images in three separate fetuses showing the normal rectum after 20 weeks gestation. The rectum (*arrows*) is closely apposed to the bladder (*dashed arrows*) and extends at least 10 mm below the bladder neck. The intraluminal signal within the rectum should be (*A*) hypointense on T2-weighted images (*A*), intermediate signal intensity on balanced steady-state free precession images (*B*), and hyperintense on T1-weighted images (*C*).

fluid (hyperintense on T2-weighted images) signal within the distal colon and rectum when a fistula is present (see **Fig. 3**A), normal signal within the distal colon and rectum when a fistula is not present, separation of the rectum from the posterior bladder wall (see **Fig. 3**B), abnormally high location of the rectum relative to the bladder base (**Fig. 4**), and enterolithiasis (**Fig. 5**) as the result of long-term mixture of urine and meconium.[21,22,24] Abnormalities of the genitourinary system are

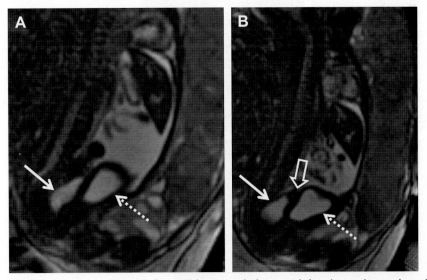

Fig. 3. Prenatal MR imaging on a 26-week fetus with prenatal ultrasound showing ascites and possible bladder outlet obstruction. The rectum is dilated and shows abnormal hyperintense fluid signal on a sagittal T2-weighted image (*A*), and there is slight separation (*open arrow*) of the rectum from the posterior bladder wall on a slightly more lateral sagittal T2-weighted image (*B*). Note also the presence of ascites and bladder wall thickening on both images. The patient was born with a cloacal malformation. Rectum (*solid arrows*), bladder (*dashed arrows*).

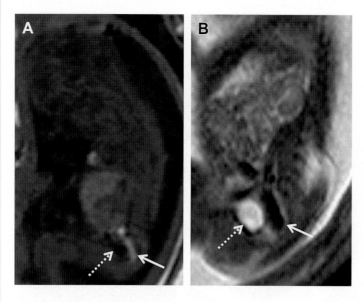

Fig. 4. Prenatal MR imaging on a 23-week fetus with a myelomeningocele (incompletely shown on these images) and an ARM. The rectum should extend greater than 10 mm caudal to the base of the bladder. In this patient, the rectum only extended approximately 4 mm caudal to the base of the bladder as seen on the sagittal T1-weighted (*A*) and sagittal T2-weighted images (*B*). Rectum (*solid arrows*), bladder (*dashed arrows*).

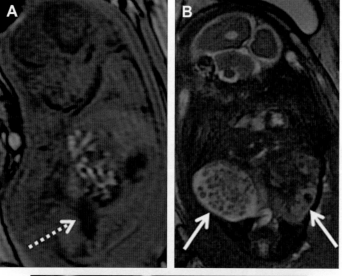

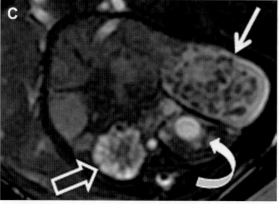

Fig. 5. Prenatal MR imaging on a 27-week fetus with multiple congenital abnormalities including an ARM with a rectourinary fistula. The sagittal T1-weighted image (*A*) shows absence of the normal hyperintense meconium-filled rectum posterior to the bladder (*dashed arrow*). The coronal T2-weighted image (*B*) demonstrates multiple dilated loops of bowel with numerous enteroliths (*solid arrows*). The axial balanced steady-state free precession image (*C*) demonstrates cystic dysplasia of the left kidney (*open arrow*), hydronephrosis of the right kidney (*curved arrow*), and again shows the dilated bowel loops with numerous enteroliths (*solid arrow*). Note the presence of oligohydramnios.

frequently encountered on prenatal MR images in patients with suspected ARM. These abnormalities include (1) abnormal bladder shape and size; (2) abnormal bladder contents; (3) bladder wall thickening; (4) renal anomalies such as agenesis, hydroureteronephrosis (see **Fig. 5**C; **Fig. 6**A), cystic dysplasia (see **Fig. 5**C), and multicystic dysplastic kidney; (5) hydrocolpos (see **Fig. 6**B); (6) presence of a common channel in cloaca patients; and (7) abnormal external genitalia.[21,24] Close attention should be paid to potential abnormalities outside of the gastrointestinal and genitourinary systems as well. In two out of four ARM patients identified by prenatal MR imaging by Veyrac and colleagues,[22] and in one out of six ARM patients identified by Calvo-Garcia and colleagues,[21] VACTERL syndrome features were present. Additionally, oligohydramnios may frequently be present on prenatal MR images in ARM patients (see **Fig. 6**B).[21]

MR IMAGING BEFORE DEFINITIVE SURGICAL CORRECTION

The postnatal management of children with ARM is predicated on accurate determination of the level and type of malformation as well as the presence and type of fistula.[26] Sometimes, in patients with an imperforate anus and a rectoperineal or rectovestibular fistula, a primary perineal anoplasty can be performed. In most other malformation types, a diverting colostomy is performed in the first few days of life. This is followed by definitive surgical repair (posterior sagittal anorectoplasty

[PSARP] with or without laparoscopy depending on the height of the rectum) later in infancy.

Imaging of the newborn with ARM before surgical correction historically relied on invertograms or cross-table lateral radiographs to determine the height of the rectal air if no fistula was evident clinically. Voiding cystourethrograms, ultrasound of the kidneys or bladder and spine, and MR imaging of the spine are mainstays in the imaging work-up of ARM patients.[26–28] High-pressure distal colostogram remains the gold-standard imaging study for determining the precise anatomy of the distal rectum. The hydrostatic pressure used fully distends the distal rectum by overcoming the compression by the pelvic muscles, thus demonstrating the anatomy accurately and helping the surgeon plan the repair.[26–28] These imaging examinations, in combination with meticulous clinical assessment and endoscopic evaluation, provide adequate information to plan the operative approach and technique.

The use of preoperative pelvic MR imaging was traditionally reserved for complex ARM or cases in which radiographic, fluoroscopic, and/or ultrasonographic findings were inconclusive. In 1988, Sato and colleagues[29] first reported the MR imaging findings on seven preoperative ARM patients, and correctly identified the level of rectal atresia. Since that time, there have been other infrequent reports of the use of MR imaging in preoperative ARM patients.[26,27,30–33] However, with the advent of faster imaging sequences and more advanced imaging techniques, MR imaging is more

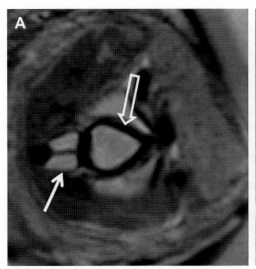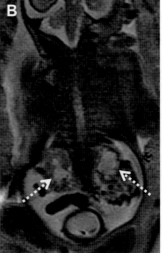

Fig. 6. Prenatal MR imaging images from a 26-week fetus with a cloacal malformation variant confirmed postnatally. Genitourinary anomalies include a septate vagina with hydrocolpos (*solid arrow*) and thick-walled bladder (*open arrow*) (*A*), as well as bilateral mild-to-moderate hydronephrosis (*dashed arrows*) (*B*). Note the presence of ascites and oligohydramnios.

frequently being relied on to aid in surgical planning. Techniques such as three-dimensional (3D) MR image reconstruction,[34] MR cloacagram-genitography,[35,36] and intraoperative MR-guided surgery[37] have been described in the literature. Even though Aslam and colleagues[32] concluded that "MRI has no role as a primary investigation in patients with high ARA [anorectal anomalies]," the authors believe that the advances in MR imaging technology, innovative MR imaging protocols, refinements in surgical techniques, and better understanding of surgical anatomy and clinical outcomes over the past 15 years since that report will result in the continued increase in the use of MR imaging before definitive surgical correction.

> MR genitography-cloacography is an MR imaging examination of the pelvis in which dilute gadolinium is instilled into the bladder, vagina, and distal colon rectum (depending on anatomy) to better depict the complex anatomy in ARM patients.

What the Referring Physician Needs to Know

The referring physician needs know

- Distal most extent of the fully distended rectum
- Presence and location of fistula
- Distance from the end of the rectum to the anal dimple
- Presence of a presacral mass and other associated congenital anomalies

Imaging Protocol

The ability of 3D reconstructions from preoperative standard MR images to improve understanding of the complex anatomic relationships in ARM patients was first shown in a rudimentary fashion by Ueno and colleagues[38] in 1995, and later by Tang and colleagues[34] using modern MR imaging equipment and sequences. In 2007, Baughman and colleagues,[36] taking advantage of these 3D reconstruction techniques, first described what they termed MR genitography. They concluded that the studies provided excellent anatomic detail and complemented the information obtained by standard pelvic MR imaging and endoscopy in complex ARM patients. Their protocol was performed on a 1.5 T magnet and consisted of routine multiplanar high-resolution T1-weighted and T2-weighted sequences through the pelvis, followed by a 3D T1-weighted spoiled gradient recalled echo (SPGR) sequence with fat saturation

acquired during active hand-instillation of dilute gadolinium through balloon catheters via the common channel, mucous fistula, and cutaneous vesicostomy (when present). The gadolinium was diluted with normal saline to a ratio of between 1:750 and 1:1000. Maximum intensity projection (MIP) and 3D volume-rendered reconstructions were performed from the SPGR data set. Coronal screening imaging of the kidneys was also performed. The investigators described a total scanning duration of approximately 30 minutes, and a total patient and scan preparation time of 30 to 60 minutes.

In 2012, Jarboe and colleagues[35] described a similar technique in which they performed MR imaging in combination with 3D rotational fluoroscopy in the same anesthetic setting. The investigators concluded that the combined fluoroscopic and MR imaging cloacagram procedure provided exceptional anatomic definition and aided with surgical planning.[35] Their protocol was performed on a 3 T magnet, and consisted of multiplanar routine T1-weighted and T2-weighted sequences, followed by a 3D T1-weighted SPGR sequence with fat saturation performed after the instillation of a dilute gadolinium solution through balloon catheters and non–balloon catheters via combinations of the mucous fistula, common channel, urinary bladder, vagina, and rectum (depending on specific patient anatomy). Because these studies were performed in combination with a fluoroscopic evaluation of the ARM, the gadolinium was diluted with iodinated contrast in a 1:200 ratio. A vitamin E capsule was placed at the site where the anus should be located to aid in MR image interpretation. 3D volume-rendered and MIP reconstructions were then created from the SPGR data set. At Cincinnati Children's Hospital Medical Center, these studies are currently performed in a similar fashion but with a more dilute gadolinium concentration of 1:600 because this concentration results in optimal contrast signal intensity. In addition, a coronal fast inversion recovery sequence is added to screen the kidneys. In many cases, screening imaging of the spine is also performed at this same sitting.

Raschbaum and colleagues[37] described the innovative use of intraoperative MR imaging in the performance of laparoscopically-assisted anorectoplasty (LAARP) in three patients with ARM, though the technique has not been widely adopted. One limitation of LAARP is the inability to visualize the narrow path of the vertical muscle fiber complex between the pelvic floor and perineal parasagittal muscle fibers, and the resultant potential for a noncentered pull-through of the rectum to the perineum. By combining intraoperative MR imaging with serial advancement of an MR-compatible needle through the central portion of the vertical muscle fiber complex (as determined with direct muscle stimulation) until the pelvic floor is penetrated, the surgeon is able to identify the needle in the peritoneal cavity and use it to ensure a centered pull-through (**Fig. 7**).

Imaging Findings

With standard multiplanar T1-weighted and T2-weighted images, the level of the ARM can be surmised, but it is critical that the radiologist recognize that without fluid distention, the distal most extent of the rectum may be underestimated. In the past, when the rectum ended above the pubococcygeus plane (an imaginary plane between the symphysis pubis and the coccyx) the malformation was regarded as a high anorectal anomaly. Although some studies have used objective measurements of the sphincteric and levator sling muscles to describe their overall quality, subjective assessment on MR imaging (good, moderate, or poor) is typically adequate.[37]

Detection and characterization of the fistula is of utmost importance for surgical correction. There

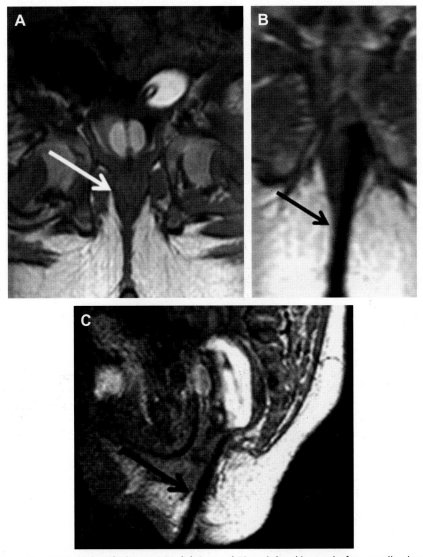

Fig. 7. Intraoperative MR imaging during LAARP. (*A*) Coronal T2-weighted image before needle placement shows the very narrow vertical muscle fiber complex (*white arrow*) in this patient with ARM. (*B*) Coronal and (*C*) sagittal T2-weighted images show the MR compatible needle (*black arrows*) being placed through the vertical muscle fiber complex into the peritoneal cavity to a point where the surgeon can see the needle laparoscopically. (*Courtesy of* Drs Grattan-Smith, Jones, and Raschbaum, Children's Healthcare of Atlanta at Scottish Rite, Atlanta, GA.)

has been varying success depicting the fistula in male ARM patients by standard MR imaging in the literature.[26,27,30,31] With the recent advent of MR cloacagram-genitography including the injection of dilute gadolinium, depiction and characterization of the fistula, if present, is readily achievable (**Figs. 8A and 9**).[35,36] Even in the absence of a fistula, these novel techniques can depict the level of rectal atresia in a distended state (see **Figs. 8B and 9**), allow for measurement of the common channel length (see **Fig. 8C; Fig. 10A, B**), demonstrate the complex anatomic relationships between the pelvic organs (see **Figs. 8 and 10; Fig. 11**), and can occasionally demonstrate vesicoureteral reflux and ectopic ureters (see **Fig. 11**).

In addition to specifically characterizing the ARM itself, MR imaging has the capability of identifying and characterizing the myriad of associated anomalies that can be found in patients with ARM,

particularly those of the skeletal system, spinal cord and surrounding structures, and genitourinary system. The overall incidence of associated anomalies in ARM patients is approximately 50%, occurring twice as often in patients with high malformations.[26] Although many of these anomalies can be identified, and even characterized, by other imaging modalities such as radiography, fluoroscopy, and ultrasound, the ability to fully demonstrate these anomalies in one imaging session without ionizing radiation is a significant advantage of MR imaging in the preoperative setting.

Spinal cord anomalies have been reported to be present in 14% to 57% of ARM patients, and significant vertebral anomalies have been reported in 54%.[39] The most frequently reported associated spinal anomaly is the tethered cord occurring in 10% to 52% of patients, with spinal lipomas and

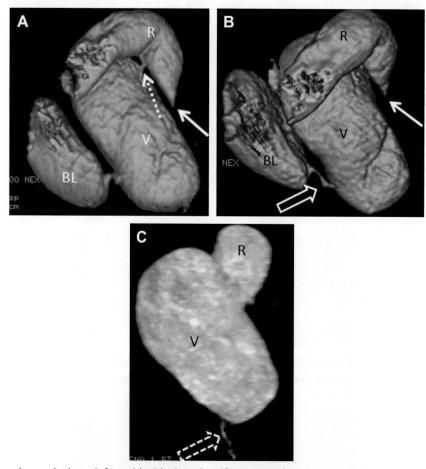

Fig. 8. MR genitography in an infant girl with cloacal malformation after diverting colostomy and before definitive surgical correction. Dilute gadolinium chelate contrast material was instilled via the mucous fistula and the common channel. 3D T1-weighted volume-rendered (*A, B*), and MIP (*C*) reconstructions were performed. There is a high rectal atresia (*solid arrows*) with a rectovaginal fistula (*dashed arrow*). The urethra (*open solid arrow*) is compressed by the distended vagina. The common channel (*open dashed arrow*) is well demonstrated. BL, bladder, R, rectum, V, vagina.

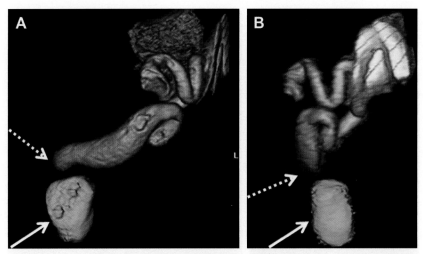

Fig. 9. MR genitography in a toddler girl with cloacal malformation after colostomy and before definitive surgical correction. Dilute gadolinium chelate contrast material was instilled via the mucous fistula and the common channel. 3D T1-weighted volume-rendered reconstructions in coronal (*A*) and sagittal (*B*) planes demonstrate no fistula between the rectum and the bladder (*solid arrows*), and clearly depict the level of the high rectal atresia (*dashed arrows*).

meningoceles commonly encountered.[39] A low-lying conus is typically defined as a conus medullaris terminating at or below the level of the L2/3 disc space (**Fig. 12**).[39] Early identification of a tethered cord before neurologic deterioration is important because surgical correction is generally advocated. A truncated or blunted spinal cord is typically seen in patients with caudal regression syndrome, a disorder composed of a spectrum of anomalies involving the lower extremities, low back or spine, genitourinary tract, and gastrointestinal tract. Although the spine anomaly in these patients is not surgically correctable, early identification can aid in management and prognosis in these patients (**Fig. 13**).[26]

> Tethered spinal cord is the most frequently reported spine anomaly associated with ARM.

Sacral abnormalities and associated presacral masses are seen in up to 50% of patients with ARM.[40] Sacral anomalies include hemisacrum or scimitar sacrum, asymmetric sacrum, posterior protruding sacrum and sacral or coccyx agenesis. In patients with an ARM, the presence of a sacral anomaly should lead to a high suspicion for a presacral mass. Sacrococcygeal teratomas (**Fig. 14**) and anterior meningoceles (**Fig. 15**) are the most frequently encountered presacral masses in ARM patients at Cincinnati Children's Hospital Medical Center. The association of sacrococcygeal teratoma with ARM has long been recognized and reported in the medical literature.[41] A foreshortened

sacrum is also a predictor of future bowel control because it is associated with poorly developed muscles and nerves of the pelvis.[1]

Sacrococcygeal teratoma is the most common solid tumor in neonates and approximately 60% are benign.[42] These tumors have typically been classified according to the Altman classification system: type I, predominantly external masses with a small presacral component; type II, external masses with a large intrapelvic component; type III, external masses with pelvic and abdominal components; and type IV, internal masses with pelvic and abdominal components.[43] The majority (~50%) of these tumors are type 1 lesions.[43] Type IV lesions are most likely to be malignant, although the other three types can be malignant.[43] Because these tumors can contain fluid, fat, calcification, and soft tissue, their imaging characteristics are varied. On MR imaging, the cystic areas will follow fluid signal on T1-weighted and T2-weighted sequences, the fat components will be hyperintense on T1-weighted images, and the calcifications will be hypointense on all sequences. The presence of a predominant solid component, hemorrhage, necrosis, distant metastases, or local invasion of adjacent structures suggest malignancy.[42] The coccyx is always involved with sacrococcygeal teratoma and is, therefore, surgically resected with the tumor.[42] When a presacral mass is encountered, it is critically important for the radiologist to recognize and report any potential spine involvement because, if present, neurosurgical assistance will be required by the pediatric surgeon during excision.

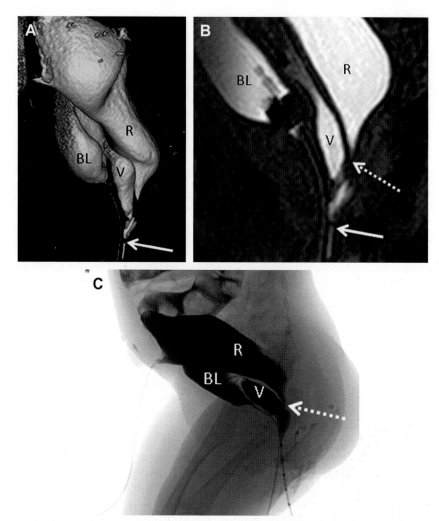

Fig. 10. MR genitography in a toddler girl with cloacal malformation after colostomy and before definitive surgical correction. Dilute gadolinium chelate contrast material was instilled via the mucous fistula and the common channel. (*A*) 3D T1-weighted volume-rendered reconstruction demonstrates the relationship between the bladder, vagina, and rectum and the common channel (*solid arrow*). (*B*) Midline sagittal T1-weighted MR image demonstrates the common channel (*solid arrow*) and the rectovaginal fistula (*dashed arrow*). (*C*) Corresponding fluoroscopic cloacagram shows similar findings to the MR imaging. BL, bladder, R, rectum, V, vagina. The *dashed arrow* indicates the rectovaginal fistula. (*Courtesy of* Dr Jonathan Dillman, University of Michigan Health System, Department of Radiology, C.S. Mott Children's Hospital, Section of Pediatric Radiology, Ann Arbor, MI.)

> Sacral abnormalities and associated presacral masses are seen in up to 50% of ARM patients.

Anterior meningoceles are another relatively commonly encountered presacral mass in ARM patients. These lesions result from herniation of the meninges and cerebrospinal fluid from the distal thecal sac through an anterior sacral defect. MR imaging is the modality of choice in evaluation of these lesions due to its multiplanar capability, and excellent depiction of the hernia sac, bony defects, and any nerve root or fat involvement.[42] Large meningoceles may cause mass effect on adjacent bowel, rectum, and bladder. Anterior meningoceles may be seen as part of the Currarino triad, a syndrome consisting of an ARM, partial agenesis of the sacrum (typically a sickle shaped sacrum), and a presacral mass.[6] The presacral mass in Currarino triad is typically either an anterior meningocele or a teratoma, although dermoid cysts, hamartomas, and enteric duplication cysts have been reported.[42] MR imaging is important in the preoperative evaluation of these patients because it exquisitely depicts the complex anomalies encountered (**Fig. 16**).

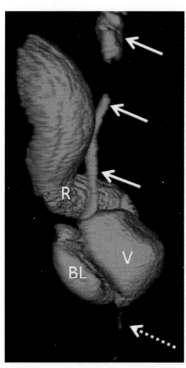

Fig. 11. MR genitography in a toddler girl with cloacal malformation after colostomy and before definitive surgical correction. Dilute gadolinium chelate contrast material was instilled via the mucous fistula and the common channel. 3D T1-weighted volume-rendered reconstruction demonstrates the distended vagina and its relationship to the bladder, vesicoureteral reflux (*solid arrows*), and the common channel (*dashed arrow*). BL, bladder, R, rectum, V, vagina.

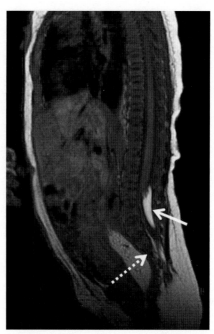

Fig. 12. Two-day-old boy with imperforate anus. Midline sagittal T1-weighted MR image demonstrates a low-lying spinal cord with an intradural lipoma (*solid arrow*). There is also sacral dysgenesis (*dashed arrow*).

Associated anomalies of the urinary system are found in approximately 30% to 40% of ARM patients.[44] These urinary system anomalies occur with much higher prevalence in patients with high ARM, but can also be seen in those with low malformations.[44] Frequently encountered congenital urinary system anomalies include absent, hypoplastic, or dysplastic kidney, horseshoe kidney, renal ectopia (see **Fig. 15**C), vesicoureteral reflux, and megaureter.[26,44] Many of these anomalies can be readily identified during preoperative MR imaging; their identification is critical because the possible resultant poor renal function is a frequent cause of morbidity and mortality in ARM patients.[45]

Duplication of the urinary bladder, which results from early embryologic duplication of the hindgut, is a rare anomaly that can be encountered in ARM patients and excellently depicted by MR imaging (**Fig. 17**).[46] Bladder duplication most frequently occurs in the sagittal plane, with two side-by-side bladders, but can also occur in the coronal plane, with the bladders resting one in front of the other.[47] Typically, each bladder will receive

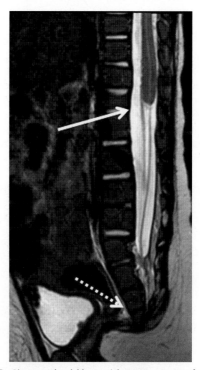

Fig. 13. Six-month-old boy with ARM as part of caudal regression syndrome. Midline sagittal T2-weighted MR image demonstrates the typical truncated or blunted distal spinal cord (*solid arrow*) seen in these patients. There is also sacral dysgenesis (*dashed arrow*).

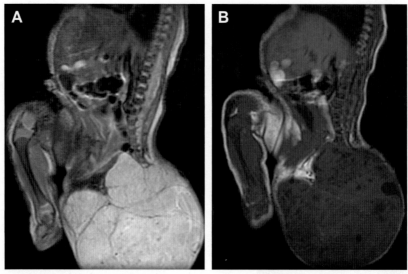

Fig. 14. One-day-old patient with ARM. Midline sagittal (*A*) T2-weighted inversion recovery and (*B*) T1-weighted MR images demonstrate a large presacral mass with a predominant external component and a small presacral component, consistent with a type 1 sacrococcygeal teratoma.

the ipsilateral ureter and is drained by its own urethra.[47] In addition to congenital urinary system anomalies, MR imaging can identify abnormalities associated with chronic neurovesical dysfunction, such as overdistended, thickened, and trabeculated urinary bladder wall.

Genital anomalies are frequently associated with ARM.[26,44] In male ARM patients, up to 52% will have abnormalities of their genitalia including undescended testes, bifid scrotum, hypospadias, epispadias, penile duplication, and penoscrotal transposition.[48,49] Cryptorchidism occurs in 10% to 40% of male ARM patients.[48,49] MR imaging is more accurate than ultrasound in detecting undescended testes, with a reported sensitivity and specificity of 96% and 100% for MR imaging,

compared with 45% and 78%, respectively, for ultrasound.[50,51] A combination of T1-weighted, T2-weighted, and postgadolinium T1-weighted images can be used to identify undescended testes. Coverage should extend from the level of the kidneys through the perineum. Coronal planes should be included because they are the best plane for detecting undescended testes.[52] On imaging, undescended testes are typically homogeneously hypointense on T1-weighted images and hyperintense on T2-weighted imaging, though their appearance may be more heterogeneous if they are ischemic or infarcted (**Fig. 18**).

Penoscrotal transposition is a rare anomaly of the external genitalia that can be seen in association with ARM. In this disorder, the scrotum is

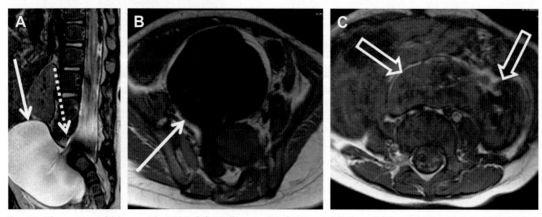

Fig. 15. Three-year-old boy with ARM. (*A*) Midline sagittal T2-weighted and (*B*) axial T1-weighted MR images demonstrate a large anterior meningocele (*solid arrow*) herniating through an anterior sacral defect (*dashed arrow*). (*C*) Axial T1-weighted MR image in this same patient showed crossed-fused renal ectopia (*open arrows*).

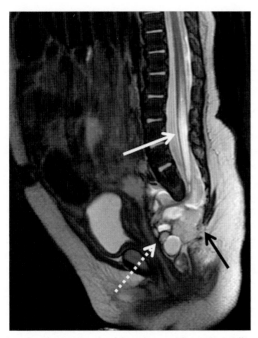

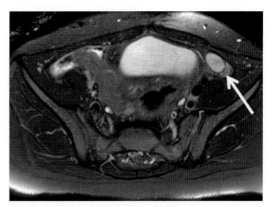

Fig. 18. Two-year-old boy ARM patient with no palpable left testis in the scrotum. Axial fat-suppressed T2-weighted MR image demonstrates a well-circumscribed, oval, homogeneously hyperintense structure in the left hemipelvis consistent with an undescended testis (*solid arrow*).

Fig. 16. Three-month-old patient with ARM. Midline sagittal T2-weighted MR image demonstrates a tethered spinal cord (*solid white arrow*), terminal myelocystocele protruding through a sacral defect (*solid black arrow*), and a presacral teratoma (*dashed arrow*). The combination of ARM, with a sacral defect and a presacral mass forms the Currarino triad.

examinations, including fetal MR imaging examinations,[54] and should be recognized by the radiologist (**Fig. 19**).

In female ARM patients, approximately 30% to 45% will have associated Müllerian abnormalities.[55–57] The paired Müllerian ducts typically undergo fusion and resorption in utero and give rise to the uterus, fallopian tubes, cervix, and upper two-thirds of the vagina.[47] In female patients with

malpositioned superior to the penis. The scrotum may entirely cover the penis (termed complete transposition) or the scrotum may not fuse completely above the penis (termed incomplete transposition).[53] Although typically easily identified on physical examination, this entity can be encountered when reviewing ARM MR imaging

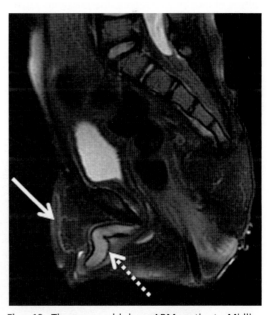

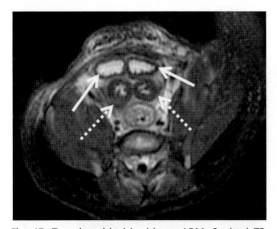

Fig. 17. Two-day-old girl with an ARM. Sagittal T2-weighted MR image with fat suppression demonstrates sagittal duplication of the urinary bladder (*solid arrows*). Two uterine horns (*dashed arrows*) are also noted as part of didelphys morphology.

Fig. 19. Three-year-old boy ARM patient. Midline sagittal fat-suppressed T2-weighted MR image demonstrates penoscrotal transposition. Note the scrotum (*solid arrow*) located superior to the corpora of the penis (*dashed arrow*). The testes are not seen on this image, but were located in the scrotum.

an ARM, this process can be disrupted, resulting in a spectrum of abnormalities that can ultimately result in hydrometrocolpos, amenorrhea, infertility, obstetric complications, and endometriosis.[58] Due to its noninvasive nature, multiplanar capabilities, high-contrast resolution, and lack of ionizing radiation, MR imaging is ideally suited for evaluation of Müllerian abnormalities. A detailed discussion of the classification of Müllerian anomalies is beyond the scope of this article; the reader is referred to several excellent articles.[58,59] Radiologists should be familiar with some of the more common anomalies of the female genital tract that are commonly encountered in ARM patients, including hydrocolpos, uterine didelphys, and bicornuate uterus.

Hydrocolpos should be suspected when there is a cystic mass located posterior to the urinary bladder in a female patient with an ARM (**Fig. 20**). The hydrocolpos can compress the trigone of the bladder and result in hydroureteronephrosis. If there is a vaginal septum present, hydrocolpos can be seen in one or both hemivaginas potentially leading to unilateral or bilateral hydroureteronephrosis. Early identification allows for decompression of the urinary system by drainage of the hydrocolpos, which decreases the risk of associated renal damage and infection.[60]

Complete failure of Müllerian duct fusion results in uterine didelphys. Each Müllerian duct develops into a uterine horn and cervix. In about three-fourths of didelphys patients, the proximal vagina will also be duplicated, with a transverse vaginal septum.[58] On MR imaging examinations, two uterine horns and two separate cervices will be encountered. If a vaginal septum is present, hydrocolpos may also be seen (**Fig. 21**). Efforts should be made to evaluate the kidneys at the same MR imaging sitting because there is a high incidence of renal anomalies in these patients.[58]

> Genitourinary anomalies are frequently found in ARM patients and consist of a spectrum of abnormalities.

POSTOPERATIVE MR IMAGING

MR imaging is being used with increasing frequency to aid in the evaluation of postoperative complications following the original corrective surgery in ARM patients.[26,27,40] Despite significant advances in surgical techniques, particularly the advent of the PSARP procedure, technical complications are not uncommon and often necessitate reoperation to correct issues such as persistent fistulae, mislocated rectum, posterior urethral diverticulum (PUD), rectal stricture, and persistent urogenital sinus. MR imaging is an ideal imaging modality to answer the clinical questions most important to the caring surgeon to help determine if reoperation is necessary and, if so, to plan surgical technique.

What the Referring Physician Needs to Know

The referring physician needs to know

- Position and trajectory of the rectum relative to the levator sling-sphincter complex
- Quality and shape of the pelvic musculature
- Presence of interposed mesenteric fat with the pulled-through rectum indicating that the original rectum was resected and the sigmoid colon was pulled-through instead
- Presence of PUD in males representing the original distal rectum attached to the urinary tract
- Presence of an initially missed presacral mass

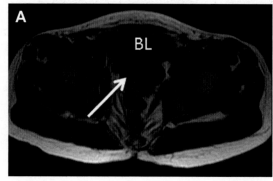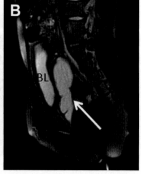

Fig. 20. Three-year-old girl with ARM. (*A*) Axial T1-weighted MR image demonstrates an oval, well-circumscribed, homogeneously hypointense mass (*arrow*) posterior to the bladder. (*B*) Midline sagittal T2-weighted image demonstrates a homogeneously hyperintense mass (*arrow*) posterior the bladder. The findings are consistent with hydrocolpos. BL, bladder.

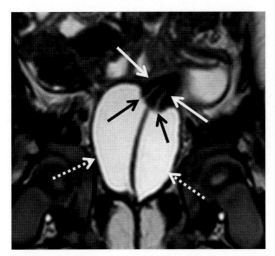

Fig. 21. Six-month-old girl with ARM. Coronal T2-weighted image demonstrates two uterine horns (*solid white arrows*) and cervices, (*solid black arrows*), consistent with uterine didelphys, as well as two obstructed vaginas with hydrocolpos (*dashed arrows*).

- Presence of initially missed associated spinal, skeletal, and genitourinary anomalies
- Presence of a persistent rectourethral fistula

Imaging Protocol

Postoperative ARM MR imaging examinations can be performed on either a 1.5 T or 3 T MR imaging system. At Cincinnati Children's Hospital Medical Center, a cardiac coil is typically used and the patient is imaged in supine position with the field-of-view optimized for the patient's size. Most examinations require sedation and appropriate fasting. To facilitate easier identification of the rectum, a 20 to 24 French Foley catheter is placed into the rectum without inflating the balloon. The urinary bladder is not typically catheterized. The protocol (**Table 2**) consists of multiplanar T1-weighted and T2-weighted images with and without fat suppression designed to optimally display the postoperative anatomy and potential complications present in postoperative ARM patients. The sequences without fat suppression are useful for highlighting the low signal intensity muscle and bowel wall against the higher signal intensity fat and mucosa. Fat-suppressed sequences better distinguish cystic structures (such as PUD and cystic components of teratomas) from surrounding suppressed fat. Postcontrast imaging is reserved for those cases in which a mass or inflammatory process is identified on the precontrast imaging.

Imaging Findings

Appropriate placement of the rectal pull-through within the levator sling and sphincter mechanism during ARM surgical correction is critical for optimal postoperative bowel continence.[29] The position and trajectory of the pulled-through rectum is best evaluated on axial and oblique coronal planes. Anterior or lateral misplacement of the pull-through relative to the sphincter complex or levator sling are the most commonly reported deviations (**Fig. 22**).[26,29,40,61,62] A pull-through with attached mesenteric fat indicates that the rectum was resected at the original surgery and the sigmoid colon was pulled-through as the neorectum. This loss of rectal reservoir is a recognized cause of postoperative fecal incontinence in ARM patients.[29,40] This fat is easily appreciated on axial or coronal T1-weighted and non–fat-suppressed T2-weighted images (**Fig. 23**).

Table 2
Postoperative ARM MR imaging protocol at Cincinnati Children's Hospital Medical Center (1.5 T)

Sequence	Plane	TE	TR	Slice Thickness/Gap (mm)	Matrix	NEX
SE T1	Coronal	Min	400	4/1	256 × 192	2
FSE T2	Axial	85	3000	4/1	320 × 256	2
FSE T2	Sagittal	85	3000	4/1	256 × 192	2
FSE T2 FS	Axial	85	3000	4/1	256 × 192	2
FSE T2 FS	Sagittal	85	3000	4/1	256 × 192	2
FSE T2	Coronal	85	3000	4/1	256 × 192	2
FSE T2	Coronal oblique to rectum (in males)	85	3000	4/1	256 × 192	2
FSE T2	Coronal oblique to uterus (in females)	85	3000	4/1	256 × 192	2

Abbreviations: FS, fat suppression; FSE, fast spin echo; NEX, number of excitations; SE, spin echo; TE, echo time; TR, repetition time.

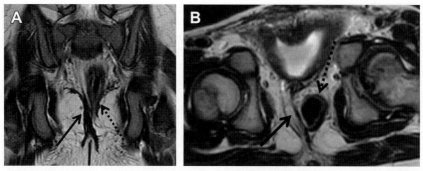

Fig. 22. Misplacement of rectal pull-through on postoperative ARM MR imaging. (*A*) Coronal T2-weighted MR image without fat suppression in a 3-year-old boy after ARM repair demonstrates eccentric location of the rectal pull-through (*dashed arrow*) relative to the levator sling (*solid arrow*). (*B*) Axial T2-weighted MR image without fat suppression in an 8-year-old boy after ARM repair demonstrates eccentric location of the rectal pull-through (*dashed arrow*) relative to the sphincter complex (*solid arrow*).

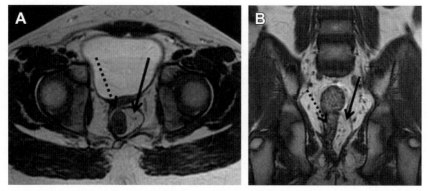

Fig. 23. Eight-year-old girl after ARM repair with complaints of fecal incontinence. (*A*) Axial and (*B*) coronal T2-weighted MR images without fat suppression both demonstrate mesenteric fat (*solid arrows*) interposed within the sphincter complex adjacent to the sigmoid colon pull-through (*dashed arrows*).

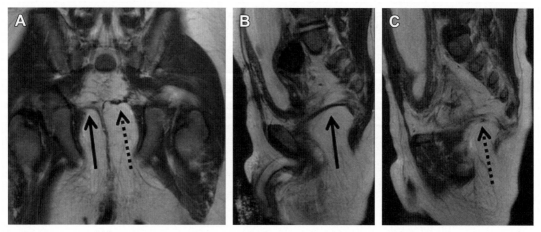

Fig. 24. Two-year-old boy status post ARM repair. (*A*) Coronal and (*B*) sagittal right and (*C*) sagittal left paramidline T2-weighted MR images without fat suppression demonstrate asymmetric attenuated right (*arrow*) levator sling musculature compared to the left (*dashed arrow*).

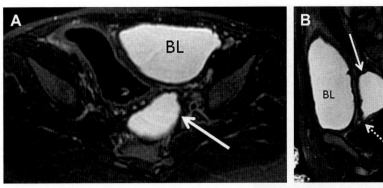

Fig. 25. Three-year-old boy with urinary dribbling after ARM repair. (*A*) Axial and (*B*) sagittal T2-weighted MR images with fat suppression demonstrate a well-circumscribed cystic structure (*solid arrows*) posterior to the bladder (BL) with the suggestion of a fistulous tract heading toward the bladder neck and posterior urethra (*dashed arrow*). The findings are consistent with a PUD, which was confirmed cystoscopically and surgically.

In some postoperative ARM patients, fecal incontinence may be due to poor pelvic musculature, for which MR imaging provides excellent diagnostic capability.[26,27,29,40] Although some investigators have described measuring the thickness of the pelvic muscles,[63] typically a subjective assessment alone is provided based on internal symmetry from side to side and comparison with normal pelvic musculature in similar aged, healthy patients (**Fig. 24**).[40] Augmentation of hypoplastic pelvic musculature with striated muscle transplantation has been described in postoperative ARM patients with poor fecal continence.[64]

> Eccentric placement of the rectal pull-through and mesenteric fat around the pull-through may explain postoperative defecatory dysfunction in ARM patients and can be identified on MR imaging.

PUD is one of the most common urologic complications in postoperative ARM patients. A rectourethral fistula is present in more than 80% of males with ARM at initial presentation. Incomplete resection of the distal rectum, leaving this segment attached to the posterior urethra, results in PUD.[65] The surgical dissection of the common wall between the rectum and urethra in ARM patients is technically challenging from an abdominal approach (abdominoperineal pull-through or laparoscopically). The advent of laparoscopy has heightened concerns about the development of PUD, particularly when a rectum that reaches below the peritoneal reflection (rectourethral [bulbar] fistula) is approached transabdominally.[66,67] In such a case, PSARP is more appropriate and avoids this complication.

Patients with PUD are at increased risk of calculus formation, recurrent urinary tract infections, urinary dribbling, difficult catheterizations, and

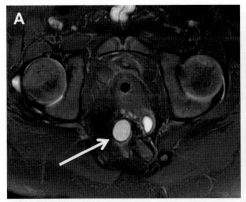
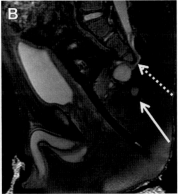

Fig. 26. Two-year-old boy after ARM repair. (*A*) Axial and (*B*) sagittal T2-weighted MR images with fat suppression and a Foley catheter in the rectum for easier identification, demonstrate a multiloculated cystic mass in the presacral space (*solid arrows*). The cystic spaces contain varying degrees of signal hyperintensity, likely due to variable proteinaceous content. Note also the hypoplastic sacrum (*dashed arrow*). The findings were suspected to represent a small teratoma, which was confirmed histopathologically after surgical resection.

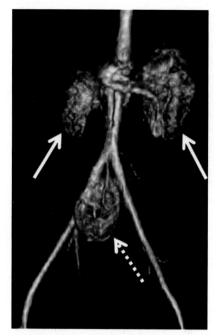

Fig. 27. Twelve-year-old boy after ARM repair. Coronal 3D volume-rendered reconstruction from an abdominopelvic MR angiogram demonstrates two normally positioned kidneys (*solid arrows*) and a third, supernumerary pelvic kidney (*dashed arrow*) located caudal to the aortic bifurcation, an extremely rare anomaly. (*Data from* Flyer MA, Haller JO, Feld M, et al. Ectopic supernumerary kidney: another cause of a pelvic mass. Abdom Imaging 1994;19:374–5.)

adenocarcinoma from long-term exposure of the colorectal mucosa to urine; therefore, their identification and ultimate resection are important.[66] Symptoms may occur many years after the initial pull-through. MR imaging is very useful in the postoperative assessment of ARM patients with suspected PUD. When a cystic lesion posterior to

the bladder neck or posterior urethra is encountered in a male patient, the interpreting radiologist should have a low threshold for advocating cystoscopic confirmation (**Fig. 25**).[66] The inability to identify the actual fistulous communication between PUD and urethra on MR imaging does not exclude PUD because it may only be apparent during voiding.

PUD is one of the most common urologic complications seen in postoperative ARM patients.

A meticulous search during postoperative MR imaging in ARM patients for unsuspected presacral masses and associated anomalies is critical to improve long-term outcomes and guide appropriate surgical management. As in the preoperative patient, spine abnormalities, sacrococcygeal teratomas (**Fig. 26**), skeletal anomalies (see **Fig. 26**), and genitourinary anomalies (**Figs. 27** and **28**) may be encountered and knowledge of their presence may have a significant impact on management in these complex patients.

SUMMARY

Radiologists have long played a key role in the evaluation of ARM patients and will continue to do so. Mainly due to advances in technical capabilities, lack of ionizing radiation, and its ability to serve as a one-stop shop for evaluation of the ARM itself and associated anomalies, MR imaging has become an increasingly important tool in the imaging armamentarium available to the radiologist in the work-up of these complex patients in

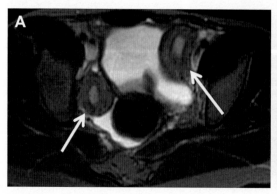

Fig. 28. Fourteen-year-old girl after ARM repair. (*A*) Axial T2-weighted MR image with fat suppression demonstrates two separate uterine horns (*solid arrows*). The patient also had two separate cervices and a vaginal septum (not shown) consistent with uterine didelphys. There was also ascites present. (*B*) Coronal T2-weighted MR image in the same patient demonstrates bilateral hydronephrosis with parenchymal thinning (*dashed arrows*).

the fetal period, before definitive surgical correction, and in the postoperative period.

REFERENCES

1. Levitt MA, Peña A. Anorectal malformations. Orphanet J Rare Dis 2007;2:33.
2. Hendren WH. Urogenital sinus and cloacal malformations. Semin Pediatr Surg 1996;5:72–9.
3. Levitt MA, Peña A. Imperforate Anus and Cloacal Malformations. In: Holcomb W, Murphy JP, editors. Ashcraft's pediatric surgery. 5th edition. Philadelphia: Elsevier Saunders; 2010. p. 468–90.
4. Boocock GR, Donnai D. Anorectal malformation: familial aspects and associated anomalies. Arch Dis Child 1987;62:576–9.
5. Currarino G, Coln D, Votteler T. Triad of anorectal, sacral, and presacral anomalies. AJR Am J Roentgenol 1981;137:395–8.
6. Belloni E, Martucciello G, Verderio D, et al. Involvement of the HLXB9 homeobox gene in Currarino Syndrome. Am J Hum Genet 2000;66:312–9.
7. Sharma S, Jana M. Teaching neuroimages: caudal regression syndrome. Neurology 2011;77:e149.
8. Solomon BD. VACTERL/VATER association. Orphanet J Rare Dis 2011;6:56.
9. Wangensteen OH, Rice CO. Imperforate anus: a method of determining the surgical approach. Ann Surg 1930;92:77–81.
10. Stevens CA. Rectum and anus. In: Stevenson RE, Hall JH, editors. Human malformations and related anomalies. New York: Oxford University Press; 2006. p. 1115–22.
11. Tourneux F. Sur les premiers développements du cloaques du tubercule génital et de l'anus chez l'embryon de mouton. J Anat Physiol 1888;24:503–17.
12. Retterer E. Sur l'origine et l'évolution de la région ano-génitale des mammiféres. J Anat Physiol 1890;26:126–216.
13. Bill AH, Johnson RJ. Failure of migration of the rectal opening as the cause for most cases of imperforate anus. Surg Gynecol Obstet 1958;106:643–51.
14. Gans SL, Friedman NB. Some new concepts in the embryology, anatomy, physiology and surgical correction of imperforate anus. West J Surg Obstet Gynecol 1961;69:34–7.
15. van der Putte SC. Normal and abnormal development of the anorectum. J Pediatr Surg 1986;21:434–40.
16. Holschneider AM, Hutson JM. Anorectal malformations in children: embryology, diagnosis, surgical treatment, follow-up. 1st edition. New York: Springer; 2006.
17. Kluth D. Embryology of anorectal malformations. Semin Pediatr Surg 2010;19:201–8.
18. Zhang T, Zhang HL, Wang da J, et al. Normal development of hindgut and anorectum in human embryo. Int J Colorectal Dis 2011;26:109–16.
19. Gordon PH. Anorectal anatomy and physiology. Gastroenterol Clin North Am 2001;30:1–13.
20. Stephens FD, Smith ED. Classification, identification, and assessment of surgical treatment of anorectal anomalies. Pediatr Surg Int 1986;1:200–5.
21. Calvo-Garcia MA, Kline-Fath BM, Levitt MA, et al. Fetal MRI clues to diagnose cloacal malformations. Pediatr Radiol 2011;41:1117–28.
22. Veyrac C, Couture A, Saguintaah M, et al. MRI of fetal GI tract abnormalities. Abdom Imaging 2004;29:411–20.
23. Warne S, Chitty LS, Wilcox DR. Prenatal diagnosis of cloacal anomalies. BJU Int 2002;89:78–81.
24. Saguintaah M, Couture A, Veyrac C, et al. MRI of the fetal gastrointestinal tract. Pediatr Radiol 2002;32:395–404.
25. Couture A. Fetal gastrointestinal tract: US and MR. In: Couture A, Baud C, Ferran FL, et al, editors. Gastrointestinal tract sonography in fetuses and children. Heidelberg: Springer; 2008. p. 1–84.
26. Nievelstein RA, Vos A, Valk J. MR imaging of anorectal malformations and associated anomalies. Eur Radiol 1998;8:573–81.
27. McHugh K. The role of radiology in children with anorectal anomalies; with particular emphasis on MRI. Eur J Radiol 1998;26:194–9.
28. Jaramillo D, Lebowitz RL, Hendren WH. The cloacal malformation: radiologic findings and imaging recommendations. Radiology 1990;177:441–8.
29. Sato Y, Pringle KC, Bergman RA, et al. Congenital anorectal anomalies: MR imaging. Radiology 1988;168:157–62.
30. Mchugh K, Dudley NE, Tam P. Pre-operative MRI of anorectal anomalies in the newborn period. Pediatr Radiol 1995;25(Suppl 1):S33–6.
31. Taccone A, Martucciello G, Dodero P, et al. New concepts in preoperative imaging of anorectal malformations. Pediatr Radiol 1992;22:196–9.
32. Aslam A, Grier DJ, Duncan AQ, et al. The role of magnetic resonance imaging in the preoperative assessment of anorectal anomalies. Pediatr Surg Int 1998;14:71–3.
33. Sachs TM, Applebaum H, Touran T, et al. Use of MRI in evaluation of anorectal anomalies. J Pediatr Surg 1990;25:817–21.
34. Tang ST, Cao GQ, Mao YZ, et al. Clinical value of pelvic 3-dimensional magnetic resonance image reconstruction in anorectal malformations. J Pediatr Surg 2009;44:2369–74.
35. Jarboe MD, Teitelbaum DH, Dillman JR. Combined 3D rotational fluoroscopic-MRI cloacagram procedure defines luminal and extraluminal pelvic anatomy prior to surgical reconstruction of cloacal

and other complex pelvic malformations. Pediatr Surg Int 2012;28:757–63.

36. Baughman SM, Richardson RR, Podberesky DJ, et al. 3-Dimensional magnetic resonance genitography: a different look at cloacal malformations. J Urol 2007;178:1675–8.

37. Raschbaum GR, Bleacher JC, Grattan-Smith JD, et al. Magnetic resonance imaging-guided laparoscopic-assisted anorectoplasty for imperforate anus. J Pediatr Surg 2010;45:220–3.

38. Ueno S, Yokoyama S, Soeda J, et al. Three-dimensional display of the pelvic structure of anorectal malformations based on CT and MR images. J Pediatr Surg 1995;30:682–6.

39. Miyasaka M, Nosaka S, Kitano Y. Utility of spinal MRI in children with anorectal malformation. Pediatr Radiol 2009;39:810–6.

40. Eltomey MA, Donnelly LF, Emery KH, et al. Postoperative pelvic MRI of anorectal malformations. AJR Am J Roentgenol 2008;191:1469–76.

41. Ng WT, Ng TK, Cheng PW. Sacrococcygeal teratoma and anorectal malformation. Aust N Z J Surg 1997;67:218–20.

42. Kocaoglu M, Frush DP. Pediatric presacral masses. Radiographics 2006;26:833–57.

43. Altman RP, Randolph JG, Lilly JR. Sacrococcygeal teratoma: American Academy of Pediatrics Surgical Section Survey—1973. J Pediatr Surg 1973;9:389–98.

44. Stephens F, Smith E. Anorectal malformations in children: update 1988. Birth Defects Orig Artic Ser 1988;24:1–604.

45. Paidas CN, Levitt MA, Peña A. Rectum and Anus. In: Oldham KT, Colombani PM, Foglia RP, et al, editors. Principles and practice of pediatric surgery. Phladelphia: Lippincott Williams & Wilkins; 2005. p. 1395–436.

46. Okur H, Keskin E, Zorludemir U, et al. Tubular duplication of the hindgut with genitourinary anomalies. J Pediatr Surg 1992;27:1239–40.

47. Berrocal T, Lopez-Pereira P, Arjonilla A, et al. Anomalies of the distal ureter, bladder, and urethra in children: embryologic radiologic, and pathologic features. Radiographics 2002;22:1139–64.

48. McLorie GA, Sheldon MA, Fleisher M, et al. The genitourinary system in patients with imperforate anus. J Pediatr Surg 1987;22:1100–4.

49. Metts JC, Kotkin L, Kasper S, et al. Genital malformations and coexistent urinary tract or spinal anomalies in patients with imperforate anus. J Urol 1997;158:1298–300.

50. Yeung CK, Tam YH, Chan YL, et al. A new management algorithm for impalpable undescended testis with gadolinium enhanced magnetic resonance angiography. J Urol 1999;162:998–1002.

51. Tasian GE, Copp HL, Baskin LS. Diagnostic imaging in cryptorchidism: utility, indications, and effectiveness. J Pediatr Surg 2011;46:2406–13.

52. Miyano T, Kobayashi H, Simomura H, et al. Magnetic resonance imaging for localizing the nonpalpable undescended testis. J Pediatr Surg 1991;26:607–9.

53. Pinke LA, Rathbun SW, Husmann DA, et al. Penoscrotal transposition: review of 53 patients. J Urol 2001;166:1865–8.

54. Nakamura Y, Jennings RW, Connolly S, et al. Fetal diagnosis of penoscrotal transposition associated with perineal lipoma in one twin. Fetal Diagn Ther 2010;27:164–7.

55. Mollitt DL, Schullinger JN, Santulli TV. Complications at menarche of urogenital sinus with associated anorectal malformations. J Pediatr Surg 1981;16:349–52.

56. Fleming SE, Hall R, Gysler M, et al. Imperforate anus in females: frequency of genital tract involvement, incidence of associated anomalies, and functional outcome. J Pediatr Surg 1986;21:146–50.

57. Hall R, Fleming S, Gysler M. The genital tract in female children with imperforate anus. Am J Obstet Gynecol 1985;151:169–71.

58. Behr SC, Courteir JL, Qayyum A. Imaging of Müllerian duct anomalies. Radiographics 2012;32:E233–50.

59. Troiano RN, McCarthy SM. Müllerian duct anomalies: imaging and clinical issues. Radiology 2004;233:19–34.

60. Bischoff A, Levitt MA, Breech L, et al. Hydrocolpos in cloacal malformations. J Pediatr Surg 2010;45:1241–5.

61. Peña A, Grasshoff S, Levitt M. Reoperations in anorectal malformations. J Pediatr Surg 2007;42:318–25.

62. Fukuya T, Honda H, Kubota M, et al. Postoperative MRI evaluation of anorectal malformations with clinical correlation. Pediatr Radiol 1993;23:583–6.

63. Arnbjörsnsson E, Malmgren N, Mikaelsson C, et al. Computed tomography and magnetic resonance tomography findings in children operated for anal atresia. Z Kinderchir 1990;45:178–81.

64. Vade A, Reyes H, Wilbur A, et al. The anorectal sphincter after rectal pull-through surgery for anorectal anomalies: MRI evaluation. Pediatr Radiol 1989;19:179–83.

65. Hong AR, Acuña MF, Peña A, et al. Urologic injuries associated with repair of anorectal malformation in male patients. J Pediatr Surg 2002;37:339–44.

66. Podberesky DJ, Weaver NC, Anton CG, et al. MRI of acquired posterior urethral diverticulum following surgery for anorectal malformations. Pediatr Radiol 2011;41:1139–45.

67. Alam S, Lawal TA, Peña A, et al. Acquired posterior urethral diverticulum following surgery for anorectal malformations. J Pedatr Surg 2011;46:1231–5.

Magnetic Resonance Imaging of Perianal and Perineal Crohn Disease in Children and Adolescents

Matthew R. Hammer, MD[a],*, Jonathan R. Dillman, MD[b],
Ethan A. Smith, MD[c], Mahmoud M. Al-Hawary, MD[d]

KEYWORDS

- Magnetic resonance imaging • Crohn disease • Pelvis • Perineum • Perianal • Fistula • Abscess
- Children

KEY POINTS

- High-resolution, especially at 3-T, magnetic resonance (MR) imaging with a small field of view allows comprehensive evaluation of the perineum in pediatric Crohn disease, including assessment of the perianal, labial, and scrotal regions.
- Crohn disease–related perianal fistulas (including complex fistulous disease) and associated abscesses, as well as cutaneous inflammation, are exquisitely depicted by MR imaging.
- Other imaging modalities (such as fluoroscopic fistulography, endoscopic and transperineal ultrasonography, and computed tomography) and physical examination can provide useful information about perineal Crohn disease; however, they frequently do not depict the true extent of perineal and pelvic inflammation as well as does MR imaging.
- MR imaging findings predict outcomes in perineal Crohn disease better than other imaging modalities and physical examination.
- MR imaging improves surgical outcomes in perianal fistulous disease by alerting surgeons to exact anatomic relationships and true extent of disease.

INTRODUCTION

Crohn disease (CD) is one type of chronic inflammatory bowel disease (IBD) affecting both children and adults that can involve any portion of the gastrointestinal tract from the mouth to the anus. This condition can also affect a variety of extraintestinal structures and body systems, including the perineum and skin. The initial diagnosis of IBD is made approximately 20% to 30% of the time during childhood, with a pediatric prevalence of 5 to 16 cases per 100,000 children.[1,2] Perianal and perineal cutaneous inflammatory involvement in the setting of IBD occurs almost exclusively with CD (rather than ulcerative colitis) and has been reported to occur in 13% to 49%

[a] Section of Pediatric Radiology, Department of Radiology, C.S. Mott Children's Hospital, University of Michigan Health System, 1540 East Hospital Drive, Room 3-220, Ann Arbor, MI 48109-4252, USA; [b] Section of Pediatric Radiology, Department of Radiology, C.S. Mott Children's Hospital, University of Michigan Health System, 1540 East Hospital Drive, Room 3-226, Ann Arbor, MI 48109-4252, USA; [c] Section of Pediatric Radiology, Department of Radiology, C.S. Mott Children's Hospital, University of Michigan Health System, 1540 East Hospital Drive, Room 3-224, Ann Arbor, MI 48109-4252, USA; [d] Section of Abdominal Radiology, Division of Abdominal Imaging, Department of Radiology, University of Michigan Health System, 1500 East Medical Center Drive, Ann Arbor, MI 48109, USA
* Corresponding author.
E-mail address: hammerm@med.umich.edu

Magn Reson Imaging Clin N Am 21 (2013) 813–828
http://dx.doi.org/10.1016/j.mric.2013.07.003

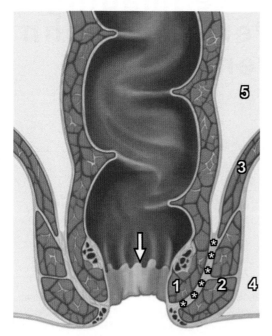

Fig. 1. Coronal illustration of the rectum and perianal region. The internal anal sphincter (IAS) (*1*) and external anal sphincter (EAS) (*2*) are separated by the intersphincteric space (*asterisks*). The levator ani muscles (*3*), along with the external sphincter, form the boundary of the ischioanal and ischiorectal fossa (*4*). The space lateral to the rectum and above the levator ani muscles is the supralevator space (*5*). The dentate line (*arrow*) represents the anorectal junction.

of pediatric CD patients.[3–5] In a small number of children with CD (up to about 4%), perineal and cutaneous inflammation may become evident before detection of bowel involvement.[3,6,7] Cutaneous inflammatory involvement by pediatric CD very commonly affects the perineal region

(perianal, labial, and scrotal regions), presenting as fistulas and fissures, associated abscesses, uncomplicated skin inflammation, and skin tags.[3,8,9]

Recent advances in magnetic resonance (MR) imaging have transformed the clinical and operative management of pediatric CD patients. MR enterography allows for dedicated nonionizing, high-quality imaging of the bowel and can detect inflamed intestinal segments characterize inflammatory disease activity, and diagnose a variety of disease-related complications, such as strictures and internal fistulas. High-resolution, small field-of-view MR imaging of the perineum, particularly at a field strength of 3-T, provides for nonionizing, multiparametric evaluation of the perianal, labial, and scrotal regions in a noninvasive manner, and allows for definitive assessment of perineal and pelvic inflammation in pediatric CD. This article provides a contemporary review of perineal MR imaging appearances of CD in the pediatric population, including fistulous disease, abscesses, and skin manifestations. The perineal MR imaging technique is also discussed.

PERIANAL ANATOMY

Understanding the anatomy of the perineum and perianal region is necessary to properly interpret imaging of these areas and to appropriately direct clinical and surgical care (**Figs. 1** and **2**). The internal anal sphincter (IAS) is a smooth muscle layer that encircles the anal canal and provides a majority of resting anal tone, although it is not necessary for maintenance of bowel continence. The external anal sphincter (EAS) is composed of striated muscle and is located peripheral to the IAS. It provides voluntary muscle contraction and a small amount of resting anal tone; disruption of the EAS can

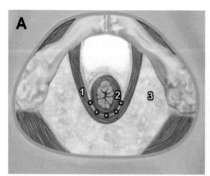
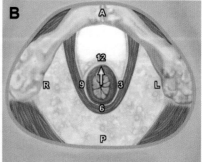

Fig. 2. Axial illustrations of the perianal region. (*A*) The EAS (*1*) and IAS (*2*) form the boundaries of the intersphincteric space (*asterisks*). The ischioanal fossa (*3*) is outside of the EAS and below the levator ani musculature (not shown, located superiorly). (*B*) The "anal clock" is used to describe the location of perianal abnormalities. The patient is supine in the lithotomy position (anterior [A] represented by 12 o'clock, posterior [P] represented by 6 o'clock, patient's left [L] represented by 3 o'clock, and patient's right [R] represented by 9 o'clock).

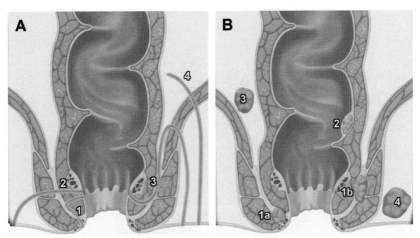

Fig. 3. Coronal illustrations of the rectum and perianal region. (*A*) Classification of fistula tracts as described by Parks and colleagues, showing the intersphincteric (*1*), transsphincteric (*2*), suprasphincteric (*3*), and extrasphincteric (*4*) fistula tracts. (*B*) The locations of perianal abscess formation, usually associated with fistula tracts, are shown: superficial intersphincteric (*1a*) and intersphincteric (*1b*), submucosal/intramuscular (*2*), supralevator (*3*), and ischioanal (*4*) abscesses.

result in bowel incontinence. The EAS attaches to the perineal body anteriorly and the anococcygeal ligament posteriorly, and is continuous with the puborectalis muscle and the levator ani musculature superiorly. The IAS and EAS are separated by a layer of loose connective tissue commonly referred to as the intersphincteric space (or plane), which represents a potential space for fistula passage and infection. Lateral to the EAS is the contiguous spaces of the ischioanal fossa and is-chiorectal fossa, which contain mostly fat as well as inferior rectal vessels and nerves.[3,10]

Description of the location of perianal abnormality in the axial (transverse) plane commonly makes use of the "anal clock" (see **Fig. 2**). When using anal-clock nomenclature, the patient is supine (in the lithotomy position) and the physician is presumed to be standing at the patient's feet looking

Table 1
Sample pediatric MR imaging perineal fistula protocol pulse sequences and key parameters at 3-T

Sequence	Plane	Fat Saturation (Yes/No)	Flip Angle (°)	TE (ms)	TR (ms)	Slice Thickness/Gap (mm)	NSA
Single-shot fast spin-echo	Coronal	No	90	80	Shortest	4/1	1
T2-weighted fast spin-echo	Axial	No	90	80	5000	4/0	2
T2-weighted fast spin-echo	Sagittal and axial	Yes	90	80	4000	4/0	4
T1-weighted fast spin-echo	Axial	No	90	11	750	4/0	2
Precontrast T1-weighted 3D-SPGR[a]	Axial	Yes	10	Shortest	Shortest	1.8	4
Postcontrast T1-weighted 3D-SPGR[a]	Coronal, axial, sagittal	Yes	10	Shortest	Shortest	1.8	4

Shortest = TE and/or TR set to be the shortest allowed by the scanner.
   Abbreviations: 3D-SPGR, 3-dimensional spoiled gradient recalled echo; NSA, number of signal averages; TE, echo time; TR, repetition time.
   [a] 50% overlap (ie, 1.8 mm slice every 0.9 mm).

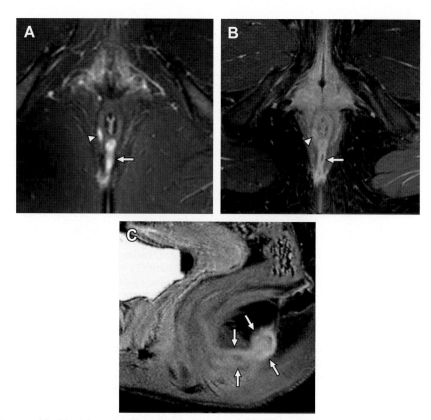

Fig. 4. A 17-year-old girl with Crohn disease (CD) and perianal discharge. (*A*) Axial T2-weighted fast spin-echo image with fat saturation shows linear hyperintense tracts in the 8 o'clock position in the intersphincteric space (intersphincteric fistula, *arrowhead*) and 6 o'clock position traversing the IAS and EAS (transsphincteric fistula, *arrow*). (*B*) Axial postcontrast T1-weighted 3-dimensional spoiled gradient recalled echo (3D-SPGR) fat-saturated image shows enhancement of the tracts. (*C*) Sagittal postcontrast T1-weighted 3D-SPGR fat-saturated image shows the blind-ending transsphincteric fistula extending into ischioanal fat.

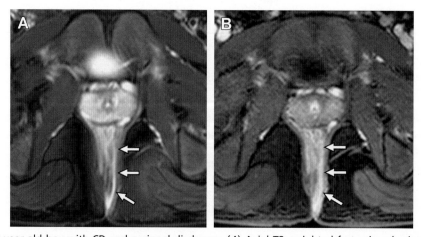

Fig. 5. A 16-year-old boy with CD and perianal discharge. (*A*) Axial T2-weighted fast spin-echo image with fat saturation shows a hyperintense fluid-filled fistula tract (*arrows*) arising from the 4 o'clock position traversing both the IAS and EAS. (*B*) Axial postcontrast T1-weighted 3D-SPGR fat-saturated image demonstrates hyperenhancement of the fistula tract (*arrows*). This transsphincteric fistula can be followed to the left gluteal skin surface.

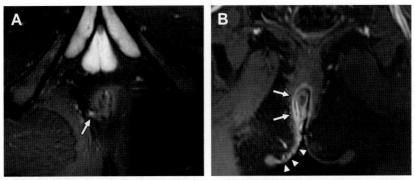

Fig. 6. A 17-year-old boy with CD and worsening perianal pain. (*A*) Axial T2-weighted fast spin-echo image with fat saturation shows a hyperintense fistula tract (*arrow*) arising from the 8 o'clock position and traversing both the IAS and EAS. (*B*) Coronal postcontrast T1-weighted 3D-SPGR fat-saturated image demonstrates hyperenhancement of the fistula tract (*arrows*), which contains fluid. Right gluteal skin thickening and hyperenhancement (*arrowheads*) is due to cutaneous CD.

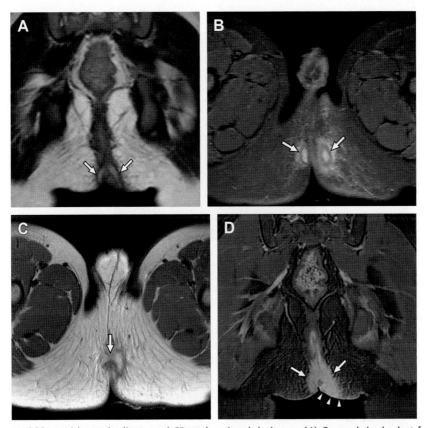

Fig. 7. A 6-year-old boy with newly diagnosed CD and perianal drainage. (*A*) Coronal single-shot fast spin-echo image shows a complex branching perianal fistula (*arrows*). (*B*) Axial short-tau inversion recovery (STIR) image confirms the presence of fluid-filled fistula tracts (*arrows*) in the bilateral gluteal regions. Adjacent subcutaneous signal hyperintensity is due to inflammation. (*C*) Axial T2-weighted fast spin-echo image confirms that the 2 gluteal fistula tracts join (*arrow*), and have a single opening from the anal canal (not shown). (*D*) Coronal postcontrast T1-weighted 3D-SPGR fat-saturated image demonstrates striking enhancement of the fistula tracts (*arrows*). Left gluteal skin hyperenhances (*arrowheads*).

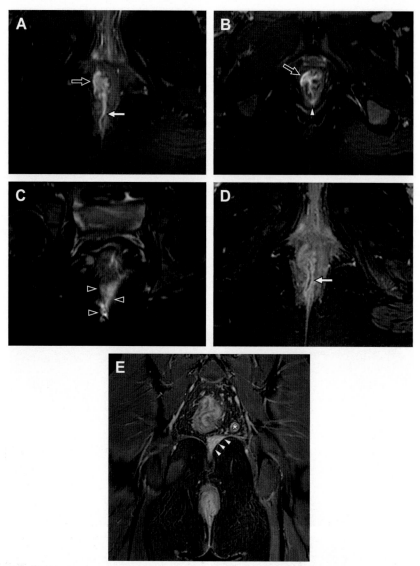

Fig. 8. A 14-year-old girl with CD and perianal drainage. (*A–C*) Axial T2-weighted fast spin-echo fat-saturated images demonstrate multiple perianal fistula tracts. A linear fluid-filled superficial perianal fistula arises from 6 o'clock (*white arrow*). An intersphincteric fistula is seen at the 10 o'clock position (*black arrow*), while an additional fistula tract (*white arrowhead*) arising from the 6 o'clock position more superiorly leads to an ill-defined fluid collection (*black arrowheads*) above the levator ani musculature. The rectum is thick-walled, and there is perirectal hypervascularity and lymph node enlargement. (*D, E*) Axial and coronal postcontrast T1-weighted 3D-SPGR fat-saturated images demonstrate a linear hyperenhancing fluid-filled superficial fistula tract at 6 o'clock (*arrow*). Abnormal enhancement is seen abutting and just superior to the levator ani musculature on the left (*arrowheads*). The rectal wall hyperenhances, and there is an enlarged perirectal lymph node (*asterisk*).

at the perineum. The anterior (toward the perineal body) and posterior (toward the intergluteal cleft) positions are represented by 12 o'clock and 6 o'clock on the clock face, respectively. The left (patient left) lateral position is represented by 3 o'clock, and the right (patient right) lateral position is represented by 9 o'clock.

CLASSIFICATION AND MANAGEMENT OF PERIANAL FISTULOUS CROHN DISEASE

The EAS joins the puborectalis muscle at the level of the dentate (or pectinate) line, a point about 2 cm deep to the anal verge where squamous epithelium transitions to columnar epithelium. At this location, longitudinal columns of mucosa

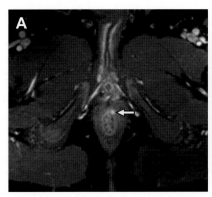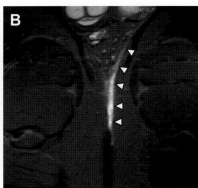

Fig. 9. A 15-year-old boy with CD and scrotal drainage. (*A*) Axial postcontrast T1-weighted 3D-SPGR fat-saturated image shows a hyperenhancing perianal fistula tract (*arrow*) arising from the 1 o'clock position. (*B*) Axial T2-weighted fast spin-echo image with fat saturation shows abnormal signal hyperintensity (fistula tract) extending inferiorly into the left hemiscrotum (*arrowheads*).

(columns of Morgagni) are present with intervening anal sinuses (or crypts), which collect drainage from the anal glands.[11,12] Obstruction and infection of the glands at this location has been hypothesized to be the cause of most idiopathic abscesses and fistulas in the "crypto-glandular hypothesis" described by Parks[13] in 1961. However, in the setting of CD, the development of perineal inflammation and infection is more complex as other routes of inflammation and infection are possible, including extraintestinal granulomatous inflammation arising primarily in the perineal skin/soft tissues, or contiguous extension of inflammation from affected bowel directly to the perineum.

Based on extensive clinical experience in adults with fistula-in-ano, Parks and colleagues[14] developed a novel classification system for describing perianal fistulas that is still used by surgeons today. This classification system more recently has been applied to both fistulas and abscesses arising in CD patients (**Fig. 3**). Although variations exist, this classification scheme has 4 major groupings based on anatomic location of the fistula:

- Type 1: Intersphincteric. Fistula crosses the IAS and extends only within the intersphincteric plane
- Type 2: Transsphincteric. Fistula traverses both the IAS and EAS, and extends into the ischioanal fossa
- Type 3: Suprasphincteric. Fistula extends superiorly within the intersphincteric space and over the top of the puborectalis muscles, then traverses the levator ani musculature and extends downward to the ischioanal fossa
- Type 4: Extrasphincteric. Fistula extends from the deep pelvis (high perirectal region) through the levator ani and into the ischioanal fossa without involving the EAS complex

Knowledge of the type of fistula and the anatomic structures involved has been shown to be crucial for proper surgical planning and good postoperative outcomes in adults. A type 1 (intersphincteric) fistula is the simplest form, and can be treated surgically by dividing the IAS (fistulotomy or fistulectomy) with very low associated risk of subsequent loss of bowel continence. More complex fistula types (types 2, 3, and 4) usually necessitate an operation involving the EAS complex for complete excision, which increases the chances of bowel incontinence. To avoid a loss in bowel control, alternative surgical therapies, such as seton stitch placement that

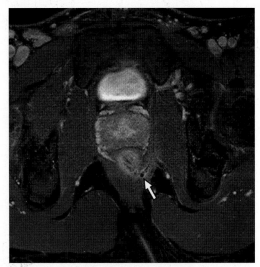

Fig. 10. A 17-year-old boy with CD and perianal drainage. Axial postcontrast T1-weighted 3D-SPGR fat-saturated image shows an intersphincteric hyperenhancing fistula. A small focus of signal hypointensity in the intersphincteric space is due to gas (*arrow*).

promotes healing by keeping the fistula tract patent for drainage of infectious material, may be used; such alternative techniques are often preferred in CD patients because of the presence of complex fistulous disease (eg, multiple or branching fistula tracts) and an increased risk of local recurrence after operations involving the EAS.[15] Rarely, diversion of the fecal stream with ostomy formation may be required to promote healing of perianal CD.

Referring physicians can often visualize fistula tracts that extend to the skin surface. By performing a digital rectal examination and probing the tract, commonly under sedation or general anesthesia, the course of a fistula tract can sometimes be established. Clinical parameters also have been developed to characterize perianal fistulas, such as the perianal disease activity index (PDAI), which evaluates a fistula for discharge, pain, restriction of activity, type of recurrent disease, and extent of disease.[11,16] Physical examination and clinical evaluation, however, often do not detect blind-ending tracts, secondary tracts, abscesses, and extension into the deep pelvis,

and therefore may underestimate the true extent of perianal inflammatory activity. Detection of such occult perineal CD manifestations directly affects patient management. Proper clinical (both medical and surgical) decision making requires precise knowledge of the true extent of disease. Such knowledge, which is now provided by high-resolution, small field-of-view perineal MR imaging, can establish the feasibility and efficacy (at follow-up) of medical management (eg, treatment with immunomodulator and/or biological therapies, which can be associated with serious side effects) as well as determine which patients will benefit from surgery.[17]

IMAGING OF PERINEAL CROHN DISEASE

Multiple imaging modalities have been used to evaluate for the presence and extent of perianal CD. Fluoroscopic fistulography was used in the past, but was often difficult to interpret, as the anal sphincter complex cannot be directly visualized and some fistula tracts or abscesses may not fill with injected contrast material.[10,18]

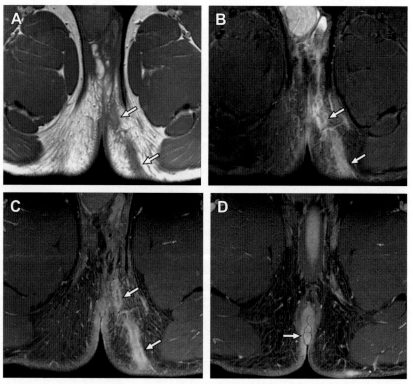

Fig. 11. An 18-year-old boy with CD and perianal drainage. (*A, B*) Axial T1-weighted fast spin-echo and T2-weighted fast spin-echo fat-saturated images shows linear signal abnormality (*arrows*) coursing through left gluteal subcutaneous tissues without an obvious perianal origin. (*C*) Axial T1-weighted 3D-SPGR fat-saturated image shows that the tract peripherally hyperenhances (*arrows*). (*D*) Axial postcontrast T1-weighted 3D-SPGR fat-saturated image more inferiorly demonstrates a large skin tag (*arrow*) in the intergluteal cleft.

Endoscopic and transperineal ultrasonography have been used and can provide useful results, although the full extent of inflammation, particularly involving the EAS and deeper structures, may not be visualized owing to the lack of sound-wave penetration.[10,19,20] The limited soft-tissue contrast resolution of computed tomography (CT) makes distinguishing perineal musculature, fibrous tissue, and fistula tracts potentially difficult, although organized fluid collections larger than about 1 cm in size generally can be readily seen. The availability of other imaging modalities that do not require ionizing radiation also makes CT imaging less desirable in this patient population, as repeat imaging is often required during the course of treatment. Recently, MR imaging has emerged as an ideal modality for assessing perineal CD. High-resolution, small field-of-view MR imaging of the perineum at a field strength of 3-T provides images with excellent spatial resolution and contrast

resolution, enabling comprehensive evaluation of the entire perineum (perianal, labial, and scrotal regions) and lower pelvis.

Perineal MR Imaging Technique

The authors presently perform perineal MR imaging exclusively at a field strength of 3-T if there is no contraindication (eg, certain implanted devices that have been demonstrated to be safe at a field strength of 1.5-T only). 3-T MR imaging systems offer increased signal-to-noise ratio (SNR) when compared with 1.5-T systems, allowing for shorter image acquisition times and/or improved spatial resolution.[21,22] A multielement torso surface coil is placed over the patient's pelvis and upper thighs anteriorly. Parallel imaging can be used to reduce scan times, although care must be taken not to noticeably diminish the SNR. In the authors' experience, the known disadvantages of 3-T MR

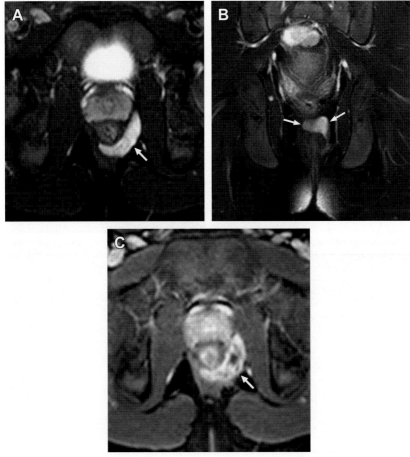

Fig. 12. A 16-year-old boy with CD. (*A, B*) Axial and coronal T2-weighted fast spin-echo fat-saturated images show a hyperintense focal fluid collection (*arrows*) located from 2 to 7 o'clock between the IAS and EAS, crossing the midline. (*C*) Axial postcontrast T1-weighted 3D-SPGR fat-saturated image confirms peripheral hyperenhancement of the fluid collection (*arrow*), consistent with intersphincteric ("horseshoe") abscess.

imaging rarely adversely affect the diagnostic quality of perineal examinations. However, on occasion, air adjacent to the perineum may cause localized susceptibility artifacts or inhomogeneous fat suppression. Endorectal coils are generally avoided in pediatric perineal MR imaging because of safety concerns, their invasive nature, and the small field of view afforded.

The authors' perineal MR imaging protocol comprehensively assesses the perineum and lower pelvis from the skin surface through the mid-to-upper rectum in the transverse plane. Coronal and sagittal images generally extend from the iliac crests through the perineal skin. Perineal MR imaging is most often performed without associated MR enterography pulse sequences, and therefore requires no specific patient preparation (other than peripheral intravenous catheter placement) if the examination is to be performed without sedation. In patients undergoing MR enterography with known or suspected perineal CD, limited high-resolution, small field-of-view imaging (eg,

axial and sagittal T2-weighted fast spin-echo with fat saturation, and postcontrast T1-weighted 3-dimensional spoiled gradient recalled echo [3D-SPGR] with fat saturation in 3 planes) may be acquired. Our routine clinical perineal MR imaging protocol is shown in **Table 1**.

Classification and Outcomes of MR Imaging

MR imaging has become the non invasive modality of choice for the evaluation of perineal CD in adults, and increasingly so in children. MR imaging has been shown to be superior to other imaging modalities in defining the extent of disease and is highly accurate, with reported sensitivities and specificities for evaluating fistula tracts and abscesses higher than 90%.[12,23–26] Moreover, when performed before surgery in adult fistula-in-ano patients, MR imaging has been shown to correlate with patient outcomes and improve operative results with an approximately 75% decrease in postoperative recurrence, which is attributable

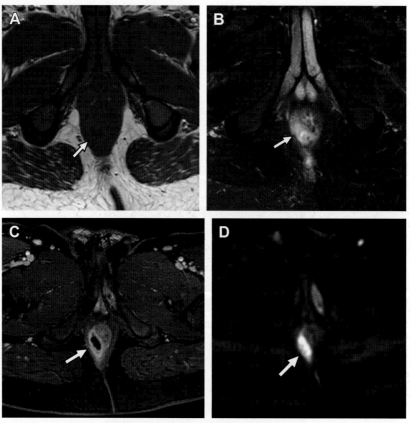

Fig. 13. A 17-year-old boy with newly diagnosed CD and perianal pain. (*A, B*) Axial T1-weighted fast spin-echo and T2-weighted fast spin-echo fat-saturated images show abnormal signal (*arrow*) located from 6 to 11 o'clock between the IAS and EAS. (*C*) Axial postcontrast T1-weighted 3D-SPGR fat-saturated image confirms the presence of a peripherally hyperenhancing intersphincteric abscess (*arrow*). (*D*) Axial diffusion-weighted image demonstrates restricted diffusion (*arrow*).

to the detection of additional fistula tracts and extensions that would go undetected in the operating room.[10,25]

A widely known MR imaging classification scheme for perianal fistulous disease was described by Morris and colleagues[10] at St James's University Hospital.

- Grade 1: Simple linear intersphincteric fistula (arises from anal canal, penetrates IAS, and courses through intersphincteric space to the skin surface)
- Grade 2: Intersphincteric fistula with intersphincteric abscess or secondary fistulous tract
- Grade 3: Transsphincteric fistula (arises from anal canal, penetrates IAS and EAS, and courses through ischioanal fossa to the skin surface)
- Grade 4: Transsphincteric fistula with abscess or secondary tract within the ischioanal fossa
- Grade 5: Supralevator and translevator disease (suprasphincteric fistulas arise from anal canal, penetrate the IAS, course through

intersphincteric space to involve the supralevator space above the levator ani musculature, then descend into the ischioanal fossa to the skin; extrasphincteric fistulas arise above the sphincter mechanism, extend through the levator ani musculature, and course to the skin)

The grades of this classification scheme correspond to clinical outcomes at the authors' institution, with grades 1 and 2 having the best outcomes while grades 3 and 4 that involve the EAS had worse outcomes in terms of bowel continence and extent of necessary surgery. Grade 5, supralevator or translevator disease, was suggestive of a deep pelvic source of infection and had the worst outcomes. Not included in this grading scheme are superficial tracts or abscesses, located in the space between the sphincter muscles and the superficial perianal skin and not involving the intersphincteric space. Submucosal or intramuscular abscesses or fistulas, which are present within the submucosa or muscular layer of the rectal wall but do not penetrate the internal sphincter or other perirectal muscles, also can occur. Finally,

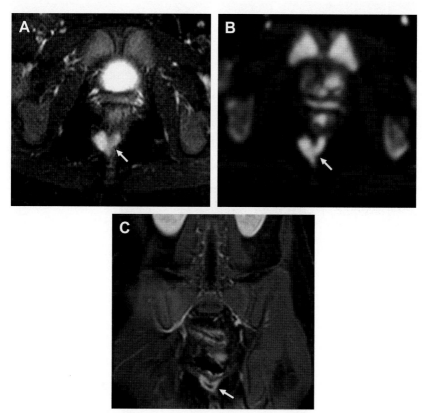

Fig. 14. A 17-year-old girl with CD. (*A, B*) Axial T2-weighted fast spin-echo fat-saturated and diffusion-weighted images show a hyperintense intersphincteric fluid collection that restricts diffusion (*arrow*). (*C*) Coronal post-contrast T1-weighted 3D-SPGR fat-saturated image confirms the presence of a peripherally hyperenhancing "horseshoe" abscess (*arrow*).

perineal fistula tracts that do not communicate with the rectal wall, and are external to the EAS and superficial to the levator ani musculature, rarely exist.

Perineal MR Imaging Findings

T2-weighted pulse sequences without and with fat saturation are critical to the assessment of perineal CD, and particularly fistula type characterization. Fat-saturated or short-tau inversion recovery (STIR) pulse sequences are most sensitive for detecting fluid and inflammation, including fistula tracts and focal fluid collections, whereas non–fat-saturated imaging is used to delineate muscular anatomy and visualize the relationships of the musculature to fistulas and fluid collections. Postcontrast T1-weighted fat-saturated sequences are used to demonstrate areas of inflammation. Both active (commonly fluid-filled on T2-weighted imaging and draining on visual inspection) and healing fistula tracts typically hyperenhance in a linear manner, whereas

abscesses show peripheral hyperenhancement. Diffusion-weighted imaging has been shown to aid in identification of perianal lesions and to confirm findings seen on other sequences.[27] In particular, perineal abscesses demonstrate restricted (impeded) diffusion of water.

Fistulas

Active fistula tracts are typically hyperintense on T2-weighted and hypointense on precontrast T1-weighted imaging because of fluid and associated inflammation (**Figs. 4–8**). These tracts can be linear or complex, with multiple branch points (see **Fig. 7**). Multiple fistulas may also be present in a given patient (see **Figs. 4** and **8**). Radiologists should describe the exact site of origin and course of fistulas as well as where they terminate (eg, where they open on the skin surface). Whereas many perianal fistulas open on the perianal or gluteal skin, some can take unusual courses terminating elsewhere on the perineum (eg, labia or scrotum) (**Fig. 9**), while others may be

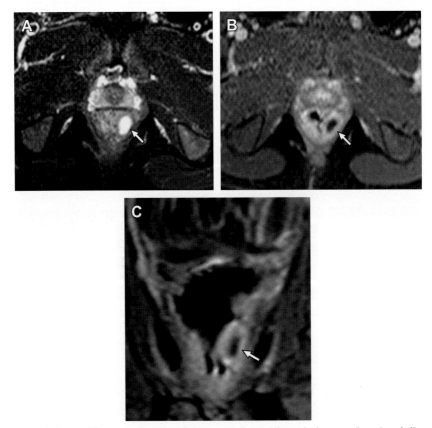

Fig. 15. A 14-year-old boy with newly diagnosed CD presenting with oral ulcers and perianal disease. (*A*) Axial T2-weighted fast spin-echo image with fat saturation shows a hyperintense focal fluid collection (*arrow*) in the wall of the rectum. (*B, C*) Axial and coronal postcontrast T1-weighted 3D-SPGR fat-saturated images show a peripherally hyperenhancing abscess in the rectal wall (*arrow*).

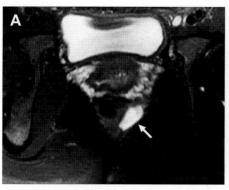
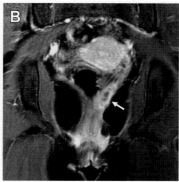

Fig. 16. A 19-year-old woman with CD and perianal pain. (*A*) Axial T2-weighted fast spin-echo image with fat saturation shows a hyperintense focal fluid collection (*arrow*) adjacent to the rectum. (*B*) Coronal postcontrast T1-weighted 3D-SPGR fat-saturated image confirms the presence of a peripherally hyperenhancing abscess (*arrow*) involving left-side levator ani musculature and the suprasphincteric space.

blind-ending (see **Fig. 4**). As fistulas heal and are replaced with granulation tissue and scar, associated inflammation decreases and T2-weighted signal and postcontrast hyperenhancement abate.[12,28] Foci of signal hypointensity within fistula tracts that are noted on all pulse sequences and that are most conspicuous on 3D-SPGR may be due to gas (**Fig. 10**). On occasion, perineal fistula tracts may appear entirely separate from the perianal region, perhaps because of extraintestinal CD (**Fig. 11**). A recent study in adult CD patients has also described the use of dynamic contrast enhancement and measurement of the slope of contrast material wash-in from time versus signal intensity curves to evaluate for early perianal fistula treatment response.[29]

Abscesses

Perianal abscesses typically arise from superinfected fistula tracts, appearing as focal fluid collections of variable size. These abscesses can reside within the musculature of the sphincter mechanism, between the IAS and EAS (intersphincteric abscess or "horseshoe" abscess if located on both sides of the midline), or in the ischioanal or supralevator spaces. Less commonly, abscesses caused by perineal CD may be located in the labia or scrotum. Like abscesses elsewhere in the body, perineal abscesses are typically T2-weighted hyperintense, T1-weighted hypointense, peripherally hyperenhance following intravenous contrast administration, and restrict diffusion (**Figs. 12–17**). Nondependent gas may be noted within these collections, appearing hypointense on all pulse sequences and demonstrating susceptibility artifact. At times, unorganized inflammatory fluid collections (phlegmons) may be associated with fistulous disease, lacking a discrete peripherally enhancing wall (see **Fig. 8**).

Cutaneous manifestations

Cutaneous inflammation can occur in CD, often affecting the perianal region, labia, scrotum, buttocks, inguinal creases, and lower abdominal wall. Skin involvement can be either contiguous with CD of the rectum or separated from the gastrointestinal tract by normal skin ("metastatic" cutaneous CD). At MR imaging, findings suggestive of cutaneous CD include skin thickening, skin and underlying soft-tissue edema (T2-weighted

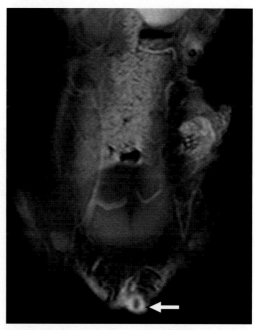

Fig. 17. An 11-year-old girl with CD and labial pain. Coronal postcontrast T1-weighted 3D-SPGR fat-saturated image shows a small peripherally hyperenhancing focal fluid collection (*arrow*) in the left labia majora, consistent with abscess. Physical examination confirmed labial CD.

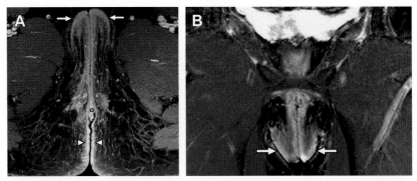

Fig. 18. A 17-year-old girl with CD and labial erythema. (*A, B*) Axial and coronal postcontrast T1-weighted 3D-SPGR fat-saturated images show extensive skin thickening and hyperenhancement of the perineal skin, including the perianal region (*arrowheads*) and labia (*arrows*). A small skin tag is present (*asterisk*).

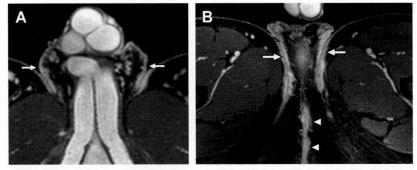

Fig. 19. A 13-year-old boy with CD, scrotal pain, and perineal bleeding. (*A*) Axial T2-weighted fast spin-echo image with fat saturation shows scrotal and inguinal crease skin thickening and signal hyperintensity (*arrows*). (*B*) Axial postcontrast T1-weighted 3D-SPGR fat-saturated image demonstrates scrotal and inguinal crease skin thickening and hyperenhancement (*arrows*). Perianal cutaneous CD is also present (*arrowheads*).

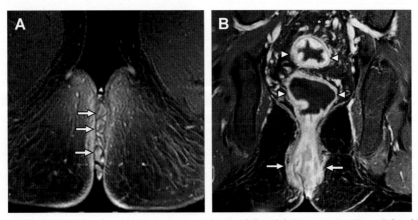

Fig. 20. A 13-year-old girl with CD and worsening rectal pain. (*A*) Axial postcontrast T1-weighted 3D-SPGR fat-saturated image shows a large, lobular mass–like structure in the intergluteal cleft (*arrows*), consistent with a skin tag. (*B*) Coronal postcontrast T1-weighted 3D-SPGR fat-saturated image demonstrates rectal wall thickening and hyperenhancement caused by active proctitis (*arrowheads*). Perirectal fat and vascularity are both increased. Complex perianal fistulous disease with several small abscesses is also noted (*arrows*).

signal hyperintensity), and skin postcontrast hyperenhancement (see **Figs. 6, 7,** and **11; Figs. 18** and **19**).[7] Perianal skin tags, which are highly associated with CD (opposed to ulcerative colitis) in the setting of IBD, are commonly seen on MR imaging, although small skin tags may go unrecognized. These skin tags are typically clinically apparent on physical examination, and appear as oval-shaped, enhancing, lobular mass–like structures arising from perianal skin and residing in the intergluteal cleft on MR imaging (see **Figs. 11** and **18; Fig. 20**).[30,31]

SUMMARY

Perineal involvement is common in pediatric CD. In some instances, perineal involvement may be discovered before the detection of bowel-wall inflammation. High-resolution, small field-of-view MR imaging of the perineum at a field strength of 3-T excellently depicts perineal inflammation caused by CD in children, including involvement of the perianal, labial, and scrotal regions. MR imaging exquisitely identifies and characterizes numerous forms of perineal CD, including fistulas, abscesses, and skin manifestations. Knowledge of the true extent of perineal CD provided by MR imaging can directly guide optimal medical and surgical management of affected patients. Perineal surgery performed following MR imaging results in improved outcomes, including fewer recurrent fistulas and lower risk of bowel incontinence.

ACKNOWLEDGMENTS

The authors thank Leslie Burrell of the University of Michigan Medical School for the medical illustrations used in this article.

REFERENCES

1. Diefenbach KA, Breuer CK. Pediatric inflammatory bowel disease. World J Gastroenterol 2006;12(20): 3204–12.
2. Hyams JS. Crohn's disease in children. Pediatr Clin North Am 1996;43(1):255–77.
3. Essary B, Kim J, Anupindi S, et al. Pelvic MRI in children with Crohn disease and suspected perianal involvement. Pediatr Radiol 2007;37(2):201–8.
4. Markowitz J, Daum F, Aiges H, et al. Perianal disease in children and adolescents with Crohn's disease. Gastroenterology 1984;86(5 Pt 1):829–33.
5. Tolia V. Perianal Crohn's disease in children and adolescents. Am J Gastroenterol 1996;91(5):922–6.
6. Horsthuis K, Lavini C, Bipat S, et al. Perianal Crohn disease: evaluation of dynamic contrast-enhanced MR imaging as an indicator of disease activity. Radiology 2009;251(2):380–7.
7. Pai D, Dillman JR, Mahani MG, et al. MRI of vulvar Crohn disease. Pediatr Radiol 2011;41(4):537–41.
8. Pinna AL, Atzori L, Ferreli C, et al. Cutaneous Crohn disease in a child. Pediatr Dermatol 2006; 23(1):49–52.
9. Corbett SL, Walsh CM, Spitzer RF, et al. Vulvar inflammation as the only clinical manifestation of Crohn disease in an 8-year-old girl. Pediatrics 2010;125(6):e1518–22.
10. Morris J, Spencer JA, Ambrose NS. MR imaging classification of perianal fistulas and its implications for patient management. Radiographics 2000;20(3): 623–35 [discussion: 635–7].
11. Szurowska E, Wypych J, Izycka-Swieszewska E. Perianal fistulas in Crohn's disease: MRI diagnosis and surgical planning: MRI in fistulizing perianal Crohn's disease. Abdom Imaging 2007;32(6): 705–18.
12. O'Malley RB, Al-Hawary MM, Kaza RK, et al. Rectal imaging: part 2, Perianal fistula evaluation on pelvic MRI—what the radiologist needs to know. AJR Am J Roentgenol 2012;199(1):W43–53.
13. Parks AG. Pathogenesis and treatment of fistula-in-ano. Br Med J 1961;1(5224):463–9.
14. Parks AG, Gordon PH, Hardcastle JD. A classification of fistula-in-ano. Br J Surg 1976;63(1):1–12.
15. Bartram C, Buchanan G. Imaging anal fistula. Radiol Clin North Am 2003;41(2):443–57.
16. Irvine EJ. Usual therapy improves perianal Crohn's disease as measured by a new disease activity index. McMaster IBD Study Group. J Clin Gastroenterol 1995;20(1):27–32.
17. Gage KL, Deshmukh S, Macura KJ, et al. MRI of perianal fistulas: bridging the radiological-surgical divide. Abdom Imaging 2012. [Epub ahead of print].
18. Kuijpers HC, Schulpen T. Fistulography for fistula-in-ano. Is it useful? Dis Colon Rectum 1985;28(2): 103–4.
19. Maconi G, Ardizzone S, Greco S, et al. Transperineal ultrasound in the detection of perianal and rectovaginal fistulae in Crohn's disease. Am J Gastroenterol 2007;102(10):2214–9.
20. Choen S, Burnett S, Bartram CI, et al. Comparison between anal endosonography and digital examination in the evaluation of anal fistulae. Br J Surg 1991; 78(4):445–7.
21. Choi JY, Kim MJ, Chung YE, et al. Abdominal applications of 3.0-T MR imaging: comparative review versus a 1.5-T system. Radiographics 2008; 28(4):e30.
22. Erturk SM, Alberich-Bayarri A, Herrmann KA, et al. Use of 3.0-T MR imaging for evaluation of the abdomen. Radiographics 2009;29(6):1547–63.
23. Beets-Tan RG, Beets GL, van der Hoop AG, et al. Preoperative MR imaging of anal fistulas: does it

really help the surgeon? Radiology 2001;218(1): 75–84.

24. Buchanan GN, Halligan S, Bartram CI, et al. Clinical examination, endosonography, and MR imaging in preoperative assessment of fistula in ano: comparison with outcome-based reference standard. Radiology 2004;233(3):674–81.

25. Halligan S, Buchanan G. MR imaging of fistula-in-ano. Eur J Radiol 2003;47(2):98–107.

26. Villa C, Pompili G, Franceschelli G, et al. Role of magnetic resonance imaging in evaluation of the activity of perianal Crohn's disease. Eur J Radiol 2012; 81(4):616–22.

27. Hori M, Oto A, Orrin S, et al. Diffusion-weighted MRI: a new tool for the diagnosis of fistula in ano. J Magn Reson Imaging 2009;30(5):1021–6.

28. Savoye-Collet C, Savoye G, Koning E, et al. Fistulizing perianal Crohn's disease: contrast-enhanced magnetic resonance imaging assessment at 1 year on maintenance anti-TNF-alpha therapy. Inflamm Bowel Dis 2011;17(8):1751–8.

29. Ziech ML, Lavini C, Bipat S, et al. Dynamic contrast-enhanced MRI in determining disease activity in perianal fistulizing Crohn disease: a pilot study. AJR Am J Roentgenol 2013;200(2):W170–7.

30. Bonheur JL, Braunstein J, Korelitz BI, et al. Anal skin tags in inflammatory bowel disease: new observations and a clinical review. Inflamm Bowel Dis 2008;14(9):1236–9.

31. Korelitz BI. Anal skin tags: an overlooked indicator of Crohn's disease. J Clin Gastroenterol 2010;44(2): 151–2.

Advanced Techniques in Pediatric Abdominopelvic Oncologic Magnetic Resonance Imaging

Ethan A. Smith, MD

KEYWORDS

- Oncology • Malignancy • PET-MR imaging • Whole-body imaging
- Dynamic contrast enhancement • Children

KEY POINTS

- The use of magnetic resonance imaging (MRI) in the setting of pediatric abdominopelvic malignancy is increasing because of concerns regarding ionizing radiation exposure, superior contrast resolution compared with computed tomography (CT), and recent technical advances.
- Many ongoing oncologic clinical trials now incorporate MR imaging in their protocols as an alternative to CT imaging.
- Advanced MR imaging techniques, such as diffusion-weighted imaging, dynamic contrast–enhanced imaging (MR imaging perfusion), and ^{18}F-fluorodeoxyglucose positron emission tomography MR imaging, provide functional assessment of abdominopelvic tumors in addition to morphologic information.
- Whole-body (WB) MR imaging has been shown to be useful in staging and surveillance of pediatric malignancy without the use of ionizing radiation, as is required for other currently used WB imaging techniques. The major disadvantage of WB-MR imaging is its lack of specificity compared with more targeted imaging strategies, such as metaiodobenzylguanidine (MIBG) scanning in neuroblastoma.
- Major weaknesses of MR imaging in pediatric oncologic imaging include difficulty evaluating the lung parenchyma for metastatic disease and detection of calcification within tumors.

INTRODUCTION

Magnetic resonance imaging (MRI) is firmly established as a useful imaging technique in pediatric patients. However, MRI use has lagged behind the use of computed tomography (CT) in pediatric abdominopelvic oncology because of a variety of factors, including issues related to cancer research protocols, concerns about the sensitivity of MR imaging, and a general lack of awareness among clinical providers as to the feasibility and advantages of current MR imaging techniques.

As abdominopelvic MRI has become more widely available, pulse sequences have become faster and more robust, and image quality has improved, the use of MRI in pediatric oncologic imaging has increased. This growth in MRI use in most instances has been as an alternative to CT imaging for morphologic evaluation, although recent technologic advances now allow functional assessment of abdominopelvic tumors as well.

This article focuses on advanced MRI techniques currently being clinically used or investigated in pediatric abdominopelvic oncologic imaging. A range

Section of Pediatric Radiology, Department of Radiology, C.S. Mott Children's Hospital, University of Michigan Health System, 1540 E. Hospital Dr., SPC 4252, Ann Arbor, MI 48109-4252, USA
E-mail address: ethans@med.umich.edu

Magn Reson Imaging Clin N Am 21 (2013) 829–841
http://dx.doi.org/10.1016/j.mric.2013.06.002
1064-9689/13/$ – see front matter © 2013 Elsevier Inc. All rights reserved.

of different techniques, including diffusion-weighted imaging (DWI), dynamic contrast-enhanced (DCE) MRI, whole-body (WB) MR imaging, and ^{18}F-fluoro-deoxyglucose (^{18}F-FDG) positron emission tomography MR (PET-MRI) imaging, are discussed. In addition, the increasing acceptance of MRI in pediatric cancer research protocols and a brief discussion of specific issues related to performing MR imaging in children, such as sedation, are addressed.

PROTOCOL AND PATIENT ISSUES

A standardized, but flexible, MRI protocol for abdominopelvic tumor imaging is important for success in pediatric oncology imaging. Standardization of the protocol, including standardized pulse sequence parameters and imaging planes, allows for signal intensity and size measurements that can be used for characterization of the lesion(s) at the time of initial diagnosis and for assessing treatment response on follow-up imaging. A large number of pediatric oncology patients, especially those with solid tumors, are formally treated and followed after therapy using specific protocols, often through the Children's Oncology Group (COG). Having a standardized, reproducible protocol is important in these patients because imaging findings commonly determine patient eligibility for clinical trials and changes in lesions over time directly affect patient treatment and follow-up decisions. Fortunately, most COG protocols are straightforward and commonly used clinical pediatric abdominopelvic MR imaging protocols often fulfill necessary imaging requirements. Our institutional routine clinical abdominopelvic mass MRI protocol is presented in **Table 1**.

MRI protocols can be altered in order to optimize evaluation depending on the clinical setting and suspected tumor type. For example, in the setting of a known or suspected primary liver neoplasm, we routinely perform dynamic postcontrast MR imaging through the liver, including arterial phase imaging. In this clinical situation we also routinely administer a hepatocyte-specific contrast agent (gadoxetate disodium; Eovist, Bayer HealthCare, Wayne, NJ) and acquire additional delayed hepatocyte phase imaging at 10 and 20 minutes following injection. Tailoring the MRI protocol to the tumor or organ of interest often provides added information, while maintaining the ability to perform routine assessments of signal intensity and size.

The use of sedation and general anesthesia is commonplace in young children undergoing abdominopelvic MRI for the assessment of suspected or known malignancy, because of several factors. Most young children are unable to remain sufficiently motionless for MRI, because imaging times are commonly in the 30 to 60 minute range. In addition, young children often have difficulty cooperating with breath-holding instructions. The physical appearance of the MRI scanner and the noises produced during imaging may also be frightening to some children, making cooperation even less likely.[1] To this end, the use of ear plugs, noise-cancelling headphones, and distraction devices (eg, music headphones, movie goggles) may be helpful, especially in school-aged children.[2] Preprocedure preparation with play therapy and other strategies have also been shown to be effective in reducing the need for general anesthesia.[1,3] Imaging studies performed under general anesthesia have been shown to require longer recovery times and are more costly than those performed without general anesthesia.[1] Some studies have shown that repeated exposure to general anesthetics may be associated with negative long-term cognitive effects, although others studies have not found such an association.[4,5] When deciding between the use of nonsedated CT and MRI performed under sedation or general anesthesia, the advantages and disadvantages of both modalities should be carefully considered, including the potential harmful effects of both ionizing radiation and general anesthesia.

DIFFUSION-WEIGHTED IMAGING

DWI uses the motion of water molecules to provide image contrast and to characterize tissues. The motion of water molecules in a glass of water is random (Brownian motion), whereas in biological tissues this random motion can be impeded (or restricted), primarily by cell membranes.[6] The first widespread clinical use of DWI was in neuroimaging, specifically stroke imaging, because the cellular swelling that accompanies acute infarction (cytotoxic edema) results in restricted water motion and signal hyperintensity. DWI is now being evaluated as an oncologic imaging biomarker for distinguishing benign from malignant lesions and for evaluating response to therapy, including in the setting of pediatric abdominopelvic malignancy. The increased cellularity of many malignant tumors compared with normal tissues impedes the motion of water and presents as restricted diffusion (signal hyperintensity) on DWI.[7] In current clinical practice, DWI sequences (with higher b values) are used for qualitative assessment, because tumors and abnormal lymph nodes are usually

Table 1
Abdominopelvic mass MR imaging protocol at 1.5 T

	T1W TSE	T2W TSE	T2W SSFSE	T2W TSE	DWI EPI	T1W In-phase FFE	T1W 3D FFE Precontrast	T1W 3D FFE Postcontrast
Plane	Coronal	Coronal	Coronal	Axial	Axial	Axial	Axial	3 planes
Slice thickness	5	5	5	5	6	5	2-3	2-3
TR (ms)	554	Shortest	Shortest	Shortest	Shortest	Shortest	Shortest	Shortest
TE (ms)	4.6	80	80	80	Shortest	4.6	Shortest	Shortest
Respiratory compensation	None	Trigger	Trigger	Trigger	Trigger	Breath hold	Breath hold	Breath hold
NSA	4	2	1	2	3	1	1	1
Fat saturation	N	Y	N	Y	Y	N	Y	Y
b values	—	—	—	—	0, 100, 750	—	—	—

Shortest means the shortest time required as determined by scanner.
Abbreviations: 3D, three-dimensional; EPI, echo planar imaging; FFE, fast field echo; Free, free breathing; IR, inversion recovery; NSA, number of signal averages; SSFSE, single-shot fast spin-echo; STIR, Short tau inversion recovery; T1W, T1 weighted; T2W, T2 weighted; TE, echo time; TR, repetition time; Trigger, respiratory triggered; TSE, turbo spin-echo.

hyperintense relative to the background, allowing increased sensitivity (**Fig. 1**). The degree of restricted diffusion can be quantified by performing DWI with multiple b values and calculating a map of apparent diffusion coefficient (ADC) values (**Fig. 2**). The number of b values required (eg, 2, 3, 4 or more) as well as their absolute values (0 to greater than 1000 m/s²) have yet to be established

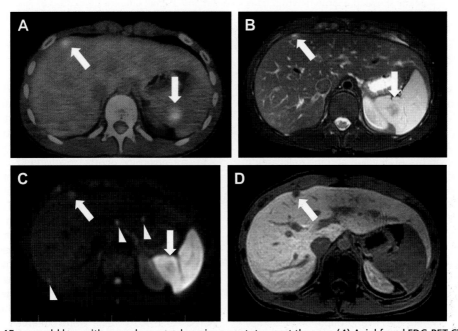

Fig. 1. A 15 -year-old boy with nasopharyngeal carcinoma, status post therapy. (*A*) Axial fused FDG-PET-CT images show focal, abnormal hypermetabolism in the spleen and liver (*arrows*). (*B*) Axial T2W fat-saturated MR image showing focal lesions in the liver and spleen (*arrows*) corresponding with the PET avid lesions. (*C*) Axial DWI (b = 800) shows hyperintense signal corresponding with the liver lesion (*arrow*). Several additional lesions are also present in the liver, none of which were visible on the other sequences or PET-CT (*arrowheads*). The splenic lesion is relatively hypointense relative to the normally hyperintense spleen (*arrow*). (*D*) Axial T1W spoiled gradient recalled echo (SPGR) 20 minutes after intravenous administration of gadoxetate disodium (Eovist) shows hypointensity of the larger liver lesion, consistent with a metastasis (*arrow*).

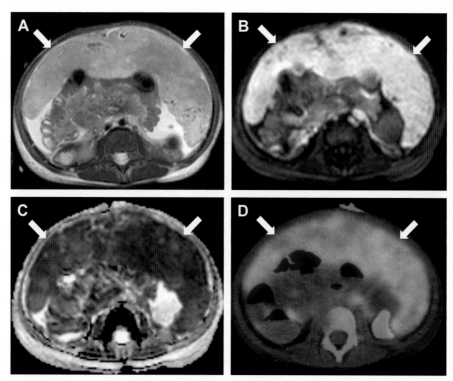

Fig. 2. A 5-year-old girl with abdominal distention caused by Burkitt lymphoma. The patient underwent MR imaging because of suspected peritoneal and omental masses based on initial ultrasound imaging. (*A*) Axial T2W fat-suppressed image showing a large omental mass (*arrows*) and a small amount of ascites. (*B*) Axial diffusion-weighted image (b = 750) shows a large omental mass that appears hyperintense because of restricted diffusion (*arrows*). (*C*) The mass appears hypointense on the corresponding ADC image (*arrows*), confirming restricted diffusion. (*D*) Axial fused ^{18}F-FDG-PET-CT image performed the following day confirms that the large omental mass is hypermetabolic (*arrows*).

for accurate, reproducible ADC calculation in pediatric oncologic imaging.

Humphries and colleagues[8] evaluated ADC values in 19 children with extracranial soft tissue masses. Although they found an inverse relationship between the ADC value and the cellularity of tissues on histopathology, there was no significant difference between benign and malignant lesions, and their final conclusion was that ADC value alone could not accurately distinguish between benign and malignant tumors. Contradictory results were observed in a study performed by Kocaoglu and colleagues,[7] who found that significantly lower ADC values were observed with malignant lesions in a group of 31 pediatric abdominal masses (15 benign, 16 malignant), although there was some overlap between the two groups. Interestingly, these studies used different methods for determining the region of interest for calculation of the mean ADC values.[7,8] More recently, Gahr and colleagues[9] retrospectively evaluated 19 pediatric neurogenic tumors and found a significant difference between the ADC values of neuroblastoma and ganglioneuroblastoma/ganglioneuroma. Their

conclusion was that neuroblastoma could be differentiated from the other less aggressive neurogenic tumors based on ADC values, and that the lower ADC values observed in neuroblastoma were caused by the greater cellularity of this neoplasm.

In a feasibility study involving 7 pediatric oncology patients with 9 tumors, McDonald and colleagues[10] analyzed ADC values before and after completion of chemotherapy. The ADC values of all tumors changed following chemotherapy, with an increase in the median ADC values seen in most lesions. The increased ADC value (indicating less impeded diffusion and less hyperintense signal on DWI images) was thought to represent decreased cellularity of the tumor, thus representing treatment response. The largest increases in ADC value were observed in those tumors that showed the greatest response to therapy on histopathologic evaluation (**Fig. 3**).

WB-DWI has recently become available on state-of-the-art MR imaging scanners. This technique can be used to complement standard oncologic MR imaging protocols or WB-MR imaging examinations, increasing the conspicuity of small

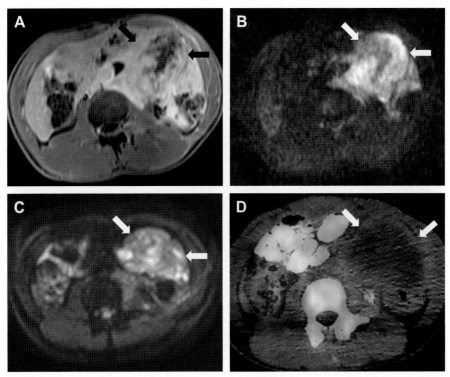

Fig. 3. A 15 year-old boy with recurrent rhabdomyosarcoma. (*A*) Axial T1-weighted postcontrast image shows a heterogeneously enhancing left-sided abdominal mass (*arrows*). (*B*) Axial diffusion-weighted image (b = 800, 1.5-T) at the same level shows increased signal within the mass (*arrows*), consistent with restricted diffusion. (*C*) Axial diffusion-weighted image (3-T) after chemotherapy shows slightly decreased size of the mass. The mass also appears less hyperintense and more heterogeneous (*arrows*). (*D*) Axial fused ^{18}F-FDG-PET-CT image performed the same day shows only a peripheral rim of ^{18}F-FDG avidity (*arrows*). Most of the mass is hypometabolic because of presumed treatment effect. Subsequent surgical resection of the mass and histopathologic evaluation showed that approximately 90% of the mass was necrotic.

lesions and possibly examination sensitivity.[11] WB-DWI can now be performed in a reasonable amount of time (20–30 minutes).[12] WB-DWI is performed using a floating table technique, similar to other WB-MR imaging techniques (such as MR angiography), and a high b value is generally chosen (eg, 800–1000 m/s²) in order to maximally suppress nonpathologic background signal from the body. One WB-DWI technique that can be performed with the patient free breathing is called DWI with background body suppression (DWIBS).[13] Acquired gray-scale images can then be inverted to resemble ^{18}F-FDG-PET images, and three-dimensional (3D) maximum intensity projections can be created to allow assessment of the entire body on a single image (**Figs. 4** and **5**).[13] Kwee and colleagues[14] compared WB-MR imaging, WB-DWI, and standard CT in the staging of lymphoma and found that a combination of WB-MR imaging and WB-DWI increased the stage at initial diagnosis of 4 of 28 patients compared with CT.

WHOLE-BODY MAGNETIC RESONANCE IMAGING

WB-MR imaging can be used to evaluate for sites of neoplasm remote from the primary tumor for staging purposes as well as to screen patients determined to be at increased risk for malignancy because of certain genetic abnormalities (eg, Li-Fraumeni syndrome). Commonly used techniques for WB (or near-WB) imaging in the setting of malignancy include radiographic skeletal surveys, CT, and a variety of nuclear medicine studies, such as technetium-99 m methylene diphosphonate (Tc-99 m MDP) bone, octreotide, metaiodobenzylguanidine (MIBG), and ^{18}F-FDG-PET scans, all of which have the disadvantage of using ionizing radiation. Several studies have shown that WB-MR imaging is useful for detecting both skeletal and extraskeletal metastases in pediatric patients.[15–18] WBMR imaging can be performed as a stand-alone examination, or WB sequences can be added to other standard MR

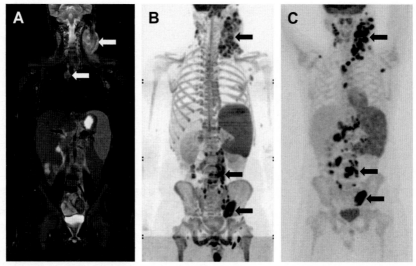

Fig. 4. A 12-year-old boy with B-cell non-Hodgkin lymphoma. (*A*) Coronal WB STIR image shows enlarged, hyperintense cervical and mediastinal lymph nodes (*arrows*). The spleen is enlarged. (*B*) 3D maximum intensity projection WB DWIBS shows widespread cervical, thoracic, and abdominopelvic pathologic lymphadenopathy (*arrows*). The spleen is enlarged and restricts diffusion. (*C*) 3D maximum intensity projection ^{18}F-FDG-PET image obtained after MR imaging and before treatment also shows widespread pathologic lymphadenopathy (*arrows*). The spleen is enlarged and hypermetabolic. The DWIBS shows a decreased number of abnormal mediastinal lymph nodes compared with the ^{18}F-FDG-PET image, in part secondary to obscuration by the overlying the spine. (*Courtesy of* Drs Thomas Kwee and Annemieke Littooij, Utrecht, Netherlands.)

protocols used to stage and follow-up pediatric oncology patients.[17,19,20]

Several advances in technology have made WB-MR imaging feasible when using state-of-the-art scanners, including floating table capabilities, improved body coils (both integrated into the scanner and surface coils), and faster imaging techniques.[20] The most commonly used pulse sequence in WB-MR imaging is short tau inversion recovery (STIR), chosen because of its

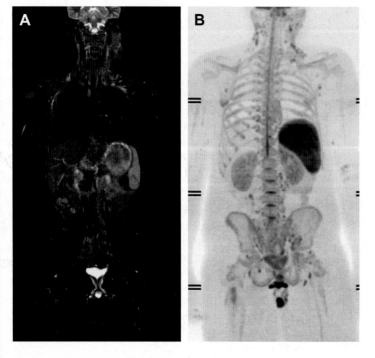

Fig. 5. A 12-year-old boy with B-cell non-Hodgkin lymphoma (same patient as in **Fig. 4**). Posttreatment WB short tau inversion recovery (STIR) image (*A*) and 3D maximum intensity reconstructed WB DWIBS (*B*) both show significant treatment response, with decreased size and number of abnormal lymph nodes. The spleen remains mildly enlarged. (*Courtesy of* Drs Thomas Kwee and Annemieke Littooij, Utrecht, Netherlands.)

sensitivity to signal from fluid (including edema, inflammation, and masses with substantial water content), relative resiliency to artifacts, and homogeneous fat saturation.[20–22] This pulse sequence takes advantage of the fact that most pathological tissues in the human body cause T2 prolongation causing conspicuous signal hyperintensity.[18,20,22] Additional pulse sequences that have been used for WB-MR imaging include T1-weighted fast spin-echo (FSE) without fat saturation (primarily used for evaluation of bone marrow), two-dimensional balanced steady-state free precession, T2-weighted single-shot FSE (SSFSE), and postcontrast 3D gradient recalled echo imaging.[20] Most investigators advocate imaging in the coronal plane because of the smaller number of images required to cover the body (compared with the axial and sagittal planes), although some also perform additional sagittal imaging to increase sensitivity for lesion detection, especially in the spine, ribs, and sternum (**Fig. 6**).[18,20,22] WB-MR imaging generally is not performed in the axial plane because of the large number of images and amount of time required to cover the body.[22]

Multiple prior investigations have examined the usefulness of WB-MR imaging in the work-up of both adult and pediatric oncology patients. Solid tumors, such as neuroblastoma and other tumors that have a propensity for osseous metastases, have been most widely studied. The staging of lymphoma has been studied as well. In addition, WB-MR imaging has been evaluated as a screening tool for patients with certain genetic familial cancer syndromes, in some nonneoplastic conditions (eg, Langerhans cell histiocytosis), and

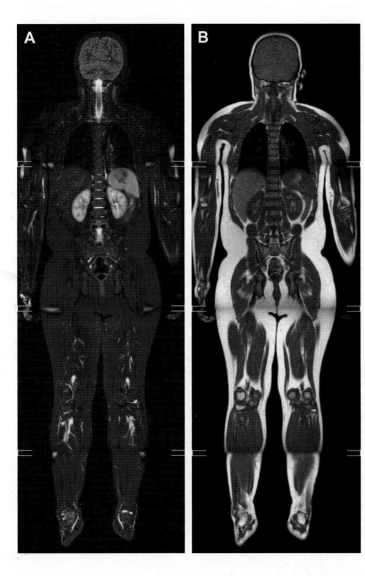

Fig. 6. WB-MR imaging examination in a 9-year-old girl with Li-Fraumeni syndrome and history of rhabdomyosarcoma. Coronal STIR (*A*) and T1-weighted turbo spin-echo (*B*) images show portions of brain, lungs, abdominopelvic viscera, spine, and extremities. No abnormalities are seen.

in certain clinical presentations of suspected infection.[20]

In a pilot study in 2002, Mazumder and colleagues[16] found that coronal STIR WB-MR imaging performed similarly to standard WB imaging techniques in the metastatic work-up in a small group of pediatric patients with small round cell malignancies. Laffan and colleagues[17] added coronal and sagittal STIR WB imaging to a group of 10 pediatric patients with suspected malignancy, but in whom a pathologic diagnosis was not known. They found distant sites of neoplasm in 8 of 10 patients and concluded that WB-MR imaging may be useful in the initial work-up of suspected malignancy.[17] Goo[19] found that WB-MR imaging was more sensitive than both Tc-99 m MDP bone scan and MIBG in a group of patients with neuroblastoma, although the positive predictive value of WB-MR imaging for metastasis was less than that of MIBG. However, this study was limited by the lack of a standardized WB-MR imaging protocol. More recently, in a large multi-institutional study sponsored by the American College of Radiology Imaging Network (ACRIN) evaluating WB-MR imaging in pediatric patients with known malignancy, Seigel and colleagues[23] were unable to show noninferiority criteria for accuracy of WB-MR imaging compared with conventional imaging methods when evaluating a combination of lymphoma, neuroblastoma, and soft tissue sarcoma. This study did find that, if lymphoma was excluded from the analysis, the diagnostic accuracy of WB-MR imaging was improved, and that it performed better than conventional imaging in the evaluation of osseous metastatic disease.[23]

WB-MR imaging does have known limitations. The most important limitation of this technique is its reduced specificity compared with more targeted imaging strategies, such as MIBG scanning in neuroblastoma. A variety of nonneoplastic processes can cause hyperintense signal on STIR images and may be confused with metastatic neoplasm, including benign infectious and inflammatory processes.[20,21] Normal red marrow shows mildly hyperintense signal on STIR images and mildly hypointense signal on T1-weighted images, and potentially can be confused for a pathologic lesion if the reader is not familiar with this appearance. Large amounts of red marrow can be present in young pediatric patients, in patients receiving certain hematopoietic medications (eg, granulocyte-macrophage colony stimulating factor), and in patients undergoing red marrow reconversion as a response to prior chemotherapy.[21] Compared with CT, both standard MR imaging and WB-MR imaging have decreased sensitivity

for detecting lung parenchymal abnormalities, including lung nodules.[24] Both normal and pathologic lymph nodes are hyperintense on STIR imaging, which means that, unlike ^{18}F-FDG-PET in which hypermetabolism is used as the primary criterion for detecting abnormal lymph nodes, the diagnosis of abnormal lymph nodes on WB-MR imaging still depends on morphology and imaging size criteria.[21] Tumoral calcifications, such as those frequently encountered in patients with neuroblastoma, often appear hypointense on both T1-weighted and STIR images, sometimes making them difficult to visualize on WB-MR imaging.[19] In addition, given the large fields of view and section thicknesses (several millimeters) used to accomplish WB-MR imaging, the sensitivity for detecting very small lesions (ie, less than 1 cm in diameter) may be diminished compared with standard MR imaging (particularly in the absence of simultaneous WB-DWI).[20,21]

DYNAMIC CONTRAST-ENHANCED MAGNETIC RESONANCE IMAGING

DCE-MRI describes a group of techniques that attempt to assess angiogenesis and perfusion in order to characterize the microvascular environment of tumors. Malignant neoplasms have been shown to have disorganized, functionally abnormal vasculature compared with normal tissues, thought to be in part secondary to an imbalance of angiogenic factors.[25] Initial studies in breast carcinoma revealed that permeability of contrast agents within malignant neoplasms is altered compared with normal tissues because of relative microvascular disorganization within the tumor.[26,27] Three different methods using different types of contrast agents have been investigated to exploit the differences in microvasculature between tumors and normal tissues: (1) macromolecular contrast agents (eg, labeled albumin) that take advantage of the increased permeability of tumor vessel basement membranes to allow larger molecules (which would normally be confined to the vascular space) to diffuse into the tumor; (2) contrast agents designed to pool at sites of angiogenesis; and (3) low-molecular-weight contrast agents.[28,29] The remainder of this section focuses on low-molecular-weight gadolinium-based contrast agents, because these are widely available and currently in use in clinical practice.

The kinetic properties of low-molecular-weight gadolinium-based contrast agents primarily depend on 3 factors: tissue perfusion, vessel wall permeability, and the rate of diffusion.[28] Tissue perfusion determines how much of the contrast agent is delivered to the tumor and depends on blood flow. Once the contrast agent arrives at the tissue, the bolus is initially confined within the vascular space, with a variable amount rapidly passing into the extravascular space. Because low-molecular-weight contrast agents do not cross cell membranes and enter cells, the site of distribution is most accurately defined as the extracellular extravascular space (EES), or v_e.[28,30] The rate of contrast passage into this space is influenced by multiple factors, including tissue perfusion, the permeability of the blood vessels within the tissue, and the surface area available.[28,31-33] These factors are described by the transfer constant, or K^{trans}, for a tissue.[30] A third variable, the rate constant, or k_{ep}, describes the flux of contrast agent between the EES (v_e) and the vascular space, and is proportional to the transfer constant (k_{ep} = K^{trans}/v_e) (**Table 2**).[30] As the intravascular volume of contrast agent is depleted (both by distribution and excretion), contrast agent begins to diffuse from the EES back into the vasculature and eventually is excreted from the body (primarily through the kidneys, and possibly the liver, depending on the contrast agent). This washout of contrast agent may be accelerated if the permeability of a tissue's vasculature is increased.[28]

DCE-MRI has been most extensively studied in breast cancer, but has been evaluated in numerous other oncologic (eg, genitourinary and musculoskeletal tumors) and inflammatory conditions (eg, Crohn disease) as well. Although both T1-weighted and T2-weighted imaging can be used for DCE-MR imaging, most studies have focused on T1-weighted imaging, exploiting the T1 shortening that occurs after the intravascular

administration of gadolinium-based contrast agents.[28,34] In pediatric patients, most reports have described the use of DCE-MR imaging in bone tumors, such as osteosarcoma.[35,36] In a series of 31 patients with primary malignant bone tumors, Reddick and colleagues[35] found that k_{ep} after completion of preoperative (neoadjuvant) chemotherapy was a statistically significant predictor of disease-free survival. More recently, Gou and colleagues[36] evaluated a group of 69 patients with nonmetastatic osteosarcoma and found that changes in several of the DCE-MR imaging parameters after preoperative chemotherapy, including K^{trans}, k_{ep}, and v_e, predicted treatment response at histology, event-free survival, and overall survival.[36]

DCE-MRI has been evaluated in several adult abdominopelvic malignancies (including cervical, prostate, and bladder cancers), but has not been widely studied in pediatric abdominopelvic cancer. There are several challenges to performing DCE-MR imaging in the pediatric abdomen. First, DCE-MR imaging techniques require multiple repeated imaging acquisitions of the same volume of tissue. Within the abdomen, movement of the diaphragm and intra-abdominal structures caused by normal respiration as well as motion secondary to bowel peristalsis make reimaging the same volume of tissue difficult.[28] Second, clinical evaluation of several abdominal tumors benefits from characterization that is achieved through imaging an organ (or even the abdomen and/or pelvis) using multiple specific phases of contrast enhancement (eg, evaluation of pediatric hepatocellular carcinoma or other arterially hyperenhancing tumors). Performance of quantitative DCE-MRI may preclude such an evaluation, unless standard postcontrast imaging is performed after DCE-MRI using a second bolus of contrast agent. However, despite these difficulties, DCE-MRI with formal calculation of perfusion parameters is possible in children with abdominopelvic malignancies and may eventually be incorporated in future clinical trials (**Fig. 7**). The knowledge gained by DCE-MRI may provide novel imaging biomarkers for establishing benign from malignant tumors, response to medical therapy, and possibly prognosis at the time of initial diagnosis.

POSITRON EMISSION TOMOGRAPHY MAGNETIC RESONANCE IMAGING

The use of fused functional and anatomic imaging in the form of PET-CT and single-photon emission SPECT-CT have become cornerstones of oncologic imaging over the past decade in both

Table 2
Definitions of kinetic factors commonly used in dynamic contrast-enhanced MR imaging

	Name	Units	Definition
K^{trans}	Transfer constant	min^{-1}	Volume transfer constant between blood plasma and EES
k_{ep}	Rate constant	min^{-1}	Rate constant between EES and plasma volume
v_e	EES	none	Volume of extracellular, extravascular space per unit of tissue

Adapted from Tofts PS, Brix G, Buckley DL, et al. Estimating kinetic parameters from dynamic contrast-enhanced T1-weighted MRI of a diffusible tracer: Standardized quantities and symbols. J Magn Reson Imaging 1999;10:223–32.

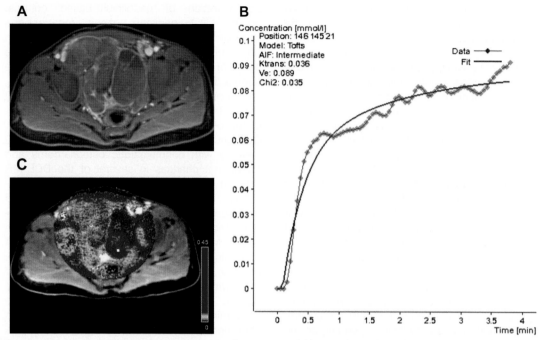

Fig. 7. Dynamic contrast-enhanced MR imaging in a 3 -year-old boy with a pelvic mass. (*A*) Free-breathing radial acquisition was performed continuously over 4 minutes during contrast injection. High temporal resolution data (less than 3 seconds) was reconstructed from small number of contiguous spokes (n = 8) with use of compressed sensing technique called Golden-angle RAdial Sparse Parallel (GRASP). The signal intensity time curve was fitted (*B*) with the generalized kinetic model to obtain K^{trans} (*C*). The pharmacokinetic modeling was performed using Siemens software Tissue 4D. Population arterial input function was used. (*Courtesy of* Dr Hersch Chandrana, New York, NY.)

children and adults. In the past, functional imaging, including metabolic imaging with ^{18}F-FDG-PET, and anatomic imaging with MR had to be performed in 2 different settings, and then images most often were fused manually or reviewed side by side. Such preliminary forms of PET-MRI were limited primarily to brain imaging, because the rigid skull and fixed landmarks made accurate fusion possible. Fusion of nonbrain PET and MR images, including abdominopelvic images, was more difficult because of a variety of physiologic and anatomic factors.[37] Techniques that obtain anatomic MR images in the same setting as PET images have recently become commercially available, creating the possibility of accurate, reliable image fusion (**Fig. 8** and **9**).

At present, there are 2 different paradigms available for PET-MR imaging. Sequential models use separate PET and MR scanners placed in sequence. The two scanners are physically separate, and the patient (on the imaging table) must be moved between the PET scanner and the MR imaging scanner. The main advantage of this technique is that the technology is less complex and is therefore less expensive. The second paradigm

involves integration of the PET and MR imaging into a single imaging unit, eliminating the need to move the patient sequentially between scanners. Although more expensive and technically complex, the main advantage of this technique is improved accuracy of fusion images, because the patient does not have to be physically moved between scanners, decreasing the risk of patient movement and misregistration.

There are several potential advantages to using fused PET-MR imaging as opposed to fused PET-CT in pediatric oncology patients. First, the inherent soft tissue contrast resolution of MR imaging is superior to both unenhanced and contrast-enhanced CT. A second advantage is that, because of its ability to perform DWI, multiphase postcontrast imaging, and imaging with unique intravascular contrast agents, such as gadoxetate disodium (Eovist; Bayer HealthCare), MR imaging can add considerably to the physiologic characterization of tissues. A final key advantage of PET-MR imaging in the pediatric population is that the MRI portion of the examination does not require ionizing radiation, unlike the CT portion of PET-CT. Although there is still exposure to ionizing radiation

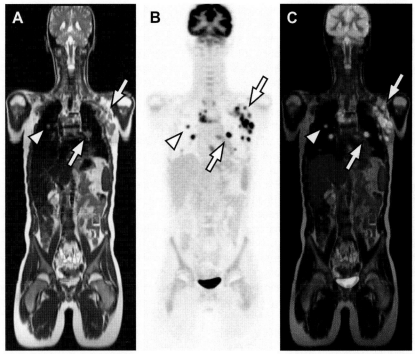

Fig. 8. PET-MR imaging in a 15 -year-old boy with relapsed Hodgkin disease. (*A*) Coronal T2W SSFSE images show enlarged left axillary and hilar lymph nodes (*arrows*) as well as pulmonary nodules (*arrowhead*). (*B*) Coronal maximum intensity projection PET image and (*C*) fused PET-MR images both show corresponding abnormal FDG uptake within the lymph nodes (*arrows*) and pulmonary nodules (*arrowhead*). (*Courtesy of* Dr Geetika Khanna, St Louis, MO.)

because of the PET portion of the MR-PET examination, the total dose of imparted radiation is less than with PET-CT. Disadvantages of fused PET-MR imaging include the decreased MR imaging sensitivity for detection of lung nodules and calcifications compared with CT as well as likely increased expense.[37,38] Another disadvantage of PET-MR imaging is that many nuclear medicine

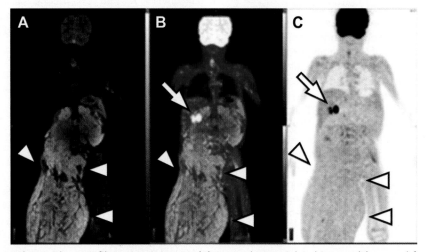

Fig. 9. Teenage boy with neurofibromatosis type 1. (*A*) Coronal T2 weighted image, (*B*) coronal fused PET-MRI, and (*C*) PET maximum intensity projection image demonstrate an extensive plexiform neurofibroma involving the abdomen, pelvis and right lower extremity (*arrowheads*), with minimal FDG uptake. A focal bilobed area of hypermetabolism (*arrow*) is present. This was considered suspicious, but not diagnostic for malignant transformation, and short term follow up was pursued. (*Courtesy of* Dr Sarah Milla and Dr Kent Friedman, MD, NYU Langone Medical Center, New York, NY.)

physicians who currently interpret and report PET-CT studies are not trained or comfortable rendering MR imaging interpretations, which may require PET-MR imaging examinations to be reviewed by both a nuclear medicine physician and a radiologist who routinely interprets clinical MRI examinations.

In a review of their early experience with PET-MR imaging in both pediatric and adult oncology patients, Antoch and Bockisch[38] described the potential advantages and disadvantages of this technique in terms of initial tumor staging. For local disease staging for which the functional/metabolic imaging is less valuable, using MR imaging in place of CT has the advantages of increased soft tissue contrast and improved tissue characterization. In terms of lymph node staging, both CT and MR imaging depend on imaging size criteria and are equivalent with regard to anatomic localization.[38] In most instances, both CT and MR imaging are inferior to metabolic imaging using ^{18}F-FDG-PET for lymph node staging. Evaluation for metastatic disease is a more complex issue. MR imaging is more sensitive than CT and may be more sensitive than ^{18}F-FDG-PET for identification of bone marrow and liver metastases, whereas both ^{18}F-FDG-PET and MR imaging have decreased sensitivity compared with CT for the detection of lung metastases.[23,24,38]

SUMMARY

At present, MRI is an important tool in the evaluation of pediatric abdominopelvic oncologic patients. Going forward, MRI will likely play an increasing role in the management of these patients, including those with abdominopelvic malignancies. The ability of MR imaging protocols to be tailored to optimally evaluate specific suspected or known neoplasms and its lack of ionizing radiation are major advantages compared with existing imaging modalities, particularly CT. Advanced MR imaging techniques, including DWI, DCE-MRI, and PET-MRI, provide functional/physiologic assessment of tumors in addition to morphologic information. Although further research into these applications is needed in the pediatric population, such imaging methods will likely keep MRI at the forefront of pediatric abdominopelvic oncologic imaging for years to come.

REFERENCES

1. Edwards AD, Arthurs OJ. Paediatric MRI under sedation: is it necessary? What is the evidence for the alternatives? Pediatr Radiol 2011;41:1353–64.

2. Harned RK, Strain JD. MRI-compatible audio/visual system: impact on pediatric sedation. Pediatr Radiol 2001;31:247–50.

3. Carter AJ, Greer ML, Gray SE, et al. Reducing the need for anaesthesia in children. Pediatr Radiol 2010;40:1368–74.

4. Bartels M, Althoff RR, Boomsma DI. Anesthesia and cognitive performance in children: no evidence for a causal relationship. Twin Res Hum Genet 2009; 12(3):246–53.

5. Flick RP, Kutasic SK, Colligan RC, et al. Cognitive and behavioral outcomes after early exposure to anesthesia and surgery. Pediatrics 2011;128: e1053–61.

6. Hagmann P, Jonasson L, Madaer P, et al. Understanding diffusion MR imaging techniques: from scalar diffusion weighted imaging to diffusion tensor imaging and beyond. Radiographics 2006;26:S205–23.

7. Kocaoglu M, Bulakbasi N, Sanal HT, et al. Pediatric abdominal masses: diagnostic accuracy of diffusion weighted MRI. Magn Reson Imaging 2010; 28:629–36.

8. Humphries PD, Sebire NJ, Siegel MJ, et al. Tumors in pediatric patients at diffusion weighted MR imaging: apparent diffusion coefficient and tumor cellularity. Radiology 2007;245(3):848–54.

9. Gahr N, Darge K, Hahn G, et al. Diffusion-weighted MRI for differentiation of neuroblastoma and ganglioneuroblastoma/ganglioneuroma. Eur J Radiol 2011;79:443–6.

10. McDonald K, Sebire NJ, Anderson J, et al. Patterns of shift in ADC distributions in abdominal tumors during chemotherapy: a feasibility study. Pediatr Radiol 2011;41:99–106.

11. Padhani A, Koh DM, Collins DJ. Whole body diffusion-weighted MR imaging in cancer: current status and research directions. Radiology 2011; 261(3):700–18.

12. Kwee TC, Takahara T, Vermoolen MA, et al. Whole body diffusion-weighted imaging for staging malignant lymphoma in children. Pediatr Radiol 2010;40: 1592–602.

13. Kwee TC, Takahara T, Ochiai R, et al. Diffusion-weighted whole-body imaging with background body signal suppression (DWIBS): features and potential applications in oncology. Eur J Radiol 2008; 18:1937–52.

14. Kwee TC, Quarles van Ufford HM, Beek FJ, et al. Whole-body MRI, including diffusion-weighted imaging, for the initial staging of malignant lymphoma: comparison to computed tomography. Invest Radiol 2009;44:683–90.

15. Daldrup-Link HE, Franzius C, Link TM, et al. Whole-body MR imaging for detection of bone metastases in children and young adults: comparison with skeletal scintigraphy and FDG PET. Am J Roentgenol 2001;177:229–36.

16. Mazumdar A, Siegel MJ, Narra V, et al. Whole-body fast inversion recovery MR imaging of small cell neoplasms in pediatric patients: a pilot study. Am J Roentgenol 2002;179:1261–6.

17. Laffan EE, O'Connor R, Ryan SP, et al. Whole-body magnetic resonance imaging: a useful additional sequence in paediatric imaging. Pediatr Radiol 2004;34:472–80.

18. Goo HW, Choi SH, Ghim T, et al. Whole body MRI of paediatric malignant tumours: comparison with conventional oncologic imaging methods. Pediatr Radiol 2005;35:766–73.

19. Goo HW. Whole body MRI of neuroblastoma. Eur J Radiol 2010;75:306–14.

20. Chavhan GB, Babyn PS. Whole-body MR imaging in children: principles, technique, current applications and future directions. Radiographics 2011;31:1757–72.

21. Kellenberg CJ, Epelman M, Miller SF, et al. Fast STIR whole-body MR imaging in children. Radiographics 2004;24:1317–30.

22. Darge K, Jaramillo D, Siegel MJ. Whole-body MRI in children: current status and future applications. Eur J Radiol 2008;68:289–98.

23. Seigel MJ, Acharyya S, Hoffer FA, et al. Whole body MR imaging for staging of malignant tumors in pediatric patients: results of the American College of Radiology Imaging Network 6660 trial. Radiology 2013;266(2):599–609.

24. Antoch G, Voit FM, Freudenberg LS, et al. Whole-body dual modality PET/CT and whole-body MRI for tumor staging in oncology. JAMA 2003;290(24):3199–206.

25. Carmeliet P, Jain RK. Angiogenesis in cancer and other diseases. Nature 2000;407:249–57.

26. van Dijke C, Brasch R, Roberts T, et al. Mammary carcinoma model: correlation of macromolecular contrast-enhanced MR imaging characterization of tumor microvasculature and histologic capillary density. Radiology 1996;198:813–8.

27. Daldrup H, Shames DN, Wedland M, et al. Correlation of dynamic contrast-enhanced magnetic resonance imaging with histologic tumor grade: comparison of macromolecular and small-molecular contrast media. Pediatr Radiol 1998;28:67–78.

28. Padhani AR. Dynamic contrast-enhanced MRI in clinical oncology: current status and future directions. J Magn Reson Imaging 2002;16:407–22.

29. Padhani AR, Husband JE. Dynamic contrast-enhanced MRI studies in oncology with an emphasis on quantification, validation and human studies. Clin Radiol 2001;56:607–20.

30. Tofts PS, Brix G, Buckley DL, et al. Estimating kinetic parameters from dynamic contrast-enhanced T1-weighted MRI of a diffusible tracer: standardized quantities and symbols. J Magn Reson Imaging 1999;10:223–32.

31. Crone C. The permeability of capillaries in various organs as determined by the use of 'indicator diffusion' method. Acta Physiol Scand 1963;58:292–305.

32. Yuh WT. An exciting and challenging role for the advanced contrast MR imaging. J Magn Reson Imaging 1999;10:221–2.

33. Taylor JS, Reddick WE. Evolution from empirical dynamic contrast-enhanced magnetic resonance imaging to pharmacokinetic MRI. Adv Drug Deliv Rev 2000;41:91–110.

34. Kershaw L, Buckley DL. Precision in measurements of perfusion and microvascular permeability with T1-weighted dynamic contrast enhanced MR. Magn Reson Med 2006;56:986–92.

35. Reddick WE, Wang S, Xlong X, et al. Dynamic magnetic resonance imaging of regional contrast access as an additional prognostic factor in pediatric osteosarcoma. Cancer 2001;91:2230–7.

36. Guo J, Reddick WE, Glass JO, et al. Dynamic contrast-enhanced magnetic resonance imaging as a prognostic factor in predicting event-free and overall survival in pediatric patients with osteosarcoma. Cancer 2012;118:3776–85.

37. Kjaer A, Loft A, Law I, et al. PET MRI in cancer patients: first experiences and vision from Copenhagen. MAGMA 2013;26(1):37–47.

38. Antoch G, Bockisch A. Combined PET/MRI: a new dimension in whole-body oncology imaging? Eur J Nucl Med Mol Imaging 2009;36:S113–20.

Magnetic Resonance Angiography of the Pediatric Abdomen and Pelvis
Techniques and Imaging Findings

Ranjith Vellody, MD[a], Peter S. Liu, MD[a],*,
David M. Sada, MD[b]

KEYWORDS

- MR angiography • Children • Vascular imaging

KEY POINTS

- Magnetic resonance angiography is particularly well suited for pediatric abdominal and pelvic vascular imaging because of its noninvasive nature and lack of ionizing radiation.
- The lack of a gadolinium-based contrast agent approved by the US Food and Drug Administration, contrast dosage restrictions, and the potential difficulty of obtaining reliable venous access render noncontrast magnetic resonance angiography a desirable modality in pediatric patients.
- Contrast-enhanced magnetic resonance imaging provides the ability to evaluate vascular anatomy and disease in multiple phases (ie, arterial, portal venous, and systemic venous phases).
- MR angiography allows for identification of various pathologic conditions and anatomic variants in the arterial, systemic venous, and portal venous systems, precluding, in some cases, the need for gold-standard catheter-based angiography.

INTRODUCTION

Advances in magnetic resonance (MR) scanner technology and pulse sequences have made magnetic resonance angiography (MRA) a clinical reality for pediatric abdominal and pelvic vascular imaging. Compared with computed tomography (CT) techniques for imaging the cardiovascular system, MRA offers several advantages, including native multiplanar capabilities, superior tissue contrast, and noncontrast angiographic imaging.[1] However, it is the lack of ionizing radiation and its noninvasive nature that make MRA such a compelling technique for pediatric use. The first half of this article focuses on the technique of obtaining high-quality MRA and the second half highlights anatomic variants and vascular diseases that can be identified in the arterial, venous, and portal venous systems.

TECHNIQUE
Pediatric MRA Protocol Considerations

There is no single correct methodology for performing MRA in the pediatric patient population. Instead, a menu of different techniques exists for radiologists to optimize angiographic evaluation in order to answer the clinical question. Broadly,

[a] Department of Radiology, University of Michigan Medical Center, 1500 East Medical Center Drive, Ann Arbor, MI 48109, USA; [b] Michael E. DeBakey VA Medical Center, Houston, TX 77030, USA
* Corresponding author.
E-mail address: peterliu@med.umich.edu

Magn Reson Imaging Clin N Am 21 (2013) 843–860
http://dx.doi.org/10.1016/j.mric.2013.07.001
1064-9689/13/$ – see front matter © 2013 Elsevier Inc. All rights reserved.

these techniques can be broken into 2 basic groups: noncontrast sequences and contrast-enhanced (CE) techniques (**Table 1**). The advent of CE-MRA techniques over the past 2 decades has largely replaced traditional noncontrast techniques for imaging most vascular territories.[2] The marked increase in signal provided by gadolinium-based contrast agents (GBCA) allows MRA to be performed rapidly, typically covering a large field of view in a single breath hold. In addition, the high signal obtained using CE-MRA allows for high spatial resolution, which often aids in depiction of subtle vascular wall abnormalities or peripheral vascular branches. Because of the high spatial resolution, a single three-dimensional (3D) data set can be obtained with CE-MRA that allows reconstruction of oblique imaging planes, along with other postprocessing techniques.[3,4] Although the advantages of CE-MRA were recognized early in adult populations, this technique has now also become standard in the pediatric population.[4,5] Nonetheless, there has also been a rejuvenated interest in modern noncontrast MRA techniques over the past several years.

Central to this renewed interest in noncontrast imaging is the recognition of an association between GBCA and nephrogenic systemic fibrosis (NSF) in patients with renal dysfunction.[6] NSF is a rare condition characterized by progressive fibrosis and swelling in the extremities of affected individuals, primarily occurring in the skin and integument.[6,7] In some individuals, the fibrotic process can be progressive, affecting visceral organs such as the lungs, esophagus, and heart, resulting in substantial morbidity or even mortality. CE-MRA is avoided in patients who have renal impairment, such as end-stage renal disease requiring dialysis, severe chronic kidney disease (estimated glomerular filtration rate [eGFR] <30 mL/min/1.73 m^2), or acute kidney injury.[7] More recently, patients who show borderline renal function (eGFR 30–40 mL/min/1.73 m^2) are increasingly urged to avoid GBCA exposure if possible. Although patients with chronic

renal disease are encountered more frequently in the adult population, many pediatric disease processes can present with chronic diminished renal function or more acute kidney dysfunction.

Beyond NSF, there are several other reasons that noncontrast MRA is useful in the pediatric population. No gadolinium contrast agent is approved by the US Food and Drug Administration (FDA) for first-pass MRA in children, so the administration of contrast agents is considered off-label use.[8] In addition, dosing for GBCA is typically achieved using a weight-based dosing scheme, typically 0.1 mmol/kg for standard doses and 0.2 mmol/kg for double doses.[9] Given the physical size of infants and children, this dosing can result in a small amount of injected contrast material, which makes accurate bolus tracking/timing challenging when CE-MRA is used. Reliable venous access in a tiny pediatric patient can be challenging because of the small blood vessel size.[10] The ability to hold the breath for 20 to 30 seconds is commonplace in adults and adolescents, allowing motion-free CE-MRA images to be obtained.[2] However, in children and infants, breath holding is not possible without the use of general anesthesia and mechanical ventilation, thereby adding substantial periprocedural complexity and the risk of sedation/anesthesia. On the other hand, noncontrast MRA techniques can be accomplished with respiratory compensation (ie, navigator pulses or mechanical respiratory tracking with a bellow) and may be more easily tolerated by pediatric patients than full anesthesia.[4,8]

Noncontrast MRA

Black blood imaging

Black blood imaging is an MRA technique that uses several inversion pulses to nullify the signal from flowing blood. An initial nonselective inversion pulse is applied broadly, followed by a section-selective inversion pulse to the area of interest, which results in signal from static tissues in the slice of interest and lack of signal from moving blood.[2,11] This situation results in a black appearance of flowing blood, most pronounced in flow that is directly perpendicular to the imaging plane. Black blood sequences are generally preferred in the evaluation of vasculitis, because wall edema/inflammation can be shown directly. The use of cardiac gating can substantially improve overall image quality by reducing pulsation artifacts.[4] Black blood techniques are generally excellent for the depiction of aortic dissection flaps or intramural hematoma, which show excellent tissue contrast versus the nullified signal in the vascular lumen.

Table 1 Pediatric MRA techniques	
Noncontrast	Black blood Time of flight Phase contrast Steady-state free precession
Contrast enhanced	Multiphase dynamic postcontrast imaging Bolus tracking or timed MRA Keyhole MRA

Time of flight

Time-of-flight (TOF) MRA is a commonly used non-contrast MRA, which offers unique information relative to CE-MRA because of its directional depiction of blood flow. TOF MRA uses several radiofrequency (RF) pulses to nullify the signal of stationary tissues within a section of interest and subsequently relies on inflowing blood to provide nonsaturated protons, which generate signal for the imaging section.[12] In addition, user-defined saturation slabs can be applied adjacent to the imaging section to purposefully eliminate flow from blood coursing into the slice from a specific direction. Therefore, when applied superior to an imaging slice, this technique causes downward flowing blood to lose signal. This situation can be helpful in identifying flow direction and results in specific arteriographic or venographic depiction.[11] The major limitation of TOF imaging is the long scan times, particularly for large coverage areas such as the extremity circulation.[2] In addition, TOF MRA works best with flow that is directed perpendicular to the imaging plane/section. TOF MRA suffers from signal loss when flow directionality is parallel or within the imaging section, which can artifactually simulate a narrowing or occlusion.[2,11]

Phase contrast

Phase contrast (PC) MRA is a unique MRA sequence that relies on the phase shift caused by moving blood when placed in a magnetic field. PC MRA results in 2 sets of images, including a magnitude image set (luminal depiction) and a phase image set (velocity/direction depiction).[2] As a result of these 2 data sets, PC MRA can quantify the flow velocity within an imaging section. By specifying the velocity encoding factor that establishes the maximum flow rate for the imaging section, the resulting PC MRA images can be interpreted quantitatively.[11] The ability to interrogate the imaging data for quantifiable flow is useful in patients with vascular shunts (such as a patent ductus arteriosus) and vascular stenosis.[11,13] PC MRA is time consuming and sensitive to disturbances in flow, resulting in overestimation of stenosis if there is substantial local flow turbulence.[2,11] Incorrect assignment of the velocity encoding parameter can result in erroneous flow data for velocities higher than this threshold. This situation results in aliasing on the obtained phase images, which may be a clue to the low velocity encoding setting.[10]

Steady-state free precession imaging

Steady-state free precession (SSFP) imaging can be used to generate bright blood MRA images. This gradient echo sequence uses RF pulses to maintain steady-state longitudinal and transverse magnetization.[11] The resultant image has a mixed image contrast, which is based on the T2/T1 ratios, with excellent signal to noise, leading to high signal intensity in both arteries and veins. With modern advances in scanner hardware, SSFP images can be obtained rapidly, which makes it an ideal solution for imaging the uncooperative or nonstationary pediatric patient.[10,14] SSFP techniques are highly sensitive to field inhomogeneities, which can cause substantial artifact at natural areas of susceptibility, such as air interfaces.[14] In addition, there is relatively poor background suppression for SSFP imaging, because of the image contrast. Therefore, if pure angiographic depiction is desired, the sequence must be modified with preparatory pulses to nullify background tissue.

Future directions

Several other new and emerging noncontrast techniques have been described for body MRA in adult patients, with potential usefulness in children. As an example, electrocardiography-gated fast spin echo (FSE) imaging has been introduced, which uses the difference between arterial signal on FSE imaging during systole and diastole to generate an arteriographic image.[11,14] In diastole, arterial flow is generally high signal intensity on T2-weighted images, because of the slow flow during this portion of the cardiac cycle. However, arterial flow during systole generally manifests as a flow void on T2-weighted images, whereas other background signal remains similar to diastole. Using image manipulation/subtraction between systolic and diastolic phase images, the arterial signal can be isolated from the data set. This technique allows depiction of flow parallel to the imaging plane, so nonaxial acquisitions may be used to increase imaging speed. Arterial spin labeling is another technique, in which arterial blood is tagged through a set of pulse sequences such that flowing blood is highlighted against a relatively nulled background.[14] Given the success of these techniques in imaging small vessels in adults (such as the renal and coronary arteries), their use in pediatric body MRA seems to be a natural extension.

CE-MRA

The use of GBCA has substantially expanded the use of MRA in clinical applications. Gadolinium chelates alter the local magnetic microenvironment around them, resulting in shortened T1 relaxation times, which translate into faster longitudinal recovery.[12] By using T1-weighted imaging sequences, high vascular signal intensity is achieved with CE imaging. Modern MR scanners use ultra-fast 3D T1-weighted gradient echo sequences, often with fat suppression, to maximize the visual impact of contrast enhancement and permit reformatting into other planes or the use of 3D reconstruction techniques.[2]

Timing the scan acquisition to coincide with the appropriate vascular phase of contrast enhancement is key in CE-MRA. In general, venous phase imaging can be obtained at a fixed delay after contrast injection, because venous opacification is related to the distribution of contrast material throughout the circulation. However, for arterial phase imaging, precise timing is required to synchronize image acquisition with the arrival of contrast material. This timing can be accomplished several ways in adults, with automatic bolus tracking techniques/software generally being preferred.[1,4] This goal can be accomplished in older children who can suspend respiration and have similar cardiovascular physiology to adults. However, in younger children who are unable to cooperate with breath holding and technologist commands, a dynamic postcontrast technique can be used, in which multiple T1-weighted data sets are obtained in rapid succession.[4,9] This strategy increases the odds that at least 1 of the data sets has a pure arterial phase. The increased speed of acquisition/temporal resolution may necessitate either using parallel imaging techniques or a decrease in spatial resolution.[5,9]

The use of multiple dynamic phase imaging sequences in the pediatric population has been termed time-resolved MRA in several studies and offers an excellent solution to arterial timing issues in children.[5,9,15] Terminology overlaps with time-resolved MRA or keyhole MRA in adults, in whom the term typically refers to techniques that highly undersample k-space to increase scan temporal resolution, and subsequently reconstructing the full k-space data using full k-space acquisitions at the beginning or end of the sequence.[16] The result of these techniques is the ability to rapidly sample the changing tissue contrast of a slice/volume during the administration of contrast and maintain spatial resolution by back-filling the spatial k-space data from other time points, because the vascular system does not move substantially during scan acquisition. Although this latter adult technique may be of benefit in the pediatric population, it has yet to gain major acceptance for pediatric body MRA applications.

Future directions

A blood pool contrast agent, gadofosveset trisodium (Lantheus Medical Imaging, North Billerica, MA), has recently been introduced in the United States for vascular imaging. Gadofosveset reversibly binds to serum albumin, leading to an elongated plasma half-life, which results in a blood pool phase of vascular imaging with a long temporal window (up to 60 minutes).[17] In addition, the contrast agent shows substantially greater relaxivity at 1.5 T than traditional contrast agents, resulting in very high signal intensity and contrast, even at reduced dosing.[18] The approved FDA indication for this contrast agent is evaluation of aortoiliac atherosclerotic disease. However, the pharmacokinetics of this contrast agent make it an excellent option for high-quality venous imaging as well.[19] This use of gadofosveset has only recently been reported in children, including for thoracic aortic imaging and high-resolution MR venography.[19,20] Future applications of this novel contrast agent in the pediatric population seem likely, particularly as the scope of pediatric endovascular therapeutic techniques continues to increase.

ABDOMINAL AND PELVIC ARTERIAL SYSTEMS
Normal and Variant Anatomy

The abdominal and pelvic arterial vasculature comprises primarily the abdominal aorta and its visceral branches and the left and right common iliac arteries and their branches. The anterior branches of the abdominal aorta include the celiac, superior mesenteric, and inferior mesenteric arteries, which comprise the principal blood supply of the viscera. There is a large amount of anatomic variation amongst these 3 vessels. The gonadal and phrenic arteries also arise anteriorly.

Laterally, the renal arteries and middle adrenal arteries come off the aorta on either side. The abdominal aorta is clinically divided into suprarenal and infrarenal segments. The renal arteries are typically seen coming off the aorta at the approximate level of L2. However, variant anatomy of renal arteries is present in up to 30% of the population, with many having multiple renal artery on one or both sides.[21,22]

Posteriorly, the lumbar arteries come off on either side of the aorta for each lumbar vertebral level. The middle sacral artery also arises posteriorly at the aortoiliac bifurcation. The aorta typically bifurcates at the L4 or L5 level into the right and left common iliac arteries, which in turn bifurcate into internal and external iliac arteries. The internal iliac artery further subdivides into an anterior and posterior division, whereas the external iliac artery continues on to become the common femoral artery and provides the primary blood supply for the lower extremity. The common femoral artery serves as the most common site of arterial access

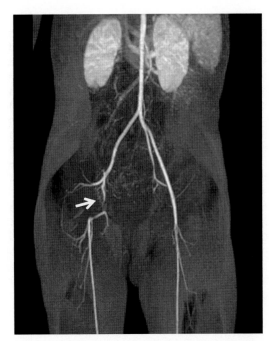

Fig. 1. Six-year-old girl with limb length discrepancy and history of multiple catheterizations. Postcontrast 3D fat-saturated T1W spoiled gradient echo maximum intensity projection image shows occlusion of the right common femoral artery (*arrow*), reconstituted distally by collaterals.

for invasive procedures, which can lead to arterial injury such as dissection, pseudoaneurysm formation, or occlusion (**Fig. 1**).

A persistent sciatic artery is a congenital variation occurring in a small percentage of the population (0.025%–0.04%), in which an embryonic lower limb axial artery (sciatic artery) fails to regress and persists as an elongation of the internal iliac artery (**Fig. 2**). The sciatic artery normally provides the major blood flow to the lower extremity during development but regresses around the sixth week of gestation into portions of the gluteal and popliteal arteries as well as the tibioperoneal trunk. At the same time that this regression is occurring, the external iliac artery and superficial femoral artery develop from a branch of the fifth lumbar artery. Persistent sciatic artery is classified as complete or incomplete depending on the level of development of the external iliac and superficial femoral arteries.[23] There is a slight male predominance, and although it can be seen bilaterally, it is most commonly noted on the right. Persistent sciatic arteries are prone to atheromatous degeneration, aneurysm formation with or without thrombosis or distal embolization, and local compression.

ABDOMINAL AORTIC NARROWING

Abdominal aortic narrowing, particularly suprarenal, typically manifests with hypertension and weakened or absent femoral pulses. This narrowing can be caused by a wide variety of diseases, such as congenital disorders, infectious or inflammatory conditions, and iatrogenic causes. Some investigators group all of these conditions together and commonly refer to them as the middle aortic syndrome. Other investigators recognize a separate specific entity called midaortic dysplastic syndrome, in cases in which suprarenal abdominal narrowing is present, but no clear underlying cause or known associated syndrome can be identified. Although the cause of midaortic dysplastic syndrome is unknown, it is believed to be a congenital arterial dysplasia, and it usually manifests in the second decade of life.[24]

Hypertension occurs as a result of suprarenal aortic narrowing or direct narrowing of the renal arteries themselves, because disease processes that narrow the aorta frequently involve branch vessels as well. The affected kidney perceives a relative hypotension secondary to the upstream

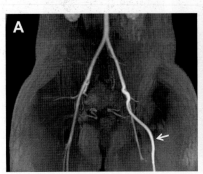
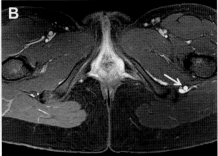

Fig. 2. Fifteen-year-old girl with left leg enlargement and pain. Postcontrast 3D T1W spoiled gradient echo coronal maximum intensity projection (*A*) and postcontrast 3D fat-saturated T1W spoiled gradient echo axial (*B*) images show a large persistent left sciatic artery (*arrow*) with a comparatively diminutive left superficial femoral artery.

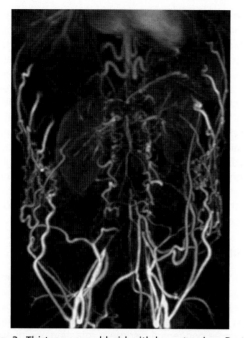

Fig. 3. Thirteen-year-old girl with hypertension. Post-contrast 3D fat-saturated T1W spoiled gradient echo maximum intensity projection image in early arterial phase shows nonvisualization of the abdominal aorta. The mesentery and lower limbs receive their blood supply from extensive collaterals involving the inter-costal, epigastric, and lumbar arteries.

stenosis, causing an increase in renin production, resulting in systemic hypertension. In general, be-tween 5% and 10% of all childhood hypertension is attributable to a vascular or renin-mediated mechanism.[25]

The MR appearance of many of these conditions is similar, with segmental (**Fig. 3**) or focal (**Fig. 4**) narrowing of the abdominal aorta and its branches (**Fig. 5**). Entities in which the arterial vasculature is narrowed secondary to extrinsic compression rather than intrinsic disease can be differentiated by MR identification of the extrinsic masses, such as in retroperitoneal neurofibromas in neuro-fibromatosis type 1. In instances in which aortic narrowing is secondary to an existing systemic condition, the clinical history or laboratory values may aid in differentiation. This information is also particularly helpful in cases in which a syndrome is present, such as in Williams syndrome (**Fig. 6**) or tuberous sclerosis.

VASCULITIS

The vasculitides are an important category of in-flammatory conditions affecting the abdominal and pelvic arterial vasculature. They are typically classi-fied as large vessel, medium vessel, or small vessel (**Table 2**). For the purposes of MR imaging, typically only large-vessel and medium-vessel vasculitides can be identified, because small-vessel disease is often below MR imaging resolution.

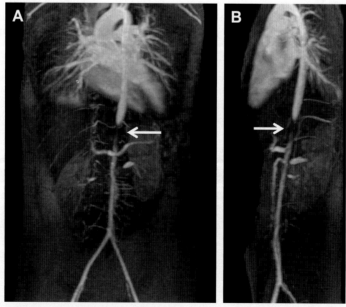

Fig. 4. Five-year-old girl with incidentally detected hypertension. Coronal (A) and sagittal (B) postcontrast 3D fat-saturated T1W spoiled gradient echo maximum intensity projection images show segmental suprarenal abdom-inal aortic narrowing (arrow), resulting in renin-mediated hypertension. There is also severe bilateral main renal artery narrowing.

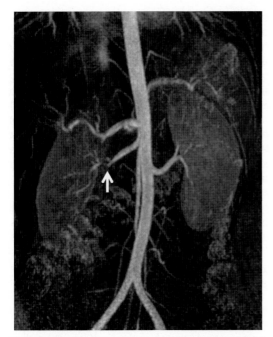

Fig. 5. Fifteen-year-old girl with hypertension. Postcontrast 3D fat-saturated T1W spoiled gradient echo maximum intensity projection image shows progressive tapering of the right renal artery (*arrow*) with narrowing proximal segments of right renal artery branches.

Table 2
Common pediatric vasculitides

Vessel Size	Vasculitis	Seen on MR
Large	Takayasu	Yes
Medium	Polyarteritis nodosa Kawasaki disease	Yes
Small	Wegener Churg-Strauss Henoch-Schönlein purpura Microscopic polyangiitis	No

Like many pediatric vasculopathies, hypertension is a common clinical sign, present in more than 90% of affected patients.[26] MR findings may include luminal narrowing of the aorta and other large arterial branches, with associated vessel wall thickening (**Fig. 7**).

Kawasaki disease is a rare systemic medium-vessel vasculitis of unknown cause. Its highest incidence occurs between the ages of 6 and 11 months, particularly in Asian populations. The diagnosis is made clinically and is characterized

Takayasu arteritis is the most common pediatric large-vessel vasculitis. Most children are diagnosed in adolescence, with a mean age of 13 years. In this granulomatous vasculitis, the most commonly affected arteries in children are the aorta, renal, subclavian, and carotid arteries.

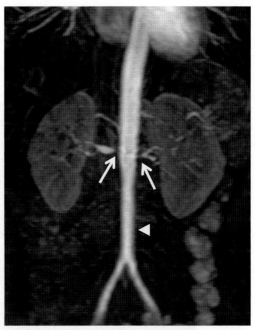

Fig. 7. Thirteen-year-old girl with hypertension. Postcontrast 3D fat-saturated T1W spoiled gradient echo maximum intensity projection image shows bilateral renal artery narrowing (*arrows*) and infrarenal aortic tapering (*arrowhead*). The appearance along with clinical history was most compatible with Takayasu arteritis.

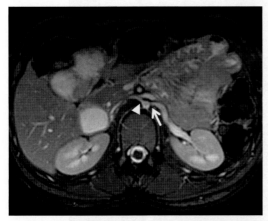

Fig. 6. Fifteen-year-old girl with documented Williams syndrome. Axial fat-saturated balanced SSFP image shows a hypoplastic abdominal aorta and right renal artery (*arrowhead*), with coexisting left renal artery stenosis (*arrow*).

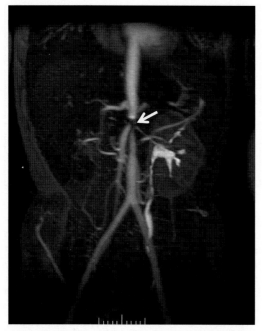

Fig. 8. Eleven-year-old boy who received abdominal radiation therapy for a neuroblastoma. Postcontrast 3D fat-saturated T1W spoiled gradient echo maximum intensity projection image shows resultant focal occlusion of the abdominal aorta (*arrow*), caused by radiation arteritis, and a severely atrophic right renal artery.

by fever of 5 days or longer with at least 4 of the following: bilateral conjunctivitis; oropharyngeal changes; cervical lymphadenopathy; polymorphous rash; and peripheral extremity or perineal

changes. Incomplete and atypical Kawasaki disease can also be diagnosed with fewer or additional atypical symptoms, respectively. Coronary artery aneurysms are the most commonly encountered vascular findings, but aneurysms involving the mesenteric arterial vasculature have also been documented.[26]

Polyarteritis nodosa (PAN) is a medium-vessel necrotizing vasculitis, with a peak age of onset at 9 years. It accounts for 3% of childhood vasculitides. PAN can affect vascular supply to any organ, although the lungs are typically spared. Arterial irregularities in PAN typically manifest as aneurysms, most commonly seen involving the distal branches of the kidneys, liver, spleen, and gastrointestinal tract.[26,27]

ARTERIAL RADIATION INJURY, INFECTION, ANEURYSMS, AND PSEUDOANEURYSMS

Inflammation of the abdomen and pelvic arterial vasculature may occur secondary to radiation therapy. Acute radiation injury affects the intima and typically spares the media and adventitia. However, several weeks after radiation injury, there is progressive medial fibrosis causing arterial luminal narrowing (**Fig. 8**).[28]

Infectious processes can cause either stenosis or aneurysmal dilatation of the abdominal and pelvic arterial vasculature. This process may manifest as narrowing of the arterial lumen because of a thickened inflamed wall in aortitis or arteritis, or as dilatation in the form of a mycotic aneurysm.

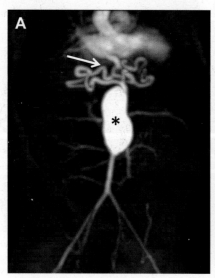
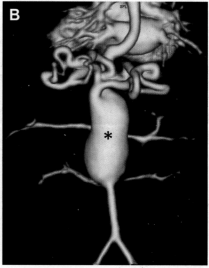

Fig. 9. Three-month-old with multiple congenital anomalies, including nephroblastomatosis. Postcontrast 3D fat-saturated T1W spoiled gradient echo maximum intensity projection (*A*) and volume-rendered (posterior view) (*B*) images show fusiform aneurysmal dilatation of the suprarenal aorta (*asterisk*), directly distal to interruption of the descending thoracic aorta with numerous collaterals (*arrow*). The proximal left renal artery was stenotic.

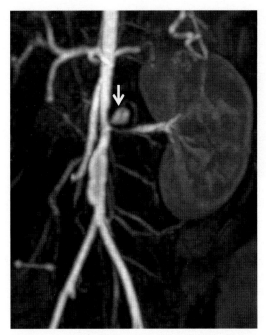

Fig. 10. Five-year-old boy after recent right nephrectomy and aortoplasty. Postcontrast 3D fat-saturated T1W spoiled gradient echo maximum intensity projection image shows development of an aortic pseudoaneurysm (*arrow*) just superior to the left renal artery, which is narrowed proximally.

Aneurysmal dilatation of the abdominal and pelvic arterial vasculature can also be noted as poststenotic dilatation downstream from stenosis secondary to arterial diseases such as those previously detailed (**Fig. 9**). Alternatively, conditions such as tuberous sclerosis may cause aneurysmal dilatation, even in the absence of an upstream narrowing or infection.[29]

Contained arterial leaks in the form of pseudoaneurysm can occur as a result of trauma or may be iatrogenic (**Fig. 10**). The risk for spontaneous rupture is greater in a pseudoaneurysm than a true aneurysm, and pseudoaneurysms require immediate treatment.[30] Although pseudoaneurysms have a greater likelihood of showing a more irregular shape than an aneurysm, it can be difficult to distinguish between the two on imaging alone. Context of trauma or other imaging signs of trauma can be helpful to make the distinction.

ABDOMINAL AND PELVIC VENOUS SYSTEM
Typical and Variant Anatomy

The normal abdominal and pelvic venous vasculature comprises primarily the inferior vena cava (IVC) and its tributaries, including the hepatic, renal, common iliac, phrenic, lumbar, and right adrenal veins. However, there are several common anatomic variants of the abdominal and pelvic systemic venous circulation.

The infrarenal IVC is typically right-sided in 97% of the population, derived from the embryonic right supracardinal vein. In 1% of the population, the left supracardinal vein fails to regress and a duplicated infrarenal IVC is present.[31] Each common iliac drains into a separate infrarenal IVC. The left-sided IVC usually drains into the left renal vein, which then drains toward the infrarenal right-sided IVC to form a common suprarenal IVC (**Fig. 11**).

In another 0.5% of the population, the right supracardinal vein regresses instead of the left, leading to a left-sided infrarenal IVC. In this situation, both common iliac veins drain into the left-sided IVC, which crosses over to the right at the level of the left renal vein.[31] Occasionally, the left-sided IVC drains into the hemiazygous vein

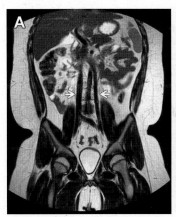
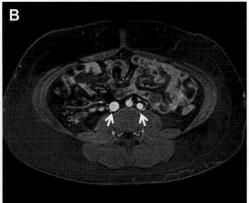

Fig. 11. Nine-year-old boy undergoing workup for undescended testes. Coronal T2-weighted single-shot FSE (*A*) and postcontrast axial 3D T1W spoiled gradient echo with fat-saturation (*B*) images show an incidentally detected duplicated IVC (*arrows*).

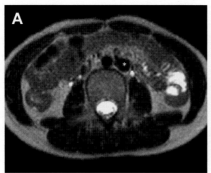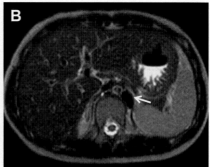

Fig. 12. Seven-year-old girl undergoing urologic evaluation with MR urography. Axial T2-weighted single-shot FSE images (*A, B*) showing an incidentally detected left-sided IVC (*asterisk*) with hemiazygous continuation (*arrow*). A right-sided IVC is not visualized.

(**Fig. 12**), azygous vein, or into the coronary sinus with a left superior vena cava.

The intrahepatic IVC is derived from the right subcardinal vein. Regression of this vein leads to interruption of the IVC in its intrahepatic portion, with azygous or hemiazygous continuation necessary to provide adequate venous drainage from the abdomen and lower extremities (**Fig. 13**).

There is some variation in renal vein anatomy. Although most of the population possesses a single renal vein on each side, multiple right-sided renal veins are present in up to 28% of patients. The left renal vein typically passes anteriorly between the aorta and superior mesenteric artery to join the IVC. However, in 3% of people, a retroaortic left renal vein is present instead, which passes posterior to the aorta. In another 7% of

people, the left renal vein has both preaortic and retroaortic components for a circumaortic left renal vein.[31]

VASCULAR ANOMALIES

Vascular anomalies can be divided into 2 broad categories: vascular neoplasms and vascular malformations. Vascular neoplasms are differentiated from malformations by the presence of increased endothelial cell turnover and proliferation, and the distinction allows a systematic approach to treatment options. Vascular neoplasm encompasses entities such as infantile hemangiomas and congenital hemangiomas (**Fig. 14**). Vascular malformations are subclassified as either slow-flow vascular malformations (**Fig. 15**) or fast-flow vascular malformations. Slow-flow malformations include capillary, venous, and lymphatic malformations, whereas fast-flow malformations are primarily arteriovenous malformations. Malformations that seem to possess elements of both slow and fast flow are considered complex-combined vascular malformations. MRI, along with ultrasonography, is the preferred imaging modality for characterizing vascular anomalies.[32] The common MR imaging characteristics of the various vascular anomalies are described in **Table 3**.

Klippel-Trenauny Syndrome

Klippel-Trenauny syndrome is a rare congenital disorder characterized by agenesis or hypoplasia of deep veins, along with capillary (port wine stain) or other slow-flow malformations, and osseous and soft tissue hypertrophy (**Fig. 16**). When arteriovenous malformations are present as well, the syndrome is classified as Klippel-Trenauny-Weber syndrome or Parks-Weber syndrome.[33] The extent of vascular malformation is best evaluated with a

Fig. 13. Three-week-old undergoing evaluation for biliary atresia. Axial T2W FSE image of a 3-week-old girl shows interrupted IVC with azygous continuation. There is absence of the intrahepatic IVC, and enlarged azygous vein (*arrow*) and associated polysplenia (*asterisk*).

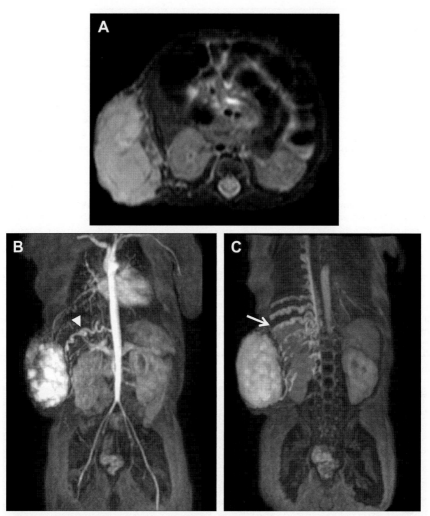

Fig. 14. Four-day-old girl with right flank mass. Fat-saturated T2W FSE axial (*A*) and postcontrast 3D fat-saturated T1W spoiled gradient echo coronal maximum intensity projection images (*B, C*) show a large congenital hemangioma of the right flank with a large feeding artery (*arrowhead*) and multiple enlarged draining veins (*arrow*), from the intercostals to the epidural venous plexus and the azygos vein.

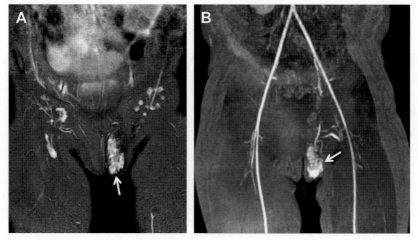

Fig. 15. Three-year-old girl with labial swelling. Coronal short tau inversion recovery (*A*) and postcontrast 3D fat-saturated T1W spoiled gradient echo maximum intensity projection (*B*) images show a slow-flow vascular anomaly comprised of many abnormal venous channels representing a labial venous malformation (*arrow*).

Table 3
MR characteristics of vascular anomalies

Vascular Anomaly	Subtype	MR Characteristics
Vascular neoplasm		Intermediate signal on T1W High signal on T2W Internal flow voids Robust contrast enhancement ± arteriovenous shunting with enlarged feeding arteries and draining veins
Slow-flow vascular malformation	Venous	Heterogeneous low to intermediate signal on T1W High signal intensity on T2W No flow voids Contrast enhancement
	Lymphatic	Low to intermediate signal on T1W High signal intensity on T2W No central enhancement on postcontrast T1W (thin internal septations and walls may enhance)
	Combined	Low to intermediate signal on T1W High signal on T2W Heterogeneous enhancement after contrast
Fast-flow vascular malformation	Arteriovenous malformation	Serpiginous signal voids on T2W No discrete mass Arteriovenous shunting with enlarged feeding arteries and draining veins

Abbreviations: T1W, T1-weighted; T2W, T2-weighted.

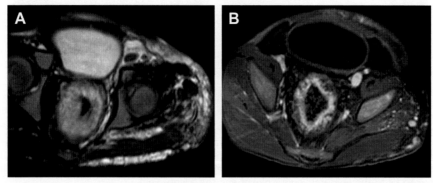

Fig. 16. Twelve-year-old boy with documented Klippel-Trenauny syndrome. T2W FSE (*A*) and postcontrast 3D fat-saturated T1W spoiled gradient echo axial (*B*) images show slow-flow vascular malformations of the subcutaneous tissues of the pelvis and proximal left thigh associated with the patient's hypoplasia of the deep venous system. Extensive rectal venous malformation is also present.

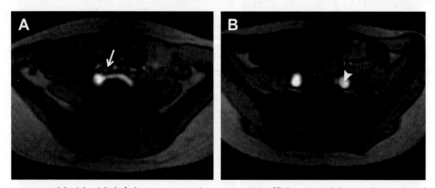

Fig. 17. Sixteen-year-old girl with left lower extremity venous insufficiency. Axial two-dimensional gradient recalled echo TOF images (*A, B*) show anterior compression of the left common iliac vein from the right common iliac artery (*arrow*), leading to May-Thurner syndrome. The caliber of the left common iliac vein is normal peripheral to the compression (*asterisk*).

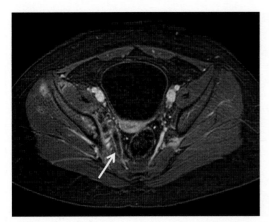

Fig. 18. Nine-year-old girl with right hip pain and multiple septic emboli. Postcontrast 3D fat-saturated T1W spoiled gradient echo axial image shows a right hypogastric branch thrombosis (*arrow*) secondary to adjacent right iliac bone osteomyelitis.

Table 4 Abernethy classification of congenital extrahepatic portosystemic shunts	
Abernethy Type	**Imaging Characteristics**
1a	Absent portal vein Separate drainage of the splenic and superior mesenteric veins into a systemic vein
1b	Absent portal vein Common trunk is formed by the splenic and superior mesenteric veins before drainage into a systemic vein
2	Normal or hypoplastic portal vein Partial shunting of blood into the IVC via a side-to-side communication to the portal vein

combination of standard MR pulse sequences and MR venography. Postcontrast imaging using gadofosveset trisodium GBCA allows for very high-resolution imaging of extremity and pelvic venous structures.

May-Thurner Syndrome

May-Thurner syndrome is a condition in which the left common iliac vein is compressed by the right common iliac artery, which crosses over it (**Fig. 17**), leading to left lower extremity swelling, varicosities, deep venous thrombosis, and chronic venous stasis ulcers. Also reported is phlegmasia cerulea dolens, a severe manifestation of deep venous thrombosis, in which massive tense edema develops because of poor venous outflow from the limb, which leads to poor arterial inflow and a cyanotic, cool, painful, and pulseless extremity. There are 3 venographic stages to May-Thurner syndrome: compression with a pressure gradient

2 mm Hg or less and no evidence of collateral filling; development of intraluminal webs or spurs; and thrombosis. May-Thurner syndrome commonly affects women in the second to fourth decade and is also termed iliac vein compression syndrome or Cockett syndrome. MR venography is helpful in diagnosing May-Thurner syndrome, because it can show the anatomic compression of the left common iliac vein and can identify suprainguinal deep venous thrombosis peripheral to the iliac vein compression, which may not be detected by Duplex ultrasonography.[34,35]

Thrombosis

Thrombus of the abdominal and pelvic vasculature can be classified into bland or tumor thrombus, and this distinction may be critically important for patient management. Bland thrombus may be

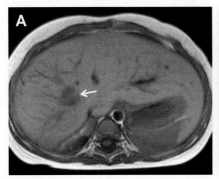
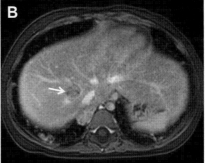

Fig. 19. Two-year-old boy with hepatoblastoma. T1W spin echo (*A*) and postcontrast 3D fat-saturated T1W spoiled gradient echo (*B*) axial images show a massive right hepatic vein tumor thrombus (*arrow*), which enhances on the postcontrast image.

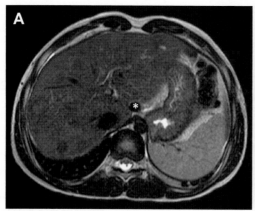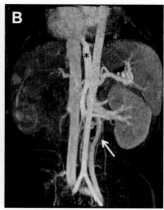

Fig. 20. Thirteen-year-old boy showing no detectable portal vein flow on ultrasonography. T2W FSE axial (*A*) and postcontrast 3D fat-saturated T1W spoiled gradient echo coronal maximum intensity projection (*B*) images show the splenic vein and superior mesenteric vein joining into a common trunk (*asterisk*) that drains into the right atrium for an Abernethy type Ib extrahepatic portosystemic shunt. The portal vein is absent. Multiple liver masses represent adenomas and regenerative nodules. Also noted is a duplicated IVC with the left-sided IVC (*arrow*) draining into the left renal vein.

secondary to adjacent infection (**Fig. 18**), stasis, or hypercoagulability. Tumor thrombus may occur when abdominal tumors invade adjacent venous structures (**Fig. 19**).[36,37] Common pediatric scenarios of tumor thrombus include invasion of the renal veins by renal tumors such as Wilms tumor or invasion of the hepatic veins by hepatoblastoma or hepatocellular carcinoma.

PORTAL VENOUS SYSTEM
Typical and Variant Anatomy

The splenic vein and superior mesenteric vein join to form the main portal vein posterior to the pancreatic neck. Other veins that contribute to main portal venous flow include the inferior mesenteric vein, left gastric vein, right gastric vein, cystic vein, and paraumbilical veins. The main portal vein travels cranially in the hepatoduodenal ligament and bifurcates into the right and left portal vein at the liver hilum. Segments I, II, III, and IV of the liver are supplied by the left portal vein. The right portal vein bifurcates again into the right anterior and right posterior portal veins. The right anterior portal vein supplies segments V and VIII, whereas the right posterior branch supplies segments VI and VII.

Alterations in the normally occurring coalescence between the vitelline and umbilical veins during development lead to variant portal vein anatomy. Major variants are rare and include portal vein duplication, preduodenal portal vein, and absent branching of the portal vein. Minor alterations are more common, including trifurcation of the main portal vein, a separate segment VI or segment VII branch of the right portal vein, and

the right posterior branch as the first branch of the main portal vein.[38]

Congenital Portal Venous Shunts

Congenital extrahepatic portosystemic shunts are rare and are grouped according to the Abernethy classification system (**Table 4**). In Abernethy type 1, there is absence of the portal vein with complete diversion of splenic and superior mesenteric venous blood return into systemic veins. Abernethy type 1 is subdivided into type 1a, in which there is separate drainage of the splenic and superior

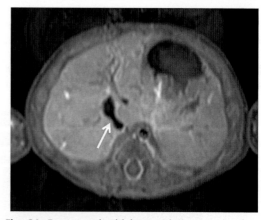

Fig. 21. Four-month-old boy with increased α-fetoprotein and an abnormal ultrasound scan showing a portocaval fistula. T1W spin echo with fat-saturation axial image shows partial drainage of the portal vein into the IVC, from a direct communication (*arrow*). Other images show hypoplastic intrahepatic portal veins, consistent with an Abernethy type II congenital extrahepatic portosystemic shunt.

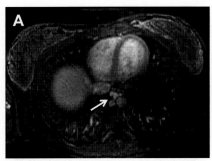
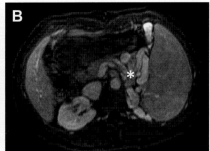

Fig. 22. Eighteen-year-old girl with a remote history of orthotopic liver transplant for biliary atresia. Postcontrast 3D fat-saturated T1W spoiled gradient echo axial images (*A, B*) show portal hypertension manifesting as esophageal varices (*arrow*), splenic hilar varices (*asterisk*), and splenorenal shunt. The spleen is also enlarged.

mesenteric veins into a systemic vein and type 1b (**Fig. 20**), in which a common trunk is formed by the splenic and superior mesenteric veins before drainage into a systemic vein. Many systemic veins may serve as the drainage for Abernethy type 1 malformations, including the IVC, renal veins, or iliac veins. Direct flow into the right atrium has also been described. An Abernethy type 2 shunt consists of a normal or hypoplastic portal vein with partial shunting of blood into the IVC via a side-to-side communication (**Fig. 21**). Abernethy malformations are also associated with other congenital anomalies, hepatopulmonary syndrome, hepatic encephalopathy, development of hepatic masses, and pulmonary arteriovenous fistulae.[39]

Acquired extrahepatic portosystemic shunts are common, usually resulting from enlargement of normally existing portosystemic communications in the setting of portal hypertension. The most commonly described shunts include coronary veins and short gastric veins draining to the azygos vein (gastroesophageal) (**Fig. 22**); left portal vein to the epigastric and external iliac veins (recanalized paraumbilical) (**Figs. 23** and **24**); splenic hilum to the left renal vein (splenorenal);

and superior rectal to the inferior hemorrhoidal branch of the internal pudendal vein and the middle rectal branch of the internal iliac vein (hemorrhoidal). Extrahepatic portosystemic shunts can be the cause of life-threatening upper and lower gastrointestinal bleeding in the setting of portal hypertension, as in the case of gastroesophageal and hemorrhoidal shunts.[40]

Intrahepatic portosystemic shunts are rare in children and typically result from a congenital vascular malformation, trauma, or portal hypertension. Four types have been described and are listed in **Table 5**. Types 2 and 3 are the most common.[40]

Arterioportal shunts may be congenital or secondary to cirrhosis, trauma, previous intervention, or tumor. Cirrhosis-related shunts on MR often show small, peripheral, subcapsular, wedge-shaped regions of homogeneous enhancement during the arterial phase, with no abnormality noted during portal venous phase. The noncontrast T1 and T2 sequences are normal in the area of increased arterial phase enhancement. Tumor-related shunting is often the result of hepatocellular carcinoma (HCC). It may be difficult to distinguish between cirrhosis-related shunting

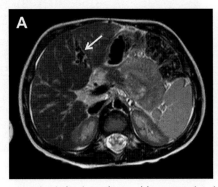
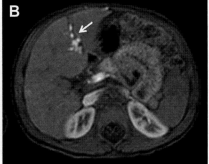

Fig. 23. Cryptogenic cirrhosis and portal hypertension in a 23-month-old boy. T2W FSE (*A*) and postcontrast 3D T1W spoiled gradient echo with fat-saturation (*B*) axial images shows recanalization of the paraumbilical vein (*arrow*).

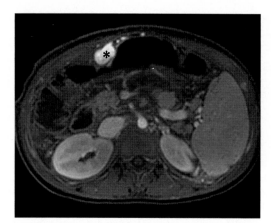

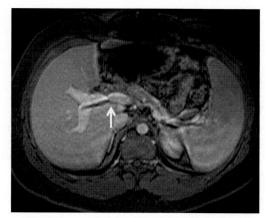

Fig. 24. Fifteen-year-old boy with hepatitis C cirrhosis. Postcontrast 3D T1W fat-saturation spoiled gradient echo axial image with fat saturation shows a large paraumbilical vein varix (*asterisk*) and splenomegaly.

Fig. 25. Thirteen-year-old boy with a history of orthotopic liver transplant and chronic increase of liver enzyme levels. Postcontrast 3D fat-saturated T1W spoiled gradient echo axial image shows portal venous anastamotic narrowing (*arrow*), with an associated linear dephasing jet.

and HCC shunting. In those cases, close surveillance imaging may be beneficial.

Portal Vein Stenosis, Thrombosis, and Cavernous Transformation

Portal vein stenosis is most often caused by tumor encasement, pancreatitis, or as a complication of hepatic surgery, including liver transplantation (**Fig. 25**). Long-standing portal vein stenosis may result in portal venous hypertension and its associated symptoms. The resultant slow flow caused by hemodynamically significant stenosis may also lead to portal vein thrombosis.

Many clinical situations are associated with portal vein thrombosis, including cirrhosis, tumors, infection, hypercoagulable states, trauma, or as a

complication of surgery or umbilical vein catheterization.[41] As in the systemic venous circulation, the distinction between tumor versus bland thrombus as well as acute versus chronic thrombus may have significant clinical applications. Acute thrombus may resolve spontaneously. Chronic extrahepatic portal vein thrombosis may lead to the development of multiple small collateral veins

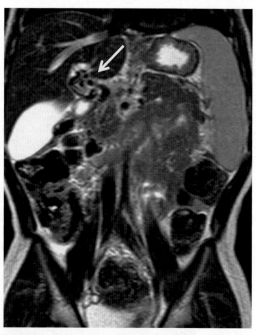

Fig. 26. Four-year-old girl with a history of splenomegaly and thrombocytopenia. T2W FSE coronal image shows multiple venous collateral structures in the porta hepatis compatible with cavernous transformation of the main portal vein (*arrow*).

Table 5 Classification of intrahepatic portosystemic shunts	
Type	**Imaging Characteristics**
1	Single shunt connecting the right portal vein to the IVC
2	Localized shunt between peripheral branches of the portal and hepatic veins in 1 hepatic segment via a single or multiple channels
3	Localized shunting between peripheral branches of the portal vein and peripheral branches of the hepatic vein with a focal varix
4	Multiple communications between the peripheral portal and hepatic circulation occurring diffusely in both lobes of the liver

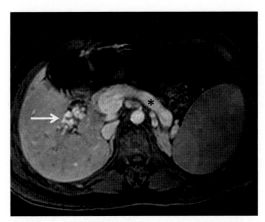

Fig. 27. Eighteen-year-old girl with Turner syndrome. Postcontrast 3D fat-saturated T1W spoiled gradient echo axial image shows cavernous transformation of the main portal vein (*arrow*) and portal hypertension manifesting as splenomegaly and splenic vein enlargement (*asterisk*).

along the thrombosed portal vein. This appearance is commonly referred to as cavernous transformation of the portal vein (**Figs. 26** and **27**) and represents the body's attempt to preserve hepatopetal flow into the liver.

SUMMARY

MRA is ideally suited to the imaging of pediatric abdominal vascular structures. The lack of ionizing radiation and noninvasive nature, coupled with the ability to obtain dynamic vascular images often without the use of a contrast agent, make MR an attractive option in this patient population. The ability to diagnose vascular variants and diseases allows for more invasive examinations to be reserved for those cases in which intervention is anticipated.

REFERENCES

1. Roberts D, Siegelman ES. Imaging and MR arteriography of the aorta. In: Siegelman ES, editor. Body MRI. 1st edition. Philadelphia: Elsevier; 2005. p. 481–507.
2. Tatli S, Lipton MJ, Davison BD, et al. From the RSNA refresher courses: MR imaging of aortic and peripheral vascular disease. Radiographics 2003; 23(Spec No):S59–78.
3. Prakash A, Torres AJ, Printz BF, et al. Usefulness of magnetic resonance angiography in the evaluation of complex congenital heart disease in newborns and infants. Am J Cardiol 2007;100(4):715–21.
4. Krishnamurthy R, Muthupillai R, Chung T. Pediatric body MR angiography. Magn Reson Imaging Clin N Am 2009;17(1):133–44.
5. Chung T, Krishnamurthy R. Contrast-enhanced MR angiography in infants and children. Magn Reson Imaging Clin N Am 2005;13(1):161–70.
6. Marckmann P, Skov L, Rossen K, et al. Nephrogenic systemic fibrosis: suspected causative role of gadodiamide used for contrast-enhanced magnetic resonance imaging. J Am Soc Nephrol 2006;17(9):2359–62.
7. American College of Radiology. Manual on contrast media, v8. 63–71. Available at: http://www.nxtbook.com/nxtbooks/acr/contrastmediamanual2012/. Accessed February 10, 2013.
8. Ley-Zaporozhan J, Kreitner KF, Unterhinninghofen R, et al. Assessment of thoracic aortic dimensions in an experimental setting: comparison of different unenhanced magnetic resonance angiography techniques with electrocardiogram-gated computed tomography angiography for possible application in the pediatric population. Invest Radiol 2008;43(3):179–86.
9. Chung T. Magnetic resonance angiography of the body in pediatric patients: experience with a contrast-enhanced time-resolved technique. Pediatr Radiol 2005;35(1):3–10.
10. Serai S, Towbin AJ, Podberesky DJ. Non-contrast MRA using an inflow-enhanced, inversion recovery SSFP technique in pediatric abdominal imaging. Pediatr Radiol 2012;42(3):364–8.
11. Morita S, Masukawa A, Suzuki K, et al. Unenhanced MR angiography: techniques and clinical applications in patients with chronic kidney disease. Radiographics 2011;31(2):E13–33.
12. Bitar R, Leung G, Perng R, et al. MR pulse sequences: what every radiologist wants to know but is afraid to ask. Radiographics 2006;26(2):513–37.
13. Wang ZJ, Reddy GP, Gotway MB, et al. Cardiovascular shunts: MR imaging evaluation. Radiographics 2003;23(Spec No):S181–94.
14. Miyazaki M, Lee VS. Nonenhanced MR angiography. Radiology 2008;248(1):20–43.
15. Muthupillai R, Vick GW 3rd, Flamm SD, et al. Time-resolved contrast-enhanced magnetic resonance angiography in pediatric patients using sensitivity encoding. J Magn Reson Imaging 2003;17(5):559–64.
16. Grist TM, Mistretta CA, Strother CM, et al. Time-resolved angiography: past, present, and future. J Magn Reson Imaging 2012;36(6):1273–86.
17. Lewis M, Yanny S, Malcolm PN. Advantages of blood pool contrast agents in MR angiography: a pictorial review. J Med Imaging Radiat Oncol 2012; 56(2):187–91.
18. Prince MR, Pearson GD, Zhang HL, et al. Advantages of blood pooling in pediatric MR angiography. JACC Cardiovasc Imaging 2010;3(5):514–6.
19. Ghanouni P, Walters SG, Vasanawala SS. Rapid MR venography in children using a blood pool contrast agent and multi-station fat-water-separated volumetric imaging. Pediatr Radiol 2012;42(2):242–8.

20. Naehle CP, Kaestner M, Müller A, et al. First-pass and steady-state MR angiography of thoracic vasculature in children and adolescents. JACC Cardiovasc Imaging 2010;3(5):504–13.

21. Spring DB, Salvatierra O Jr, Palubinskas AJ, et al. Results and significance of angiography in potential kidney donors. Radiology 1979;133:45–7.

22. Halpern E, Mitchell D, Weschler R, et al. Preoperative evaluation of living renal donors: comparison of CT angiography and MR angiography. Radiology 2000;216:434–9.

23. van Hooft IM, Zeebregts CJ, van Sterkenburg SM, et al. The persistent sciatic artery. Eur J Vasc Endovasc Surg 2009;37:585–91.

24. Sebastia C, Quiroga S, Boye R, et al. Aortic stenosis: spectrum of disease depicted at multi-section CT. Radiographics 2003;23:S79–91.

25. Ghabril R. Renovascular hypertension in children. J Med Liban 2010;58(3):146–8.

26. Weiss P. Pediatric vasculitis. Pediatr Clin North Am 2012;59:407–23.

27. Scuccimarri R. Kawasaki disease. Pediatr Clin North Am 2012;59:425–45.

28. Modrail J, Sadjadi J. Early and late presentations of radiation arteritis. Semin Vasc Surg 2003;16(3):209–14.

29. Salerno AE, Marsenic O, Meyers KE, et al. Vascular involvement in tuberous sclerosis. Pediatr Nephrol 2010;25(8):1555–61.

30. Belli AM, Markose G, Morgan R. The role of interventional radiology in the management of abdominal visceral artery aneurysms. Cardiovasc Intervent Radiol 2012;35(2):234–43.

31. Borsa JJ, Patel NH. The venous system: normal developmental anatomy and congenital anomalies. Semin Intervent Radiol 2001;18:69–82.

32. Lowe L, Marchant T, Rivard D, et al. Vascular malformations: classification and terminology the radiologist needs to know. Semin Roentgenol 2012;47(2):106–17.

33. Berry SA, Peterson C, Mize W, et al. Klippel-Trenauny syndrome. Am J Med Genet 1998;79:319–26.

34. O'Sullivan GJ, Semba CP, Bittner CA, et al. Endovascular management of iliac vein compression (May-Thurner) syndrome. J Vasc Interv Radiol 2000;11:823–36.

35. Patel N, Stookey KR, Ketcham DB, et al. Endovascular management of acute extensive iliofemoral deep venous thrombosis caused by May-Thurner syndrome. J Vasc Interv Radiol 2000;11:1297–302.

36. Macartney CA, Chan AK. Thrombosis in children. Semin Thromb Hemost 2011;37:763–71.

37. Galli R, Parlapiano M, Pace Napoleone C, et al. Neoplastic caval and intracardiac thrombosis secondary to reno-adrenal tumors. One-stage surgical treatment in deep hypothermia and cardiocirculatory arrest. Minerva Urol Nefrol 1994;46(2):105–11.

38. Gallego C, Velasco M, Marcuello P, et al. Congenital and acquired anomalies of the portal venous system. Radiographics 2002;22(1):141–59.

39. Alonso-Gamarra E, Parrón M, Pérez A, et al. Clinical and radiologic manifestations of congenital extrahepatic portosystemic shunts: a comprehensive review. Radiographics 2011;31(3):707–22.

40. Lee WK, Chang SD, Duddalwar VA, et al. Imaging assessment of congenital and acquired abnormalities of the portal venous system. Radiographics 2011;31(4):905–26.

41. Schettino GC, Fagundes ED, Roquete ML, et al. Portal vein thrombosis in children and adolescents. J Pediatr (Rio J) 2006;82(3):171–8.

Index

Note: Page numbers of article titles are in **boldface** type.

Magn Reson Imaging Clin N Am 21 (2013) 861–864
http://dx.doi.org/10.1016/S1064-9689(13)00116-5
1064-9689/13/$ – see front matter © 2013 Elsevier Inc. All rights reserved.

mri.theclinics.com

United States Postal Service

Statement of Ownership, Management, and Circulation
(All Periodicals Publications Except Requestor Publications)

1. Publication Title	2. Publication Number	3. Filing Date
Magnetic Resonance Imaging Clinics of North America	0 1 1 - 9 0 0 9	9/14/13

4. Issue Frequency	5. Number of Issues Published Annually	6. Annual Subscription Price
Feb, May, Aug, Nov	4	$357.00

7. Complete Mailing Address of Known Office of Publication (Not printer) (Street, city, county, state, and ZIP+4®)

Elsevier Inc.
360 Park Avenue South
New York, NY 10010-1710

Contact Person: Stephen R. Bushing
Telephone (Include area code): 215-239-3688

8. Complete Mailing Address of Headquarters or General Business Office of Publisher (Not printer)

Elsevier Inc., 360 Park Avenue South, New York, NY 10010-1710

9. Full Names and Complete Mailing Addresses of Publisher, Editor, and Managing Editor (Do not leave blank)

Publisher (Name and complete mailing address)

Linda Belfus, Elsevier, Inc., 1600 John F. Kennedy Blvd. Suite 1800, Philadelphia, PA 19103-2899

Editor (Name and complete mailing address)

Pamela Hetherington, Elsevier, Inc., 1600 John F. Kennedy Blvd. Suite 1800, Philadelphia, PA 19103-2899

Managing Editor (Name and complete mailing address)

Adrianne Brigido, Elsevier, Inc., 1600 John F. Kennedy Blvd. Suite 1800, Philadelphia, PA 19103-2899

10. Owner (Do not leave blank. If the publication is owned by a corporation, give the name and address of the corporation immediately followed by the names and addresses of all stockholders owning or holding 1 percent or more of the total amount of stock. If not owned by a corporation, give the names and addresses of the individual owners. If owned by a partnership or other unincorporated firm, give its name and address as well as those of each individual owner. If the publication is published by a nonprofit organization, give its name and address.)

Full Name	Complete Mailing Address
Wholly owned subsidiary of	1600 John F. Kennedy Blvd, Ste. 1800
Reed/Elsevier, US holdings	Philadelphia, PA 19103-2899

11. Known Bondholders, Mortgagees, and Other Security Holders Owning or Holding 1 Percent or More of Total Amount of Bonds, Mortgages, or Other Securities. If none, check box ☑ None

Full Name	Complete Mailing Address
N/A	

12. Tax Status (For completion by nonprofit organizations authorized to mail at nonprofit rates) (Check one)
The purpose, function, and nonprofit status of this organization and the exempt status for federal income tax purposes:
☐ Has Not Changed During Preceding 12 Months
☐ Has Changed During Preceding 12 Months (Publisher must submit explanation of change with this statement)

PS Form 3526, September 2007 (Page 1 of 3 (Instructions Page 3)) PSN 7530-01-000-9931 PRIVACY NOTICE: See our Privacy policy in www.usps.com

---

13. Publication Title	14. Issue Date for Circulation Data Below
Magnetic Resonance Imaging Clinics of North America	August 2013

15. Extent and Nature of Circulation			Average No. Copies Each Issue During Preceding 12 Months	No. Copies of Single Issue Published Nearest to Filing Date
a. Total Number of Copies (Net press run)			1,475	1,332
b. Paid Circulation (By Mail and Outside the Mail)	(1)	Mailed Outside-County Paid Subscriptions Stated on PS Form 3541. (Include paid distribution above nominal rate, advertiser's proof copies, and exchange copies)	961	889
	(2)	Mailed In-County Paid Subscriptions Stated on PS Form 3541 (Include paid distribution above nominal rate, advertiser's proof copies, and exchange copies)		
	(3)	Paid Distribution Outside the Mails Including Sales Through Dealers and Carriers, Street Vendors, Counter Sales, and Other Paid Distribution Outside USPS®	233	210
	(4)	Paid Distribution by Other Classes Mailed Through the USPS (e.g. First-Class Mail®)		
c. Total Paid Distribution (Sum of 15b (1), (2), (3), and (4))			1,194	1,099
d. Free or Nominal Rate Distribution (By Mail and Outside the Mail)	(1)	Free or Nominal Rate Outside-County Copies Included on PS Form 3541	62	83
	(2)	Free or Nominal Rate In-County Copies Included on PS Form 3541		
	(3)	Free or Nominal Rate Copies Mailed at Other Classes Through the USPS (e.g. First-Class Mail)		
	(4)	Free or Nominal Rate Distribution Outside the Mail (Carriers or other means)		
e. Total Free or Nominal Rate Distribution (Sum of 15d (1), (2), (3) and (4))			62	83
f. Total Distribution (Sum of 15c and 15e)			1,256	1,182
g. Copies not Distributed (See instructions to publishers #4 (page #3))			219	150
h. Total (Sum of 15f and g)			1,475	1,332
i. Percent Paid (15c divided by 15f times 100)			95.06%	92.98%

16. Publication of Statement of Ownership
☐ If the publication is a general publication, publication of this statement is required. Will be printed in the November 2013 issue of this publication.
☐ Publication not required

17. Signature and Title of Editor, Publisher, Business Manager, or Owner

Stephen R. Bushing – Inventory Distribution Coordinator

Date: September 14, 2013

I certify that all information furnished on this form is true and complete. I understand that anyone who furnishes false or misleading information on this form or who omits material or information requested on the form may be subject to criminal sanctions (including fines and imprisonment) and/or civil sanctions (including civil penalties).

PS Form 3526, September 2007 (Page 2 of 3)